# Seeing through the Smoke

## A Cannabis Specialist Untangles the Truth about Marijuana

### Peter Grinspoon, MD

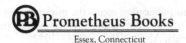

**Prometheus Books**

Essex, Connecticut

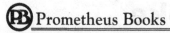

**Prometheus Books**

An imprint of Globe Pequot, the trade division of
The Rowman & Littlefield Publishing Group, Inc.
4501 Forbes Boulevard, Suite 200, Lanham, Maryland 20706
www.rowman.com

Distributed by NATIONAL BOOK NETWORK

British Library Cataloguing in Publication Information Available

**Library of Congress Cataloging-in-Publication Data**

Names: Grinspoon, Peter author.
Title: Seeing through the smoke : a cannabis specialist untangles the truth about
    marijuana / Peter Grinspoon.
Description: Lanham, Maryland : Prometheus, [2023] | Summary: "Seeing
    through the Smoke is an unflinching examination at the grossly
    misunderstood drug that uses data-driven medical science and a critical
    historical perspective to reveal the truth behind cannabis. In this
    balanced and measured investigation, Cannabis specialist and Instructor
    in Medicine at Harvard Medical School Dr. Peter Grinspoon untangles the
    reality behind cannabis, revealing how we ended up with radically
    divergent understandings of the drug and pointing a way toward a middle
    ground that we can all share"— Provided by publisher.
Identifiers: LCCN 2022034515 (print) | LCCN 2022034516 (ebook) | ISBN
    9781633888463 (cloth) | ISBN 9781633888470 (epub)
Subjects: LCSH: Cannabis—Therapeutic use—Popular works.
Classification: LCC RM666.C266 G755 2023  (print) | LCC RM666.C266  (ebook)
    | DDC 615.7/827—dc23/eng/20220913
LC record available at https://lccn.loc.gov/2022034515
LC ebook record available at https://lccn.loc.gov/2022034516

♾️™ The paper used in this publication meets the minimum requirements of
American National Standard for Information Sciences—Permanence of Paper
for Printed Library Materials, ANSI/NISO Z39.48-1992.

To my mom Betsy—the kindest of souls—without whom legalization truly would not be happening.

To my older brother David—a brilliant writer and generous mentor—without whom none of my books would have come into existence.

To my twin brother Josh—always keeping me out of trouble—thank you for all of your emotional support during this grueling process.

The illegality of cannabis is outrageous, an impediment to full utilization of a drug which helps produce the sensitivity and insight, serenity and fellowship so desperately needed in this increasingly mad and dangerous world.

—Carl Sagan, 1971

More people need to see "medical marijuana" for what it is: a cynical fraud and a cruel hoax. . . . Legitimizing smoked marijuana as a "medicine" is a serious threat to the health and safety of all Americans.

—Testimony of Robert L. DuPont, MD, first head of the National Institute of Drug Abuse (NIDA), 2004

Convictions are more dangerous enemies of truth than lies.

—Friedrich Nietzsche

# CONTENTS

# FOREWORD
## Dr. Andrew Weil

I first met Dr. Lester Grinspoon, Peter's father, when I was a medical student at Harvard, stirring up controversy by trying to study medical cannabis in an objective and legitimate manner. Harvard Medical School, following the lead of the U.S. government at the time, frowned upon that effort. Nevertheless, I managed to conduct the first randomized, double-blinded human research experiments with cannabis. Lester also got into hot water, almost continuously, during his distinguished fifty-year career on the faculty of HMS, for his work on cannabis and other drugs of misuse, as well as for his prescient criticisms of the War on Drugs. Though Lester's work brought retaliation from the Harvard establishment, it has been fully and forcefully validated by history.

It is impossible to overstate the role that Dr. Lester Grinspoon played in the progress of drug policy reform, with *Marihuana Reconsidered* reviewed on the front page of the *New York Times Book Review* in 1971, with his seminal work *Marihuana, the Forbidden Medicine* in 1993, with his 180 or so scientific papers, and with his numerous congressional and courtroom testimonies and effective media appearances. He was an intellectual leader of the cannabis legalization movement, who helped move popular opinion for legalization from 13 percent when his book came out to 67 percent when he passed away in 2020, in no small part due to his fifty years of scholarship and advocacy.

His son, Dr. Peter Grinspoon, also has a deep understanding of and broad experience with cannabis. He grew up in a household where legalization was constantly being discussed and debated by academics and luminaries. Peter watched his brother Danny derive great relief from cannabis as he struggled, unsuccessfully, with childhood leukemia and the ravages of chemotherapy. Peter spent his entire childhood, adolescence, and adulthood observing his father in action—arguing, speaking, testifying—all with the intent of reversing our government's nonsensical policy on cannabis.

After college, Peter spent five years working as a campaigner for Greenpeace before entering medical school. His experience as an activist helped him refine the skills that he would apply to cannabis reform efforts later in life, including his work with the advocacy group Doctors for Cannabis Regulation.

Peter has a vast clinical knowledge of cannabis. As a primary care doctor, he has incorporated it into his practice from the very beginning of his career, treating thousands of patients with it over the years. He has been a prominent spokesperson for legalization and an energetic debunker of the often scientifically unsound arguments against it. We saw him demonstrate his expertise at Yale Law School during his 2019 debate on the dangers of cannabis with reporter Alex Berenson.

Like his father, Peter has the courage and honesty to admit and discuss his personal experience with cannabis. It informs his discussions of both benefits and risks in a way that allows him to question, and at times satirize, cannabis "experts" whose efforts to describe a marijuana "high" reveal that they have never been within ten feet of a burning joint. I know few doctors who are as comfortable in medical grand rounds at Harvard as they are at the Boston Freedom Rally (an annual anti-prohibition event that both Dr. Grinspoons have spoken at) or at the Cannabis Cup.

Peter brings his unique viewpoint to this critically important book, which in some ways reads as the third part of a trilogy, concluding a journey started with *Marihuana Reconsidered* and furthered with *Forbidden Medicine*. He points out that we, as a society, still have a pot problem. If a person today were to walk up to a random doctor, lawyer, legislator, or policy maker and ask them about cannabis, they would likely get one of two wildly different answers. They might be informed that it is a beneficial, relatively nontoxic aid to wellness with great, untapped medical utility. Or they might get a stern warning that it is a highly dangerous, addictive drug being peddled to teenagers by criminals, to be avoided at all costs.

Peter traces the evolution of these two different realities about cannabis, the political landscapes and social forces that produced them—including the racism and the turbulent counterreaction to the 1960s counterculture—the commercial interests involved, and the pressures of the War on Drugs. These influences warped public opinion as well as scientific research and continue to do so today. Historically, the most egregious influence has been the U.S. government, which has selectively funded scientists willing to find and exaggerate the dangers of cannabis. Peter disentangles what is actually true from the nonsense and the propaganda—not an easy task.

We know that cannabis is useful in ways that are well established, and likely in many others that need to be researched, including those having to do with wellness and lifestyle enhancement. There is also the potential for harm that still needs to be studied. That potential is perhaps more than many cannabis proponents will admit, but it is clearly much less than conservative medicine would have us believe.

The ways that both sides get it wrong are profoundly illuminating. The medical establishment dismisses patients' stories and experiences and rejects information that goes against orthodoxy. Too often, its objectivity has been compromised by the economic interests of Big Pharma and the political interests of the conservative National Institute on Drug Abuse.

On the other hand, many passionate marijuana advocates have been too quick to romanticize their substance of choice and reject science altogether. For example, as far as we know, cannabis does not, by itself, "cure" cancer, as some claim. Their eagerness further alienates the mainstream medical establishment.

Decades of blatant U.S. government propaganda and lies about cannabis have intensified this dynamic, conditioning proponents to reflexively reject findings of possible harm. We need to study, evaluate, and understand potential risks as well as benefits.

More than fifty years after *Marihuana Reconsidered*, Peter Grinspoon ties it all together, helping us all see through the smoke, by taking account of multiple agendas, viewpoints, and biases. He takes the emotion out, even while acknowledging his own emotions, which stem from watching his dying brother benefit from cannabis. From this broad perspective, he addresses flash-point issues, such as impaired driving, cognition, adolescent health, the likely effects of legalization, the lifestyle benefits of cannabis, and exciting future directions of research. The length and breadth of Peter Grinspoon's experience, along with the depth of his scientific knowledge, results in a book that is an invaluable contribution to our attempts, as a society, to come to a much-needed common understanding of cannabis.

# PROLOGUE

It was 1973, two years after Nixon started his War on Drugs, when I first inhaled cannabis smoke. I was seven years old. I remember following my teenage brothers, Danny and David, as little brothers tend to do, like paparazzi, around the driveway of our childhood home. Our parents were out, and they somehow thought the teenagers would responsibly supervise me. Danny, fourteen at the time, casually pulled a thin white twig out of his pocket, lit it with a match in a practiced manner, and started sucking on the end of it, producing sickly sweet fumes. Normally an engaged and dedicated older brother, at this moment his teenage self must have assumed command because, with a mischievous grin, he handed me the white object and instructed me to put the tip into my mouth and breathe in, just as he had done. I would have jumped off a cliff if he'd asked me to. I spent the next five minutes coughing and gagging as Danny went inside to get me a glass of water, clearly feeling guilty about his poorly thought-out prank.

Danny's act of smoking a joint at age fourteen wasn't as blatantly delinquent as it sounds, as cannabis was helping to sustain him. It was the only thing that allowed him to keep food down given the aggressive chemotherapy regimen he was on during his losing battle against acute lymphocytic leukemia. My parents, after quite a bit of soul searching— and then some actual cannabis searching—eventually sanctioned his usage. I believe that they knew by that point that he was dying, and they had decided to minimize his suffering at all costs.

This culminated in my law-abiding mother going to the field next to the high school in our Boston suburb and asking Danny's best friend, Mark, to sell her some weed. Mark was so shocked and worried he almost spontaneously combusted. "Oh, Mrs. Grinspoon, I wouldn't know anything about that." Mark's loyalty as a friend and empathy for how sick Danny was must have won out over any fear of potential repercussions. Later that night, Danny announced to my mother, "Oh, Mom, guess what? I have a pipe with some grass in it in my jacket pocket."

The use of cannabis may only have added months to a year to Danny's life, but the improvement in his quality of life was incalculable. Instead of barfing, he was eating. Instead of lying in bed, he was playing with his little brothers, inventing intricate board games, and strumming on his Fender Stratocaster. Yes, cannabis was illegal. Yes, it was front and center in the culture wars in Nixon's America. Yes, if detected by the wrong people, my brother Danny and my parents could have been arrested. Their jobs as teacher and doctor could have been jeopardized. Yes, the medical establishment, which included my father, a Harvard psychiatrist, was ideologically programmed to be opposed to this.

But when push comes to shove, most parents will do almost anything to help their children. This was a simple calculus: no cannabis, no appetite, no food, no Danny.

What would you do if it were your child?

The healing power of cannabis became folkloric in my family, and the lived experience of its powers to alleviate suffering, and to prolong and sustain life, was seared into me at an early age and carried through to a career in medicine.

# INTRODUCTION

You don't have to be stoned to be dazed and confused by the current discord in our society around cannabis. Depending on which doctor you speak with, which websites you read, or which radio show host you listen to, cannabis could be an appealing, low-risk medicine—even an aid to wellness—or an insidiously addictive drug rotting the brains of our youth. At times it feels as if one is reading descriptions of two entirely different plants, grown on different worlds, nourished by different suns.

It is dysfunctional for our society to have these two different, largely contradictory narratives. This dissonance confuses teens, distresses patients, and paralyzes politicians. It invites in dubious sources of information and results in uninformed choices, enhanced polarization, and a fragmented, incoherent national policy.

The two narratives tend to radicalize each other over time. Some proponents of cannabis are loathe to admit any dangers, however real, such as the risk of fashioning cannabis edibles into delicious gummy bears that a small child might gladly eat until the bag is empty and possibly end up in the emergency room. Apparently, one's right to get stoned by gummy bear is sacrosanct. On the other hand, some cannabis opponents automatically dismiss any studies that show benefit, even though some of the stuffiest bastions of mainstream medicine are now reporting that cannabis helps people with conditions such as chronic pain.

How did we end up with these radically divergent understandings of cannabis? Is there a middle ground—a common belief system about cannabis—that we can all live with? After examining how we arrived at two separate realities about cannabis, I will focus on questions that have become the most critical flash points. Is cannabis addictive? Is it safe to use if you are pregnant? Does it help autism? Can it help cure cancer? How does it affect memory? How dangerous is it for teens? I also explore what is so alluring about its recreational uses that people risk going to jail in order to use it.

I don't have all the answers to these questions. What I do have is an unusually long perspective on this issue. I've had a front row to the legalization movement my entire life due to my dad's leadership and my brother's illness. I have two decades of clinical experience treating patients with cannabis. I have as much personal experience with the drug as many Rastafarians. I live with one foot in both worlds, just as comfortable passing a joint around at a café in Amsterdam as I am presenting grand rounds on the subject of cannabis at some of our most prestigious hospitals.

Cannabis has united Americans across the political spectrum yet divided doctors into hostile intellectual camps. The plant's history is intricately interwoven with the last ten millennia of human history as food, sacrament, fabric, and medicine. Yet for the last century or so, its legal restriction has been a vehicle for racial degradation and control. Finally, we seem to be emerging from this dark period. Yet in 2020 alone, there were more than three hundred thousand cannabis-related arrests in the United States.

Cannabis is a unique drug on every level. All of the paradigms and categories that have been transposed onto it—or imposed on it—from other drugs fall short. It is not "heroin light" or "sort of like alcohol." I feel that has been grossly misunderstood and misrepresented by the mainstream of the addiction and medical communities for the last half century. Instead of starting out neutral, they assumed cannabis is a negative and have spent the last fifty years proving this to be the case—useful helpers of our government's War on Drugs.

The medical profession has largely missed the boat with respect to cannabis and is currently out of step with the 94 percent of Americans who are in favor of legal access to medical cannabis. Patients expect their doctors to know something about cannabis but are often disappointed—if not downright discouraged—by the judgmental, snooty attitudes they can encounter. This quick dismissal masks tremendous gaps in knowledge. Doctors urgently need to get up to speed on this issue, because at this point patients simply aren't considering them useful sources of information, or aren't informing them of their cannabis use, which is dangerous to the care of these patients. In one study of over one thousand medical cannabis patients, only 2.6 percent of patients selected cannabis products with input from a medical professional, although 54.9 percent relied on advice from dispensary employees (aka "budtenders").[1] With cannabis, if doctors want to earn their relevance back, they need to update and evolve their attitudes and knowledge. They can't complain about people seeking out information from budtenders if they don't have anything helpful that they themselves can provide.

Societal knowledge changes over time, but in response to conflicting political and economic pressures, our society's understanding of cannabis started to bifurcate in the 1930s as the campaign to make it illegal in the United States kicked into high gear. We now have two disturbingly contradictory truths that need to be refashioned back into one whole. It is time to take stock (or stalk!) of what we know, sift the seeds from the buds, and reunite around one set of understandings of the basic truths of cannabis. Only in this way can we fruitfully reintegrate cannabis back into our society in a sane and sensible manner after its eighty-year exile.

**Part I**

# HOW DID WE GET HERE?

# CHAPTER ONE
# WHY AM I THE ONE WRITING THIS?

I t is difficult to find anyone who is truly objective about cannabis. How would any of us even recognize such a viewpoint? Objective according to whom? To start, there isn't yet an established expert truth about many aspects of cannabis from which to construct or defend an objective position. Further, the very discussion of cannabis, more than the use of the drug itself, elicits strong emotional reactions. According to my late dad, Dr. Lester Grinspoon, "there is something very special about illicit drugs. If they don't always make the drug user act irrationally, they certainly cause many nonusers to behave that way."

When I originally conceived of this book, I intended—as a doctor, a writer, and an activist—to embody the omniscient, objective voice that would neutrally and dispassionately tell the rousing tale of how our understanding of cannabis became fractured into two different narratives and how we might reunite them again. The only problem is that I do have strong feelings about this issue, as I've been immersed in it my entire life.

I believe that we can overcome our biases by being open and honest about where we are coming from. Cannabis has been so heavily propagandized against for almost a century and has become so politicized that it's impossible not to have a bias. Not even the scientific literature is objective when it comes to cannabis—much of it was influenced by the War on Drugs, with funding heavily allocated toward vilifying the plant and with most research on its benefits prohibited, unfunded, or curated.

I try to separate my emotional reactions to the political components of the cannabis issue, such as the Drug War–fueled mistreatment of millions of Americans, predominantly with dark skin color, from the scientific data that is coming out. As a physician, I need to separate the hopes and wishes that a treatment will work for my patients from the need for credible evidence that it does, and in an acceptably safe manner. Understanding harms is obviously just as important as understanding benefits—for all of us.

I'd ask anyone reading this to attempt to conjure up the insight and humility to evaluate their own preconceived notions about cannabis and to try to leave their emotional reactions to this subject at the door, at least for a little while, so that we can collaborate on working through these thorny problems and come out the other side of this process with solutions, or at least the best possible educated guess as to how to move forward.

One can't control what life one is born into. I was born into a front-row seat for our nation's struggle for legalization, where I've remained for the last half century. I joke that my interest and training in medical cannabis began before birth, while my twin and I were hanging out in the amniotic sac, wrestling and insulting each other, as twin boys do, listening to my father, Dr. Lester Grinspoon, a legend in the cannabis world, and those around him wax poetic about the benefits and challenges of cannabis legalization. The words were quite muted through the amniotic fluid, but we were able to intuit the gist of what the adults were saying at that impressionable age.

A good deal of my childhood revolved around my father's scholarship on cannabis and other criminalized drugs. Risking his career, he wrote two seminal books urging a reevaluation of cannabis. His 1971 book *Marihuana Reconsidered* was reviewed in glowing terms on the front page of the *New York Times Book Review*. This process led to his belief in legalization in order to better exploit the medicinal and other benefits, as well as to stop the utter madness of the War on Drugs. He is widely considered to have been one of the intellectual leaders of the legalization movement due to his scholarship and stature.

A typical scene in the living room of my childhood home would involve proponents, and some detractors, of cannabis legalization, either heatedly debating each other or peaceably sharing a joint. Or, if memory serves, they might be puffing from the long stem of a golden hookah that astronomer Carl Sagan and his wife Annie Druyan brought back for my parents from the South Pacific. This hookah was arguably the most beautiful object in my parents' home. I remember "Uncle Carl" waving away an offer of a second hit from my dad because he was carefully reading an

English paper I was proudly showing him from one of my classes—he always had helpful feedback. Growing up, I was largely unaware that other middle-class homes didn't billow cannabis smoke.

The conversations around the hookah, or the pipes, or the joints, were more mind blowing than the smoke would have been had I inhaled. It wasn't just Carl Sagan hypothesizing, in the way that only he could do, about the likelihood of finding life in the universe, or why we hadn't found any yet, and whether that was because technological species tend to destroy themselves before they can do any major outreach into space. These conversations, formed by a shifting group of academics—whoever happened to be visiting—were, in essence, ongoing symposia about philosophy, literature, and, mostly, how to solve the most intractable social problems of the day: hunger, pollution, propaganda. There was so much laughter and bonhomie! As I was growing up, these conversations were so much more impactful to me than what I was learning at school, and they motivated me beyond belief to read, to learn, and to study everything and anything. You've never seen a more motivated kid.

The associations I made with cannabis use at home vastly contradicted what we were taught at school, which was that cannabis makes you lazy, dull, and somehow morally deficient. I grew up in a white, wealthy suburb where the population had been conditioned to lionize alcohol, but marijuana was considered to be something only druggies would use. In school, they warned us over and over about the "amotivational syndrome," an insidious change in personality brought about by chronic cannabis use.

Teenagers are known to be judgmental at times. The people who usually warned us about the amotivational syndrome appeared, *through teenage eyes*, to be these dim-witted policemen who, themselves, seemed to barely have the motivation to finish their stale presentation in order to make it back to Dunkin' to secure more donuts. If we had defunded the donuts, these cops would probably still be alive today. In any case, this wasn't nearly as compelling or appealing a message as I was receiving at home. Compared with the constant stream of doctors, lawyers, professors, and activists that were populating my living room, I couldn't help but wonder who was truly amotivational here, and who was paving the way for a better future.

None of this is to say that I became "pro" (or "anti") cannabis at an early age. It's a plant, a medicine, and a psychoactive drug with vast potential benefits and harms. There's no reason to be "pro" or "anti." It can be used wisely or harmfully. The points are that, first, I learned that one has to think for oneself on this issue. I didn't know what the truth was yet (and I still don't . . . this subject is like quicksand), but I knew, starting in grade school, that what they were feeding us was pure, unadulterated nonsense. Following my dad, I became intensely engaged with this issue and followed it as closely as I could for as long as I can remember.

Far more emotionally resonant in retrospect was the fact that my older brother Danny was dying of acute lymphocytic leukemia, and that cannabis helped him weather the nausea and vomiting associated with chemotherapy. Weed enabled him to hold down food and, as such, almost certainly extended his life. His struggles, in the offhand glimpses that my parents were unsuccessful at hiding from me, taught me, at such a young age, that cannabis can vastly alleviate suffering. What could possibly be more powerful than seeing your sibling suffer less? I came to associate the sickly sweet odor with healing, with intelligent conversations, with good-natured humor, and with medicine.

Without cannabis, Danny would be lying in his room with a towel over his head and a barf bucket next to his bed at the ready. With cannabis, he would be downstairs playing board games and wrestling with his younger twin brothers. We preferred the "with cannabis" Danny, even if we didn't, as little kids, understand any of the complexity of what my parents were doing: risking criminal charges and their professions, during Nixon's War on Drugs, to provide comfort and relief for their son.

Cannabis didn't stop or slow the cancer in the end. But what it did do was enable him to eat and maintain his weight, it lessened his suffering, and it vastly increased his ability to participate in the last year of his life. As such, it gave us some of the most precious memories my twin and I have, playing with our older brother, when he otherwise would have been curled up in bed, not wanting to deal with his noisy, boisterous little brothers.

The visceral experience of watching my brother benefit from medical cannabis affected my trajectory in several ways. It obviously didn't do wonders for my respect for authority given that my parents had to break the law to obtain it and given that I knew we were being misled about it in school. The injustice of it all, and the intensive exposure at a young age to activists of all stripes, put social justice at the forefront of my future plans. Later, it gave me valuable perspective on my medical education as I knew that cannabis was an effective medication, even when my expensive medical education at Boston University and, later, at Harvard Medical largely stuck to the party line—that it was a dangerous and useless drug.

The political culture of our household always seemed to land me and my brothers in stoner circles despite my dad's firm rule, modeled on the drinking age at the time, that no one is allowed to smoke cannabis until they are eighteen years old. I didn't quite make it to eighteen (or fourteen), but despite all the smoking and fraternizing with other stoners, I can truthfully say that there wasn't a single academic class—all difficult, honors classes—that I didn't get an A in, from the time I took my first puff until I was accepted into Swarthmore College. In fact, it contributed to many of those good grades in high school once I discovered that it could improve my writing.

As a consequence of the particular life I've lived, I have accumulated a good deal of "lived experience" with cannabis. Having used it over four decades, on four continents, I understand how this drug affects different people, at different doses, in different circumstances. Lived experience is unusually helpful for this particular subject. I can't imagine how one could fully understand how it helps people or accurately gauge the harms—amid all the nonsense and propaganda—unless you have some personal experience with what the drug does and doesn't do. How could you possibly know what to believe, what to discard, and how much to weight each component of the debate? You can't. It is a question of being able to *contextualize* complex, contradictory, and agenda-driven information. This "real world" experience needs to be a complement to a rigorous, if skeptical, familiarity with the scientific literature. I'm also fortunate to have access to a wealth of clinical experience, treating my patients as a (very) early adopter.

In my humble opinion, this lack of lived experience is a major handicap for many people who study cannabis. They understand a particular parameter or facet of a cannabis-related topic that they are studying, based on other studies—many of which are biased—and then extrapolate to cannabis itself as a whole. At a certain point, if the conversation strays, it becomes clear that they are on thinner ice. For example, I was recently watching the local news on television, and a modestly prominent cannabis "expert" came on. He was explaining that you can have one drink socially, but once you start using cannabis you are "off to the races." The TV anchor agreed.

What? You can't just take one puff and enjoy a conversation, a dinner, a walk, or a movie? That was news to me, and likely to every other cannabis user on earth. One puff was all I usually took, as I didn't like the effect if it was too strong. It dawned on me that this expert had almost certainly never been in the same room as a lit joint.

Or another prominent cannabis authority, who, in a 2016 *National Affairs* piece, "The Real Dangers of Marijuana," in which he labors mightily to prove that cannabis is more dangerous than alcohol, states,

> Part of the difference [between alcohol and cannabis] may be that most people who use marijuana do so with the express purpose of getting intoxicated, whereas many people drink occasionally just to quench their thirst or to complement their dinner.[1]

My second thought was, "Why quench your thirst with water or Gatorade when you can grab some bourbon off the shelf?" My first thought was, "Have you ever actually been in the presence of someone who is using cannabis?" I thought of the dozens (hundreds?) of dinner parties that I've been to where a joint has been passed around and it only heightened and intensified the conversation, as opposed to some parties I'd been at with drunken people bellowing at each other and vastly overestimating their own ability to fascinate. (I've also, of course, been to plenty of dinner parties with people pleasantly buzzed and energized on wine and others with people far too stoned on weed to make the slightest sense on the simplest topics of conversation, such as "What is your name?" or "Please pass the butter," so it can cut both ways.)

It reminds one of the exchange between Nixon and television personality Art Linkletter almost fifty years earlier,

> LINKLETTER. There's a great difference between alcohol and marijuana.
>
> NIXON. What is it? The president wants to know!
>
> LINKLETTER. When people smoke marijuana, they smoke it to get high. In every case, when most people drink, they drink to be sociable.
>
> NIXON. That's right, that's right, a person does not drink to get drunk. A person drinks to have fun.[2]

8

Another example of missing the forest for the cannabis plants is found in a book by several cannabis policy wonks which asks, "Does marijuana use enhance creativity? Maybe. Maybe not. The scholarly literature offers no definitive answer."[3] That's like saying, "Is a Picasso painting beautiful? Maybe. Maybe not. The scholarly literature offers no definitive answer." We don't need the "scholarly literature" to tell us everything like it's the Oracle of Life. Most people learn the answer to the question of creativity after taking their first puff or two. They are using the wrong lens. "Does sex feel good? The scholarly literature says . . ." Give me a break!

Listening to a description of being "stoned" by a cannabis researcher who hasn't ever been stoned is like listening to a food critic describe a restaurant they've never been to, or a travel writer describe a destination they've never seen. There are spiritual, interpersonal, and intellectual textures surrounding the cannabis experience that these descriptions invariably lack. I fear that the lack of lived experience, or the lack of incorporation of people with lived experience, in government and policy formation has contributed to the split between two sides of the cannabis debate. We aren't sharing a common reality.

Another pet peeve of mine is that "intoxicated" is such a crude approximation of what cannabis does. Inherently judgmental, it misses all the nuance, and all of the positives. There's really no excuse for not knowing what cannabis does or how it affects people if you are wearing the mantle of an "expert" or if you are deciding policy for others.

I've also seen, and had, my share of cannabis disaster stories. Like the time my cousins and I, in our midteens, were enjoying the electric excitement of the beach in Orleans on Cape Cod under a full moon, sucking on watermelon-flavored Jolly Ranchers, and looking for adventure. On the beach at night were thousands of stars above, the forlorn sound of distant foghorns, dune grass that tickled your thighs, giggling couples making out in the dunes, and other gangs of teenagers who could be friendly or hostile.

Gradually, my cousin Lonna started to feel increasingly nervous and unsteady. We laid her down on a bench on a bluff that happened to have a spectacular view overlooking the entirety of Nauset Harbor. We tried to calm and reassure Lonna, but she started to panic and shake. "Things keep speeding up and slowing down." She hadn't smoked any more or less than the rest of us, who had been pleasantly high and alert, though alertness was rapidly turning into concern and then to panic. Lonna chose that moment to inform us that when her mom had tried pot, she had hallucinated too. *Now* you tell us! Twelve years before I received my medical degree, I received a painful lesson on how important it is to take an accurate family history. She probably didn't tell us because we would have limited and monitored her intake.

Under a sky intermittently illuminated by the Pleiades showers, we were faced with a cosmically unpalatable decision: get help and be assassinated by our parents—especially my dad—for using cannabis at age fifteen, in *direct* defiance of him, or don't get help and risk having Lonna's freak-out escalate. Not getting help was becoming increasingly untenable as Lonna was getting worse by the minute.

We skulked back to the adults. "Um . . . er . . . hello? Hi, guys . . . are you having a nice evening? Sorry to interrupt, but we were . . . um . . . I hope you won't be upset . . . we were experimenting by trying some marijuana, and Lonna is completely freaking out. We need some help here." Jaws all drop. A vein on my dad's forehead, which I'd never noticed before, began to bulge. Luckily for us, he was under social pressure to behave like an enlightened liberal in front of his guests. This was *exactly* what he didn't want to happen with cannabis: teenage use and bad outcomes. We were fucking up the plan.

The immediate commotion was focused on Lonna's well-being, which improved uneventfully as the cannabis wore off. We were relieved to see that she was fine, if a little envious that she clearly was going to be spared punishment. Soon my brother and I were shut in our small room with a terse pronouncement from my dad, imbued with all the guilt that a psychiatrist at Harvard Medical can muster: "You've disappointed me beyond words; we'll discuss this in the morning. I don't want to hear a peep." *Slam!* It was a long summer.

Finally, as to "Why me?" I've been treating people with medical cannabis for several decades. I've been glued to the literature as someone else might be glued to a scary movie. I have always integrated medical cannabis into my own primary care practice. This became significantly easier and more aboveground when Massachusetts legalized medical cannabis in 2012 and, further, when we legalized recreational cannabis in 2014. I proudly participated in both campaigns.

Before it was legal in the state where I practice, I was more subtle about it. If a patient had migraines, I'd include, as part of my spiel to my patients (if it was appropriate, depending on the context), "and some patients report that with a small amount of cannabis, their migraines resolve." I knew this worked for patients, both from the literature and from personal experience when I suffered from blistering migraines after a thirty-six-hour shift in the hospital during my training. With my patients, I'd take close mental notes of both successes and failures, and the relatively rare occasions when someone had a bad reaction. Over time, you build experience and connect with other doctors who are practicing the same medicine.

Both cannabis worlds are equally real to me. I'm just as comfortable in grand rounds listening to the speaker present new data on why cannabis is (purportedly) detrimental to the teenage brain, causes heart attacks, harms your memory, causes psychosis, and is highly addictive—all of these we will review—as I am sharing a joint with members of the Grateful Dead at a rooftop party (yes, this happened, when I worked for Greenpeace) or with a bunch of fellow concertgoers in rural Zimbabwe.

I can see that neither side has a monopoly on the truth. My struggle for objectivity will mirror the struggle for objectivity that anyone reading this will go through, readers who come to this issue from the entire spectrum of beliefs—and feelings—on this issue. I'm not a robot and obviously have my own biases.

I am asking those reading this book to separate out their feelings and to try to discard their stigmas and judgments about cannabis—pro or anti—so that we can have an open discussion about what we, at this point in history, believe to be true about cannabis, issue by issue. There's no rule that we have to swallow either the "pro" or the "anti" ideologies whole— we can pick and choose what we find convincing about each stance.

I'm not a specialist in any one area. I am a clinician-educator with a strong background in science, political activism, and the liberal arts, but I am not an epidemiologist, a cultural anthropologist, or a primary researcher. I am a primary care doctor of cannabis—I have a long and broad view of it, but I know I don't have all the answers, and that's OK, because this is mainly about starting a conversation. We are leaving Plato's cave, and we are going to stroll around.

## CHAPTER TWO

# THE BRANCHING OF
# CULTURAL PERCEPTIONS
## Reefer Pessimism

C annabis has been documented as a medicine that humans have used for at least five thousand years, and possibly much longer. Some of the oldest known human artifacts are a ten-thousand-year-old piece of hemp fabric that was found in ancient Mesopotamia and some shards of pottery with hemp cord woven into them that were discovered in what is now Taiwan, which date back at least twelve thousand years.

Starting in the 1840s, cannabis was an increasingly common and accepted medication in the United States, often in the form of tinctures, produced by mainstream pharmaceutical companies such as Parke-Davis and Eli Lilly. It is easy to Google a picture of these medications, which look like . . . ordinary medications. Cannabis was used for a wide variety of maladies, such as tetanus, neuralgia, alcoholism, convulsions, dysmenorrhea, and rheumatism. It was officially listed in the *U.S. Pharmacopoeia*, which is an official compendium of active medications, in 1851. Sir William Osler, considered by medical historians to be the father of modern medicine, claimed that "cannabis indica is probably the most satisfactory remedy for migraines." Cannabis was widely embraced by medical institutions of the day, such as the medical societies, and between 1840 and 1900 more than one hundred papers were published in the Western medical literature discussing and often recommending its clinical use for various ailments.

In the United States, over the last eight decades, despite the fact that humans have cultivated and migrated with cannabis for millennia, cannabis was criminalized. This has led to the arrests of millions for pursuing activities that humans have been doing since the dawn of agricultural society. If we use the five thousand years as our denominator, cannabis has been criminalized for 1.6 percent of the time that it's been used as a medicine on this planet. Criminalization was accomplished in the United States in 1937 over vigorous protests from the American Medical Association (AMA). At the time, cannabis was frequently used to treat the same variety of symptoms and illnesses that millions of Americans still use it for today. According to the head of the AMA testifying against the criminalization before Congress in 1937,

> there is nothing in the medicinal use of Cannabis that has any relation to Cannabis addiction. I use the word "Cannabis" in preference to the word "marihuana," because Cannabis is the correct term for describing the plant and its products. The term "marihuana" is a mongrel word that has crept into this country over the Mexican border and has no general meaning, except as it relates to the use of Cannabis preparations for smoking . . . .
>
> To say, however, as has been proposed here, that the use of the drug should be prevented by a prohibitive tax, loses sight of the fact that future investigation may show that there are substantial medical uses for Cannabis.[1]

In 1942, almost a century after it was added, cannabis was stripped from the *Pharmacopoeia* in response to political pressure from the Federal Bureau of Narcotics. It had now become an illicit, forbidden medicine. Health and safety weren't what was driving this—it was driven by the early drug warriors and the moral panic they created.

After cannabis was criminalized, patients who needed a pharmaceutical solution to their medical or social ills were largely left in the hands of the pharmaceutical or alcohol industries. Due to the outsized global influence of the United States, this "medical prohibition" was expanded globally.

As a result of two pieces of legislation, the Boggs Act in 1952 and the inclusion of cannabis in the 1956 Narcotics Control Act, a first-time offense for cannabis possession carried a penalty of two to ten years in prison, with a fine of up to $20,000 (about a quarter of a million dollars in today's money). The Boggs Act made no distinction between users and sellers—the penalties were draconian. States enacted their own punitive legislation as well. The use of medicinal cannabis was forced underground or was successfully suppressed.

A complex crescendo of cultural and societal forces contributed to the criminalization of cannabis in the United States in the 1930s. Prohibition of alcohol had recently ended, in 1933, and the massive law enforcement bureaucracy that had sustained it was desperately in need of justification and funding. You just finished one war, and what do you do with a huge army? Either dissolve it or start another war. Cannabis was the perfect target.

Various commercial interests had a shared goal of removing hemp as a competitor. These included the paper, nylon, and petrochemical industries. It is difficult to conceive of how much less polluted our climate and oceans might be had we gone the hemp route.

Other equally important factors contributing to criminalization included virulent racism and xenophobia. Concerns about health and safety associated with cannabis use were not prominent in the discussions leading up to its prohibition. At this point in time, the doctors were among the victims of the Drug War, along with their patients—they had a vital caregiving tool banned from the toolbox, for nonmedical reasons, and were facing intensive pressure to modify their long-held opinions.

To so drastically change public policy, over the objections of doctors and patients alike, required a dramatic shift in public opinion. This transpired through a massive propaganda campaign that was carried out, with gusto, by Harry Anslinger, the first director of the newly created Federal Bureau of Narcotics, in league with the media empire of William Randolph Hearst.

Together, Anslinger and Hearst exploited racist stereotypes and fears of immigrants from the southern border, many of the exact same fears being exploited today. These immigrants were supposedly corrupted and debauched by the "loco weed," so lock your white daughters up! Blacks were the other source of danger. The authorities disseminated specious stories of cannabis-induced violence. They hammered on the theme of vulnerable white women innocently using cannabis and then being taken advantage of by Black men. This succeeded in whipping up public fears. They even renamed the plant from "cannabis" to "marihuana" to make it sound more foreign and threatening, which is what Dr. Woodward was objecting to in his testimony ("The term 'marihuana' is a mongrel word that has crept into this country over the Mexican border and has no general meaning").

With the combined, coordinated organs of industry, government, and the media fully exploiting racial fears, this rebranding campaign was effective. There was no counterbalancing "cannabis lobby" back then to provide a counterargument. This is difficult to imagine in today's world of sparkling dispensaries and sleek, articulate "ganjapreneurs." A few conscientious doctors spoke up, but that was about it.

Building up to this critical historical juncture, a narrative about cannabis was begun that persisted and evolved to this day. Let's call this narrative the "Reefer Pessimism" narrative. This is the first of two major, and largely discordant, belief systems that bifurcated as cannabis became illegal. The other narrative is that of the Cannatopians, which will be discussed shortly.

While all people have their own beliefs and nuanced views of each of the issues raised below, a summary of a moderate, modern-day Reefer Pessimism might go as follows:

"By legalizing cannabis, we are conducting an uncontrolled experiment on our children. As we legalize, teenagers (and adults) get the message that cannabis is natural, safe, and harmless. Teen usage of cannabis will increase with legalization, and teens are using stronger products than previously. Decades of credible studies have shown that adolescent cannabis use lowers IQ and can damage the teenage brain's structure and function, particularly memory and executive functioning. This in turn affects their education, job prospects, and future successes.

"It doesn't matter if members of our generation used cannabis when we were younger, because we now know more about the harms involved. Cannabis is much more concentrated—about five times, on average—than it was 'back in the day,' not to mention the new concentrates that are up to 99 percent THC—so it isn't 'your grandparents' weed.' This superstrong marijuana is leading to more disability and mental health problems, such as depression, suicide, and psychosis. Emergency room visits are up for pediatric exposures because people leave 'edibles' lying around, as well as for acute psychotic reactions due to increased availability and potency. As it is, 9 percent of adults and 17 percent of teens get addicted—this will only go up as it gets stronger and more available.

"The diminishment of negative perceptions around cannabis use that come with legalization is also giving pregnant and breast-feeding women the idea that cannabis is safe and helpful. Rates of use are going up by orders of magnitude. Decades of studies have shown severe, lasting damage to the offspring, including birth complications like low birth weight, as well as negative neurodevelopmental consequences, potentially including autism and epigenetic changes.

"Big Marijuana is a ruthless industry that is mostly made up of people from the alcohol and tobacco industries. They can't wait to start targeting teens with their advertisements; in fact, some already have. They don't seem to mind pregnant and breastfeeding moms using cannabis—it's all about the money to them. They are happy to create addicted people; it is the same 'addiction for profit' industry that they created for tobacco and alcohol. Most cannabis is used by heavy, daily users; the industry literally has *every* incentive to get people increasingly addicted to weed. They talk about social justice a lot, but it is the poor and minorities who are going to suffer the most as marijuana addiction spreads. Minority neighborhoods are where they try to locate the dispensaries, so as to better target disadvantaged people. Speaking of social justice, the cannabis industry uses tons of energy and is not at all environmentally friendly, with its obscenely high water and electricity use.

"Most medical societies are against 'medical marijuana,' which we all know is largely a hoax to get recreational marijuana legalized. At a time when the American public didn't support recreational legalization, cannabis activists pulled on heart strings to sneak 'medical' through. Doctors get stuck as gatekeepers. There is minimal if any regulation of this process, or of the products or the labeling. Anyone can pretend to have a backache, call it 'chronic pain,' and get a marijuana card. There are no conditions that medical marijuana treats that safer, regulated, approved medications can't alleviate. In fact, using cannabis to treat mental health conditions is highly misguided, as it can increase suicide and worsen depression and anxiety. It harms our veterans to give them cannabis for PTSD. There are hardly any randomized controlled studies showing the benefits of cannabis—what benefits people think they are getting are likely just the placebo effect or an 'expectancy' effect. The use of medical marijuana is going up in elderly patients, which can cause falls, memory loss, and confusion.

"Drugged driving is on the rise, with more drivers who are involved in fatal car crashes testing positive for THC. Astoundingly, some people think they drive better while stoned. The cannabis industry does nothing to discourage these dangerous notions.

"The tax revenues from legalizing cannabis have been disappointingly small and don't come close to covering the 'hidden' costs of legalization, such as more crime, more addiction, and more accidents.

"Marijuana has not been approved by the FDA, it is largely unregulated, and people don't know what dose or product they are getting. It is nonsense that cannabis can help with the opioid crisis—the last thing we need is more addictive drugs floating around. People say that marijuana helps with things like creativity, but there is absolutely no evidence of this.

"There are many possibilities between keeping cannabis fully illegal and legalizing it with no restrictions, so we get the free-for-all we are seeing today. For example, it could be decriminalized and distributed through nonprofit, state-owned stores.

"We are in favor of more research into cannabis—both harms and purported benefits, and we certainly don't believe in putting people in prison for marijuana use."

As this book progresses, we will look at the origins and assess the validity of many of these claims. The Cannatopians would be quick to point out that the Reefer Pessimists have always enjoyed a tremendous advantage in spreading their gloomy and sanctimonious message due to the backing of virtually all of the organs of power, including dozens of different agencies in the U.S. government, particularly NIDA, the DEA, SAMHSA, and the ONDCP (Office of National Drug Control Policy). There are many other ways in which bias has entered the discussion.

The medical profession was quickly frog-marched into allegiance with Reefer Pessimism by direct pressure by Anslinger and the Federal Bureau of Narcotics on institutions such as the American Medical Association. Over time, doctors, being the politically passive species of sheep that we are, gave up our clinical knowledge about cannabis and started parroting the government's position, even if it contradicted our clinical experience. As far as cannabis goes, "do no harm" became "be good sheep." Or, in sheep language, "Bah! Bleet! Bah!" The curriculum concerning cannabis in most medical schools—if they mentioned it at all—has been focused on scaremongering and has largely ignored the robust history and potential of medical usage. This is still true today.

Most scientists who have been studying cannabis are just trying to get to the truth about it. But in the aggregate, over the last half century, their jobs have been performed under the biased funding requirements, the political pressures, and the constant propaganda stream of the War on Drugs. This *has* to have had a monumental effect on what researchers think about cannabis and must have had an enormous impact on what people decided to study, as well as on how the studies are framed, interpreted, and explained.

As a thought experiment, imagine what our current scientific canon about cannabis would look like if our government had been aggressively pro-cannabis all along. Imagine that Richard Nixon was a happy stoner. Imagine if billions spent on the "War for Drugs" were spent trying to prove the benefits of cannabis, while studies of harm were rejected. Imagine if researchers searching for benefits were the ones whose careers were funded and supported. If you were a young researcher interested in the harms of cannabis, no one would fund you, and you would eventually either have to find something else to pursue, or you might start investigating some potential benefit. Imagine if our government, along with corporations and the media, had spent the last fifty years telling teachers, parents, scientists, and doctors how helpful and safe cannabis is. Our society's understanding of cannabis would be vastly different. It would already have been re-legalized. We might be in the opposite position that we are in today: trying to achieve balance by educating ourselves about potential harms.

As it stands, we have this vast scientific canon, spanning fifty years, that was performed under subtle and overt pressure to find harm, not benefit, in cannabis. We have these quasi-ingrained beliefs such as "cannabis lowers IQ" that haven't actually been established (see chapter 12). We have things like "amotivational syndrome," which started out as government propaganda points but then were so heavily researched and repeated that they ended up stuck in the minds of many doctors. What do we do with all of this accumulated literature? We can't just throw it all out, but we also can't just ignore the context in which virtually all of our cannabis research was performed—with an agenda.

It's difficult to imagine the War on Drugs taking off at all, or gaining much traction, without the stigmatization and demonization of cannabis, which was the most commonly used and culturally symbolic of the illegal drugs. All crusades need simple messages with clear delineations of who is good and who is bad. Nixon and Reagan wouldn't have gotten anywhere with a more nuanced, and more truthful, message like "cannabis has some harms, especially for teens, but generally is a softer drug, with medical uses, but drugs like heroin, cocaine, and alcohol have more dangers." Rather, they had to go all in with cannabis to make the broader agenda appear coherent and sufficiently scary to be effective.

Many people earn buckets of money, on both sides of the cannabis debate. Corporate support for prohibition never let up and continues into the present. The $40 billion rehab industry handles the bulk of our country's residential addiction treatment. This industry has fattened itself on referrals from the criminal justice system for "cannabis addiction"—even though many of these unfortunates were "caught by the law and sent to rehab" rather than being "addicted to cannabis."

It should come as no great surprise that the private prison industry has also bellied up to the prohibition bar, as their economic model depends on prisons being full. In my opinion, the idea of a "private prison" is one of the low points of American capitalism and of our society in general. It sounds like something from a dystopian Philip K. Dick novel: spend money to keep laws in place that allow law enforcement to lock people up for nonviolent drug offenses, for a profit, so you have more money with which to lobby. Philip K. might call this novel *Do Prohibitionists Dream of Electric Fences?* It brings to mind the Dostoyevsky quote, "The degree of civilization in a society can be judged by entering its prisons." What would he have thought of a for-profit prison? It represents Dostoevskian-grade evil.

The alcohol industry has been worried for a long time that cannabis would cut into their sales, especially low-cost beer. Market analyses have shown that the cost per hour of intoxication is less for cannabis, and thus, for a certain demographic, inexpensive beer gets replaced with weed. Additionally, there's evidence that binge drinking goes down with legalization. While the evidence is mixed, there is data to suggest that in some states, post-legalization, people are substituting cannabis for alcohol. I expect more people to do so as there is increasingly, for the first time, a legitimate choice between two recreational drugs. The alcohol industry, after opposing legalization, is now adopting an attitude of "if you can't beat them, join them" and is fashioning cannabis-infused beverages.

Over the last few decades, Big Pharma has been a steadfast opponent of legalization and has contributed lavishly to torpedoing state cannabis referendums. Their ideal situation is maintaining the illegality of medical cannabis so that, to obtain relief, people must buy their exorbitantly priced cannabinoid formulations. For example, as concisely summarized in a *Washington Post* article,

> Insys Therapeutics, a pharmaceutical company that was one of the chief financial backers of the opposition to marijuana legalization in Arizona last year, received preliminary approval from the Drug Enforcement Administration this week for Syndros, a synthetic marijuana drug.[2]

How cynical! Insys also got into hot water for the kickbacks they provided to doctors for overprescribing their fentanyl lollipops to kids as well as for a rap video they did promoting this fentanyl product.[3] Good people.

More recently, Big Pharma seems to be going along more with legalization, focusing on developing improved drugs via the endocannabinoid system.

Law enforcement, in particular, has always been a superfan of the anti-cannabis narrative, amplifying and embellishing it for decades, as they have profound financial interests in continuing prohibition, as well as ideological interests. For them, cannabis is easy, low-risk work compared to other (actual) crimes they might be involved with. It gives them immense leverage over certain subsets of our population, with their "stop and frisk" policies or their using the smell of cannabis as "probable cause" to search and harass. Guess what demographic usually ends up in their crosshairs.

Local police departments have made a fortune from "asset forfeiture" as a source of revenue. Under broad circumstances, as a result of draconian drug laws that are still on the books in many places, they are allowed to confiscate the assets of people they suspect (or claim to suspect) of drug dealing. These assets end up in the departmental piggy bank. Most criminal justice reformers view this as theft, pure and simple. At best, it is a spectacular conflict of interest.

The racial disparities in arrests and imprisonment for cannabis possession, perpetrated by law enforcement, constitute one of the most shameful
chapters in our nation's history. Blacks and whites use cannabis at about
the same rate, yet Blacks get arrested almost four times as often. This has
resulted in millions of racially biased arrests. It may be difficult to point
to this in order to say that any particular member of law enforcement is
racist, but, as an institution, law enforcement has perpetrated this horren-
dous racial crime on our society. All members of law enforcement need
mandatory trainings on racial sensitivity as well as strict, broad oversight
to put a lid on this type of systemic racism seeping into their activities.

The cannabis component of the U.S. government's War on Drugs has
always had both a high-profile side and a less visible side. During the
late 1960s and early 1970s, much of America was watching on television
the spectacle of hippie protesters enjoying the summers of love, prancing
around in flamboyant garb, challenging conventions, "letting their freak
flags fly," and trying to widely spread their message of peace and love. In
response, they were chased, gassed, beaten, and arrested. Or they were
drafted for the Vietnam War. Nixon's assistant for domestic affairs, John
Ehrlichman, later admitted that the marijuana arrests had been intended
to target leaders of the antiwar left and the African American community.
"Did we know we were lying about the drugs? Of course we did."[4]

There were quieter and gentler ways in which the U.S. government
controlled hearts and minds. Through agencies such as the National Institute for Drug Abuse (NIDA), founded in 1974, the federal government
has exclusively controlled the funding of medical and scientific research.
As NIDA was in charge of the purse strings, as well as of growing and
providing the actual cannabis, for virtually all studies related to benefits and
harms of cannabis, it is legitimate to ask if they were neutral on this topic.

Their first leader, starting at NIDA's inception in 1974, Dr. Robert
DuPont, set the tone. In hearings in 1977, before the Select Committee on
Narcotics Abuse and Control in the U.S. House of Representatives, he said,

> We also want to do much more in the areas of problems associated with
> marihuana use, particularly use among the very young and in populations
> that use marihuana very heavily. Much of our past research has been in
> the areas of more intermittent or occasional use of marihuana. As you

know, the findings there haven't identified serious health consequence associated with marihuana use. *Part of the problem* has been we haven't looked hard enough at the very heavy or long-term users of marihuana—that's something we will do more of in the future. (emphasis added)

It is, indeed, a "problem" if you are running a War on Drugs, are desperately trying to demonize a drug, and the studies don't show it is unhealthy. NIDA, under DuPont, intended to orient its funding toward finding harm, one way or another. For the next fifty years, they would sidetrack or just reject any attempts to investigate benefits. DuPont would later, famously, claim that "marijuana is the most dangerous of all drugs." Personally, he owned drug-testing companies and made a fortune from drug-testing cannabis users and other drug users. He goes on, in 2004:

More people need to see "medical marijuana" for what it is: a cynical fraud and a cruel hoax. . . . Legitimizing smoked marijuana as a "medicine" is a serious threat to the health and safety of all Americans.

This is the person in charge of all of our drug funding? You see the problem—this doesn't exactly provide for a neutral body of research.

One final quote, from 2004: "If an enemy nation were to plan to undermine America's fortune, they could not think of a more effective strategy of poisoning our youth. Marijuana is such a poison."[5]

Fifty years after he was appointed the head of NIDA, he is still fighting the good fight. His website for his "Institute for Behavior and Health" claims, "Marijuana is not needed for any of the illnesses commonly cited by proponents." His institute is supported by a group with a logo that says, "Random Student Drug Testing" (Hmm . . . I wonder who they buy the drug tests from). At least he's consistent.

DuPont established the mind-set, and subsequent directors of NIDA were similarly antagonistic to the need to evaluate the benefits of cannabis. NIDA funds about 85 percent of the world's research on drug misuse and addiction. As we'll see, NIDA blatantly misused this position to deny cancer and other researchers the opportunity to study the medical effects of cannabis.

In defense of sabotaging medical cannabis research, NIDA's director, Nora Volkow, claimed, it's "not NIDA's mission to study the medicinal use of marijuana or to advocate for the establishment of facilities to support this research." Yet for decades they controlled both the purse strings and the actual weed so that no one could legally do substantive research into the benefits. According to journalist and activist Jag Davies,

> the National Institute on Drug Abuse (NIDA) has a monopoly on the supply of research-grade marijuana, but no other Schedule I drug, that can be used in FDA-approved research. NIDA uses its monopoly power to obstruct research that conflicts with its vested interests.[6]

As the *Boston Globe* reported in 2006,

> It's not in NIDA's job description—or even, perhaps, in NIDA's interests—to grow a world-class marijuana crop. . . . Since NIDA's stated mission "is to lead the Nation in bringing the power of science to bear on drug abuse and addiction," federally supported marijuana research will logically tilt toward the potential harms, not benefits, of cannabis.[7]

Very recently, the toxic monopoly NIDA had on being the only source of research weed has been overturned.

The bias in funding, toward harms, persists to this day. According to a 2018 study cited in *Science*, "research on the potential harms of cannabis received more than 20 times more funding than research on cannabis therapeutics, according to an analysis of cannabis research grants from 50 public agency and charity funders."[8] This is now, in our "enlightened" age, with most Americans supporting legalization. Imagine what things were like in the dark days of Nixon's War on Drugs, or Reagan's.

You could write a whole book on the sometimes gruesome experiments our government supported and performed to "prove" the dangers of cannabis. In a 1973 experiment, "Comparison of Acute Oral Toxicity of Cannabinoids in Rats, Dogs and Monkeys," they literally tried to kill dogs and monkeys with cannabis to show that cannabis is deadly. None of the dogs or monkeys died despite receiving phenomenal dosages of cannabis. The monkeys were given as much as 42,300 milligrams of THC. A regular dose is anywhere from five to twenty. This is calculated to be the equivalent of more than eight thousand five-milligram gummies. "In dogs and monkeys, single oral doses of Δ9-THC and Δ8-THC between 3000 and 9000/mg/kg were nonlethal." For an average seventy-kilogram person, that would translate into 630,000 milligrams, or 126,000 five-milligram gummies. The highest edible doses I typically took were twenty milligrams for comparison. I don't think the monkeys or dogs had a particularly good time, as this level of THC makes you very sick and disoriented—add "cruelty to animals" to the long list of abuses during the War on Drugs. Paradoxically, instead of generating the intended headlines, "Cannabis Is Deadly," these experiments did demonstrate that it's virtually impossible for higher mammals (much higher in this case) to overdose on cannabis.

As a consequence of our government's agenda, for the last half century, until fairly recently, the only careers to be made in the field of cannabis were if you studied or found some harm of cannabis. To get a study funded or a dissertation approved, you had to lower IQ, sperm count, motivation, educational achievement, or something else with cannabis. Or you had to find psychosis, delinquency, cancer, depression, depravity, debauchery, or deficits in something important. It became heresy to discuss benefits or even to question harms.

The approval of the DEA was also needed for research. The DEA was so regressive that they at times managed to make even NIDA look like Cheech and Chong by comparison. They obstructed the hell out of any cannabis research that wasn't potentially usable as fodder for the Drug War. This is epitomized by the noble efforts of Dr. Lyle Craker, who is now an emeritus agriculture professor at UMass Amherst. Dr. Craker specializes in medicinal plants. He first applied for a research license to grow and study cannabis in 2001 at the University of Massachusetts. According to Craker,

> It would be nice to be able to develop plant material that would be specific for glaucoma, specific to inhibit vomiting and all those other things that the plant is credited with doing. Currently, people with ailments are . . . going to illegal sources, which I suspect most of them are.[9]

The DEA stonewalled on providing its approval for years, but in 2007, six years later, an administrative law judge for the DEA agreed that it would be "in the public interest" to grant Craker a license to grow cannabis for federally regulated research. But in 2009 an administrator for the DEA overruled their own judge's ruling and rejected the license, *eight years* after it was filed—a decade wasted by the DEA obstructing vitally important research into medicinal cannabis, solely to maintain the narrative that cannabis was harmful, not beneficial. Craker was celebrated as a hero for cannabis, for medicine, and for the right to research, but his decadelong effort wasn't successful.[10]

When the U.S. government says, "There isn't enough research in favor of using or approving medical marijuana," the case of Lyle Craker, one of many, shows us why this is the case. It is a scarcity that was manufactured by NIDA and the DEA.

This obstructionism still goes on today. Cannabis researcher Dr. Sue Sisley has been trying to research the role of cannabis in alleviating PTSD in veterans. She has treated vets for decades. Veterans share a widespread knowledge that cannabis helps their PTSD, and Dr. Sisley wanted to see if there was objective validity to these claims, as well as nuances that could be exploited to improve their treatment. To say she has faced an uphill battle would be to understate the case.

She managed to get NIDA approval for the study in early 2014. Then, a few months later, she was fired from the University of Arizona, almost certainly for working on cannabis. This is an example of what my dad called "psychopharmacological McCarthyism" and is reminiscent of the way Harvard Medical retaliated against him as well for working with cannabis, documented in the piece by the *Harvard Crimson* called "Grinspoon, Reconsidered."[11]

Sisley's work was then supported by the Multidisciplinary Association for Psychedelic Studies (MAPS), which had also supported Lyle Craker (and Dr. Donald Abrams, who comes in later), and which supports rigorous research and education on psychedelic drugs under the dogged, forward-thinking leadership of Rick Doblin. In 2016, the DEA approved of Sisley's work and provided her with the necessary cannabis. A happy ending?

The cannabis that arrived was from NIDA's farm in Mississippi, and it was, as it is rumored to be, profoundly substandard. Remember, NIDA at this point is the only place allowed to grow weed for medical studies, even though many researchers could walk out their door in major cities and legally purchase the beautiful buds that patients are actually using.

Our government prohibits dispensary weed from being used in studies. Sisley described the cannabis she received from NIDA as a "powdery mishmash of stems, sticks and leaves." I've seen pictures and would have turned this down with a snide, disdainful comment if my ninth-grade drug dealer had offered it to me. It tested positive for mold and was about 8 percent THC, when dispensary weed is twice that. Genetically, it was found to be closer to hemp than to marijuana. How are you supposed to demonstrate benefit with this? If you gave it a strain name, it would be called Moldy Mush.

Under pressure, the DEA had been promising for years that it was going to open up more places to grow and provide cannabis to researchers so that researchers don't have to use Moldy Mush, which wouldn't cure your basic need to get stoned, let alone any medical problems under investigation. Dr. Sisley suspected that the DEA was still playing games to foil medical cannabis research, as they have been doing since their inception, in this case by dragging their feet. She sued them for their legal justification to prevent researchers from accessing better pot.

Sisley's case was ultimately dismissed, but it moved the ball forward in many ways. To start, she educated many on the specific mechanisms by which the U.S. government has been deliberately preventing research on medical marijuana. By 2021, the DEA was forced to consider applications from other growers. As poetic justice, one of these applications was from Dr. Sue Sisley's lab.

With concerted efforts from citizens and scientists, the U.S. government's stranglehold on medical cannabis research is finally weakening. We are a half century behind where we would have been without this Drug War mentality, and we are behind other countries, but better late than never. Thank you, Dr. Sisley, Dr. Lyle Craker, Dr. Donald Abrams, MAPS, and thousands of others for your dogged advocacy!

# CHAPTER THREE
# CANNATOPIANISM

Another narrative started branching off as cannabis was criminalized in 1937. I'll call this other narrative "Cannatopianism" to capture its idealism, often accompanied by its own quality of quasi-religious zeal. We didn't hear too much about a cannabis underground when it was criminalized in the late 1930s. People continued to use cannabis, or there wouldn't have been the perceived need to add additional criminal statutes, such as the Boggs Act in 1952 and the inclusion of cannabis in the 1956 Narcotics Control Act.

In the 1970s, in response to the renaissance of cannabis use, Nixon went after cannabis with evangelical enthusiasm. This strengthened the already-growing movement for legalization. During the 1980s with Reagan's all-out "this is your brain on propaganda" campaign, the cannabis movement was on the defensive but still managed to plant the seeds for eventual medical legalization in California in 1996. The need for legalization was publicly illustrated by the suffering of the victims of the War on Cannabis (see chapter 6). With each pointless arrest, each needless imprisonment, and widespread stories of people just trying to treat infirm family members or neighbors and being raided by the police—with each of these outrages, the Cannatopian movement grew stronger.

Like any ideology, Cannatopianism spans a wide range of denominations, but it generally refers to a belief in cannabis as a medicine, a wellness aid, and a lifestyle enhancer, not a problematic, seductive drug that needs to be eradicated.

One phenomenon that helped legitimize this narrative from the beginning is that most people's lived experience with cannabis had no resemblance to the picture that was being painted about cannabis by the

U.S. government. For example, in the poster for the 1936 movie *Reefer Madness*, there is a hypodermic syringe. Have you ever seen or heard of anyone injecting cannabis? Is it even possible? "Hey man, do you have a kit I can borrow? I need to mainline some weed." The only person I know of who has injected anything similar into people is a researcher at an Ivy League institution who injected people with relatively large doses of 99.6 percent pure THC in a profoundly unnaturalistic laboratory environment and then opined, in effect, "Look, these twenty people are anxious and disoriented, therefore the use of the cannabis plant causes psychosis and schizophrenia and therefore should not be legalized." (This is quite representative of the research our government was funding to support the narrative it was trying to spin.)

With the 1937 Marihuana Tax Act, the U.S. government was determined to prevent doctors from dispensing, and patients from legally utilizing, cannabis as a remedy for their ills—but this didn't mean that cannabis stopped having medicinal value. The commonly purchased tincture bottles may have disappeared from the shelves, but criminalization of the plant itself didn't change its chemical composition. Cannabis remained a potent biological factory producing hundreds of chemicals, which are particularly adept at hijacking and magnifying our natural endocannabinoid systems. In response to racist appeals and Harry Anslinger's urgent proscriptions against the ills of cannabis, human physiology didn't change, with its widely distributed networks of cannabinoid receptors that can block pain and facilitate sleep.

Anslinger, followed by many others in his place, utilized the organs of government and the press to taint cannabis. In many ways, the War on Cannabis over the last century is a case study in both the power and limits of propaganda, as well as in how governmental pressure can affect the process of scientific discovery.

Cannatopians were not without sporadic glimmers of encouragement from mainstream institutions. In 1944, a report from the LaGuardia Committee, which was prepared by the prestigious New York Academy of Medicine, condensed five years of research into thirteen points, all along the lines of,

> The practice of smoking marihuana does not lead to addiction in the medical sense of the word. . . . The use of marihuana does not lead to morphine or heroin or cocaine addiction and no effort is made to create a market for these narcotics by stimulating the practice of marihuana smoking. . . . Marihuana is not the determining factor in the commission of major crimes. . . . The publicity concerning the catastrophic effects of marihuana smoking in New York City is unfounded.[1]

Anslinger was apoplectic. This prestigious panel of doctors had the potential to whisk away the propaganda house of cards he had been meticulously erecting, including such cornerstones as the "gateway theory" that cannabis use leads to addiction to other drugs and the "marihuana causes violence and crime" narrative. Anslinger forced the medical journals to retract their initial praise for this report and publish criticisms of it. One might reasonably ask why these doctors went along with this—there is no flattering answer. Anslinger took steps to ensure that few if any independent medical studies came out under his watch that concluded anything except that marijuana is harmful.

Almost three decades after the LaGuardia Committee undermined Anslinger's attempts to exaggerate the dangers of cannabis, a similar thing happened to a more familiar drug crusader, Richard Nixon. A committee that Nixon appointed to gear up for his reinvigorated War on Cannabis, called the Shafer Commission, named after former Pennsylvania governor Raymond Shafer and formally known as the National Commission on Marihuana and Drug Abuse, concluded in 1972 that the concerns and fears about marijuana were vastly overblown. It concluded,

> From what is now known about the effects of marihuana, its use at the present level does not constitute a major threat to public health. . . . We believe that experimental or intermittent use of this drug carries minimal risk to the public health, and should not be given overzealous attention in terms of a public health response.[2]

It called for the decriminalization of cannabis and a selective focus on the very small percentage that become heavy users.

After blowing a gasket or two, Nixon proceeded to flat-out ignore the recommendation of his own committee. He doubled down on his crackdown as if nothing had happened. The damage to his credibility was already done. Nixon the scientist responded to his own Shafer Commission:

> As you know, there is a Commission that is supposed to make recommendations to me about this subject; in this instance, however, I have such strong views that I will express them. I am against legalizing marijuana. Even if the Commission does recommend that it be legalized, I will not follow that recommendation. . . . I can see no social or moral justification whatever for legalizing marijuana. I think it would be exactly the wrong step. It would simply encourage more and more of our young people to start down the long, dismal road that leads to hard drugs and eventually self-destruction.[3]

This, of course, raised the question of why he commissioned a group of top experts to make recommendations if he was going to do the exact opposite of what they recommended. I guess they weren't being sufficiently sensitive to his political need to fight a racially based War on Drugs.

The Shafer Commission provided sustenance and ammunition to the Cannatopians in several ways. First, it gave official backing to their stance that the government's position on the harms of cannabis was largely a fabricated construct, not a legitimate medical stance. The Shafer Report validated their lived experience that cannabis was more of a medicine and a wellness and lifestyle enhancer than a deadly drug. Finally, Nixon's nonresponse to the Shafer Commission evidenced the notion that there was a government conspiracy to keep cannabis illegal regardless of what the facts revealed and the experts concluded.

Not to be left behind in pure mindlessness, Canada had a similar thing happen. Its Le Dain Commission was a governmental commission that concluded in 1972 that the fears about cannabis were being grossly exaggerated and that cannabis should be decriminalized and researched. The (first) Trudeau administration ignored its conclusions as nothing more than an inconvenient annoyance distracting from their attempts to parrot U.S. drug policies.

Cannatopian culture was a natural fit with the antiwar left of which Richard Nixon was so fond. People were beaten, arrested, and jailed. This, as we've seen countless times in so many political struggles across time and history, is a great way to strengthen a cause or a symbol. In 1970, the

Controlled Substances Act passed, which entirely outlawed any usage of marijuana as a medicine or recreationally, putting it into Schedule I, along with heroin and LSD, drugs that are defined as having "no currently accepted medical use and a high potential for abuse." Of course, LSD and heroin both also have important medical uses, but that is sort of off topic right now. Once a substance is labeled "Schedule I," it becomes notoriously burdensome to research.

Were doctors willing to stand up for the Cannatopian point of view during the tumultuous time of the Vietnam War? It would have greatly helped so many of the young people who had lost faith in the "system" if even a significant minority of adult role models spoke up against the nonsense and helped validate their beliefs. A few doctors stood up, but too many hid, sheeplike, in their suburbs, not lifting a finger in the face of exponentially increasing cannabis possession arrests. These went from a few thousand per year in the mid-1960s to nearly half a million per year by the mid-1970s.[4]

There was immense professional pressure to not challenge the orthodoxy on this issue. Being pro-cannabis had echoes of bucking McCarthyism. Only a few doctors showed integrity and courage—including my father. This provided an invaluable ballast and credibility to the Cannatopians. My dad paid a price in terms of denied promotion and other disapproval from Harvard Medical.[5]

After cannabis was ostracized from doctors' offices, it, by default, became allied with the "naturalistic" healing camp. From the strict Cannatopian perspective, using cannabis to help you sleep, instead of a pharmaceutical sedative like the barbiturates or the benzodiazepines they were using at the time, is like eating fresh blueberries instead of McDonald's, so natural medicine wasn't entirely a bad fit for cannabis. In truth, cannabis has been around for millennia, and who knows what Benadryl, Ambien, Belsomra, trazodone, or Valium (diazepam) actually do to your brain over the long term (we don't use barbiturates for sleep anymore because they are too dangerous).

Despite severe criminal penalties, the use of cannabis was never extinguished. The very underground nature of pot surely added to its allure, with hippies passing pipes around VW vans, getting baked on the way to a Jimi Hendrix concert, in the face of "square" adults droning on and on about how dangerous marijuana is. Cannabis became a powerful symbol not only of countercultural rebellion and freedom, but also of naturalistic health and healing. Unfortunately, it also contributed to the unsound reasoning that goes along the lines of, "Because it's natural it's safe," which often isn't true (think of poisonous mushrooms). The fact that doctors, along with other civic leaders, were saying things about cannabis that were so obviously contradicted by the lived experience of young cannabis users helped cement the pervasive distrust of authority at the time.

What was it about cannabis that landed it front and center as the symbol of resistance in the sixties, the seventies, and beyond? Did it just happen to be the symbol, due to being at the right time and place, as well as having powerful cultural associations, like the image of the Ukrainian fighter saying, "Russian warship: F*ck off" (or the symbols of the tractors towing destroyed tanks off the battlefield)? Or is it because cannabis itself had some psychopharmacological properties that brought out, and were related to, the actual changes in people and in society that the counterculture wanted to see? It's not hard to imagine that young people coming from the mind-numbingly boring, conservative, and conformist 1950s would be tempted to smoke something that stimulated creative thought, facilitated social connection, and lessened the brainless monotony of our culture.

Cannabis seemed to bring out exactly the types of brainwaves the authorities of the time didn't want to have emphasized or propagated. It seems plausible that the creativity, sexual freedom, heightened sensations and perceptions, mindfulness, independent thinking, and awe and sense of newfound wonder in the world—all of the things that cannabis fosters—could uncoincidentally have landed it in the center of the fray. It was more convenient for the government when people merely drank themselves into oblivion. They might throw punches or crash cars, but they weren't talking about revolution. Now cannabis was fomenting dangerous thoughts and was fertilizing a countercultural explosion of art, music, and activism.

Are these reasons related to why some people remain so opposed to cannabis to this day? Maybe the fight between the Reefer Pessimists and the Cannatopians comes down to societal echoes of the 1960s rift between the hippies and the straights, or simply to how people believe that members of society should think, feel, and behave.

Throughout the 1970s, there were hundreds of thousands of arrests per year for cannabis possession. However, despite the steady drumbeat of anti-cannabis propaganda from the government, the political climate started to improve for Cannatopia by the mid to late 1970s. This was largely in response to the legalization movement. There was state-level progress toward legalization as a dozen states decriminalized cannabis and many others reduced their penalties. In 1973, Oregon became the first state to decriminalize, reducing the penalty for up to one ounce to a $100 fine. Other states passed medical cannabis laws, the first of which was New Mexico in 1978.

There were more prominent national advocates coming forward, including President Jimmy Carter in the White House. He stated the problem quite eloquently:

> Penalties against possession of a drug should not be more damaging to an individual than the use of the drug itself; and where they are, they should be changed. Nowhere is this more clear than in the laws against possession of marijuana in private for personal use. . . . Therefore, I support legislation amending Federal law to eliminate all Federal criminal penalties for the possession of up to one ounce of marijuana.[6]

This doesn't mean that the arrests stopped; the curve merely flattened out, hovering around four hundred thousand a year. That's more than one in a thousand Americans getting arrested each year for cannabis possession. There is no way to quantify this cost in terms of economic, social, or emotional pain. The damage caused by involving millions of young Americans with the criminal justice system cannot be understated. A criminal record often follows a person for life, affecting student loan applications, college admissions, job prospects, social standing, and housing.

This legacy of widespread and purposeless criminalization of people is why one so frequently hears the words "expungement" (i.e., removing or erasing a criminal record so they can go on with their lives) and "reparations" in the context of discussions of how the plant should be legalized. This is especially relevant to Black and brown Americans, who have withstood the brunt of the arrests and who need to be made whole again.

For a variety of reasons, the legalization movement fizzled out in the late 1970s. Support for legalization was around 12 percent in 1971 when my father's book came out, shooting up to around 30 percent over the next eight years. Then, starting in 1980, support began to decline, dropping down to the mid-twenties by the end of the Reagan years.

This reversal of fortunes in the legalization movement comes down to several factors: missteps by the legalization movement, the declining popularity of President Carter, and a movement rightward in the national sentiment on drugs. One debacle in the legalization movement, in particular, both epitomized and catalyzed this change in momentum. It involved not just cannabis, but some cocaine molecules and a high-profile nose.

I remember, when I was around twelve years old, my usually mild-mannered father was furious, storming around the house and muttering to himself. My twin and I were like, "What did we do now?" But for once this had nothing to do with us. It had to do with what the *Washington Post* labeled the "cocaine-sniffing incident." Who was doing the sniffing? Unfortunately, it was President Carter's director of drug abuse policy, Dr. Peter Bourne. According to a 1978 article in the *Post*, "Dr. Peter Bourne publicly used two illegal drugs, cocaine and marijuana, at a party given for 600 people by the National Organization for the Reform of Marijuana Laws." Whoops.

Dr. Bourne denied the cocaine use, but once the media frenzy gets going, it is difficult to quell. Apparently there were witnesses. Dr. Bourne subsequently got into hot water for a prescription he wrote for a staffer. According to a *Frontline* interview with Dr. Bourne,

> [the staffer] said she didn't want it on her record, and she'd rather that I use a pseudonym or something, so I used a pseudonym for her. I signed my own name to the prescription and used a pseudonym for her, which is common in normal medical practice.[7]

What? No it isn't! I can write prescriptions for controlled substances, for anyone and everyone, using fake names for them, and then have anyone pick it up? Absolutely not. My previous opioid-addicted self would have loved this loophole!

In any case, Bourne was forced to resign. This was not a good look for the architects of the liberalized cannabis policy, and it helped bring the momentum of cannabis legalization to a screeching halt.

With the election of Reagan, a new sheriff was in town, one who wanted to stigmatize and persecute drug users. First Lady Nancy Reagan launched her national, stigmatizing "Just Say No" campaign, which whipped up hoards of parents, who didn't know anything about drugs, into a "parent's movement," which was essentially a genteel, misinformed lynch mob. Cannabis arrests doubled under Reagan, reaching almost a million per year. Reagan did exactly what Carter wisely warned not to do by creating "penalties against possession of a drug [that are] more damaging to an individual than the use of the drug itself." Kids were even encouraged to turn in their parents. The War on Drugs had lost its mind.

This renewed aggressive prosecution of cannabis possession drove the active Cannatopians underground. Many cannabis growers were forced either indoors or overseas, or they were imprisoned. The 1986 "Anti-Drug Abuse Act" included vicious mandatory minimum sentences for many drug-related infractions and dumped another $1.7 billion into the War on Drugs ($5 billion in today's dollars). This law "led to a massive increase in incarcerations for nonviolent drug offenses, from 50,000 in 1980 to 400,000 in 1997."[8]

The sustained pressure that the DEA placed on cannabis growers caused the plant itself to evolve. It became too dangerous for growers to continue to cultivate the sativa varieties (e.g., Acapulco Gold, which gives an energetic, euphoric high), as these were tall and expansive plants—and thus too easily seen by snooping DEA agents in helicopters. In response, the cultivators interbred them with indica varieties (e.g., Afghani; more of a relaxed, calming type of high; indica = "in-da-couch"), which are short and bushy. These "hybrids" made outdoor growing much more difficult to detect. It also leaves us today with mostly "hybrid" varieties of cannabis available, which contain aspects of both varieties.

Under the market pressures of prohibition, the THC content of cannabis steadily climbed, as this made for the most economical smuggling. Unfortunately, the levels of the more medicinal cannabinoids, such as cannabidiol (CBD), dropped in a proportional manner. The variety of different strains, or, technically, "chemovars," proliferated, as did the quality and variety for recreational purposes, as breeding was elevated to an underground art form. The War on Drugs ruined countless lives, but it greatly improved the quality and augmented the potency of the recreational weed—while making all weed less medicinal. Ironic.

Soon, large-scale outdoor cultivation became too dangerous altogether, and breeders went indoors and started to grow hydroponically. This became a cult science, with many brilliant people contributing to the evolution of profoundly powerful and more enjoyable (and potentially more addictive) cannabis. Not to be deterred, the DEA started staking out and targeting customers at hydroponics stores. They subpoenaed the customer lists and used them to target people with raids (see chapter 6). On numerous occasions they raided and terrified innocent people who had no connection to cannabis. For example, during Operation Constant Gardener, there was an ill-fated 2012 raid in Kansas of two retired CIA officers, during which law enforcement barged in with assault rifles, utterly traumatizing the parents and kids alike, only to find a small hydroponic tomato garden.[9] The DEA also monitored electrical bills looking for spikes in usage that would suggest the use of indoor grow lights, and they used infrared sensors from helicopters to find the thermal signatures of indoor grow operations.

Meanwhile, the movement for medical access was accelerating, fueled by the AIDS epidemic, as cannabis was thought to be particularly effective at treating the severe pain and weight loss/wasting that often accompanies a diagnosis of AIDS. It was too visibly cruel to deny cannabis to these patients—the U.S. government was getting justifiably annihilated in the public relations war. Who could possibly support, in good conscience, the sending of dying AIDS patients—or those who supply them with misery-sparing cannabis—to prison? This is your conscience on drugs.

To blunt this seemingly unstoppable momentum toward the legalization of medical cannabis, the U.S. government legalized Marinol in 1985. Marinol is pure, synthetic THC, the main psychoactive component of cannabis. Marinol does have medical utility. However, as THC is only one of five hundred or so molecules in the cannabis plant, if people just use THC alone (i.e., Marinol), they don't benefit from the "entourage effect," which results from the synergistic effect of all the molecules in cannabis working together to produce a "whole that is greater than the sum of its parts" effect. The entourage effect speaks of evolutionary precision, and to find therapeutic benefit, patients often require more than just the main THC molecule. I don't believe there have been many patients who have found that single-molecule THC (Marinol) is as effective as cannabis itself for alleviating symptoms. Also, it doesn't have the pleasing, creative effects of cannabis. I've tried Marinol once (for scientific purposes . . .), and it just made me feel fuzzy and dull—a huge disappointment. It didn't help my migraine, which whole-plant cannabis reliably does. Legalizing Marinol wasn't particularly effective in slowing medical cannabis legalization.

Throughout the 1990s, collectives called "buyers' clubs" were at times tolerated in California and other places, and at other times were raided by the feds. Each raid cemented and broadened the movement to legalize and provided a PR black eye for the DEA. This was especially true when they terrified and menaced terminally ill or elderly patients who were using medical cannabis. Desperately ill patients would show up in court in wheelchairs and handcuffs. Typically the judge would respond, "What are you doing here? Go home and suffer in peace."

The most prominent advocacy group for the Cannatopians was NORML, the National Organization for the Reform of Marijuana Laws. NORML has been fighting doggedly for legalization for half a century, with lots of victories under their belt. My dad, and many of the guests who peopled my childhood home, were early, influential members of NORML. I remember a beautiful poster hanging in our porch my entire childhood, a piece of artwork with the NORML logo. It featured a quote from Spinoza:

> He who seeks to regulate everything by law is more likely to arouse vices than to reform them.

I read that quote almost every day when I was growing up. At some point, its wisdom starts to sink in.

In 1972, NORML petitioned to reschedule cannabis. Having it in Schedule I, with "no medical utility and high abuse liability," made cannabis almost impossible to study, so that the government could continue to say "there's no evidence" of benefit. After years and years of stalling and litigation, the DEA was finally forced to hold public hearings. In 1988, more than a decade after the original petition, the DEA's own administrative law judge, Francis Young, after an extensive review of the literature, sided with NORML, stating, "Marijuana, in its natural form, is one of the safest therapeutically active substances known to man." Judge Young continued,

> The evidence in this record clearly shows that marijuana has been ac-
> cepted as capable of relieving the distress of great numbers of very ill
> people and doing so with safety under medical supervision. It would
> be unreasonable, arbitrary and capricious for DEA to continue to stand
> between those sufferers and the benefits of this substance in light of the
> evidence in this record.[10]

The War on Cannabis could have ended in 1988, yet, for political, ideological, and budgetary purposes, the DEA overrode their own administrative law judge. They refused to reschedule cannabis. It remains locked in Schedule I to this day. Think of the lives that might have been spared from harm had they listened to Judge Young! The DEA has incalculable misery, and some blood, on its hands.

The citizens of our country were starting to have enough of this nonsense. Support for legal access to medical cannabis had been steadily growing. Awareness was spreading about the different medical benefits and the relief it was providing to suffering patients. The stories and images of terminally ill people getting raided and arrested put the cruelty of the illegality of medical cannabis in sharp relief. In the face of all this, the government was having trouble sustaining an adequate level of mass hysteria and moral panic about the harms of cannabis with the public. Increasingly, lived experience was trumping gaslighting.

Decades of governmental stonewalling, combined with a steady increase in public support for legal access to medical cannabis, paved the way for the states to take their own decisive action. California was the first, legalizing medical use in 1996 by ballot initiative. Proposition 205 easily passed, with 57 percent voting in favor, and only about a third of people voting against. It passed in California by more than a million votes under the brave leadership of activist Dennis Peron.

When the medical marijuana law passed in California in 1996, Clinton's drug czar, Barry McCaffrey, called California's law, which has provided safe and humane comfort to millions and which is still active and popular almost three decades later, "a falsely labeled, cynical initiative," and he stated, "We should ask ourselves whether we really want Cheech and Chong logic to guide our thinking about medicine." It is astounding that someone in this high a position of authority could have such a cartoonish, fantastical picture of medical cannabis. It was almost as if he actually read and believed his own department's nonsense! They threatened to yank the licenses of any California physicians who provided cannabis for their patients. They even threatened them with criminal charges. The feds were forced to back down by the full weight of public disapproval, as well as by Dr. Marcus Conant, who clubbed them senseless, repeatedly, in the federal court system.[11]

Dr. Marcus Conant was a clinical professor in dermatology at the University of California, San Francisco. He was the one who first discovered Kaposi's sarcoma in AIDS patients—an enormous contribution that saved countless lives. He was the lead on a lawsuit, brought about on behalf of patients and doctors, to stand up for their rights to discuss the use of medical cannabis openly, without government censorship.

The lawsuit contended that doctors and patients have a First Amendment right to discuss treatments without fear of governmental interference. The first judge agreed: "The First Amendment allows physicians to discuss and advocate medical marijuana, even though use of marijuana itself is illegal," and ruled in favor of the doctor and the patients. Seems reasonable.

The case was appealed by the feds, who then tried to argue that there is a national standard for the practice of medicine, and individual doctors shouldn't be allowed to depart from that by recommending cannabis. Once again, the government's position was shot down. According to the judge, "Who better to decide the health of a patient than a doctor?" Case dismissed.

The Department of Justice appealed again, yet were met with criticism and skepticism from the next judge they encountered:

Why on earth does an administration that's committed to the concept of federalism . . . want to go to this length to put doctors in jail for doing something that's perfectly legal under state law?

In a 3–0 ruling, the government lost, with this judge noting that the government's attempt to bar doctors from recommending medical marijuana

does . . . strike at core First Amendment interests of doctors and patients.
. . . Physicians must be able to speak frankly and openly to patients.[12]

Amen to that.

The Department of Justice took this to the Supreme Court, which refused to hear the case, giving all cannabis patients, and all doctors, regardless of their stance on cannabis, a final victory. This paved the way for other states to legalize medical marijuana. Anslinger and the feds were kicked out of the exam room once and for all, at least for the cannabis issue.[13]

As they say, "the rest is history," though it's a living history that we are still in the middle of. California was the first crack in the dam in 1996, followed by other states voting on ballot initiatives. Now, twenty-five years later, almost all of the other states have instituted some sort of medical cannabis laws or provisions. At the time of this writing, nineteen states have fully legalized recreational use as well. The narrative is now shifting from "Should we legalize it?" to "How can we most effectively legalize it?"

Is there truth to the Reefer Pessimist claim that medical cannabis is just a Trojan horse for legalizing recreational cannabis? Of course, some people will fake or exaggerate symptoms to get cannabis, just like they do for opioids or benzos, or for handicap plates. Some doctors just sign off on medical cards for the cash and don't really evaluate the patients. These scenarios aren't ideal, but they by no means invalidate the entire endeavor, which is to provide safe medical marijuana to millions of patients. To claim this is to speciously dismiss the history of the profound suffering of medical patients and the vast relief they have found with cannabis, which is what ultimately fueled the legalization movement.

Several states have simultaneously legalized medical and recreational, so even if "first medical, then recreational" was the paradigm in the past, it's sort of moot now. In chapter 21, we discuss how very fine, and possibly illusory, the line is between "medical" and "recreational" or "adult use" cannabis.

One main problem with the "first legalize medical then recreational" structure is that it puts doctors in the role of gatekeepers. The three problems with this are, first, that doctors know less about cannabis than almost any other group—so how does it make sense for them to be the gatekeepers? Second, people don't view doctors as reliable resources on this issue. And third, this is the absolute last thing that most overtaxed doctors wish to deal with.

How well is legalization going so far? It depends on whom you ask. As far as I can tell, arrests are dropping, fewer Black and brown lives are being needlessly harmed, and we are wasting less money on enforcement and imprisonment. Neither crime, driving accidents (see chapter 11), nor teen rates of usage have climbed. Opioid and other prescriptions are down (see chapter 15), as well as Medicare D prescriptions across the board, for conditions that medical cannabis can treat, as shown in Colorado. Records are being expunged. The quality of regulated cannabis that users are exposed to, now routinely tested for mold, heavy metals, and other contaminants, is much safer. Tax revenue is robust. For example, in 2021 in Massachusetts, tax revenue from cannabis, for the first time, was higher than tax revenue from alcohol: $74 million versus $51 million.[14]

Reefer Pessimists claim that the tax revenue we are collecting from cannabis sales will be dwarfed by all the "hidden costs" of legalization, such as future addiction, crashes, and crime, though I haven't seen any solid, consistent evidence for this from sources that are independent of law enforcement.

More medical patients now have safe access to a safer product. A large proportion of people can now buy cannabis without legal or employment risk. The use is more out in the open, and thus it's easier to get help if you run into difficulty. It appears to be a win all around. Law enforcement, itself, is freed up to investigate and safeguard against actual criminal behavior that is harmful to society.

It's much too early to see longer-term trends, like whether the rates of addiction or other harms, such as mental health issues, will go up, as the Reefer Pessimists are concerned about. Indeed, there are some areas for concern. It would be better if we had an accurate way to monitor, detect, and prevent stoned driving. ER visits appear to be going up for pediatric exposures, though it's possible that this is partly an artifact secondary to people now being able to tell the truth about why they are there at the ER without criminal or social penalties. I believe that this particular problem would be easy to fix if people would just accept some reasonable limits around not making edibles into candies or chocolates so that kids don't stumble into accidental exposures. Another valid concern is that many people are inappropriately receiving medical advice from medically untrained budtenders, though this has a straightforward fix as well—educate doctors and nurses about cannabis so that they can provide legitimate education for patients. Use in pregnant and breastfeeding women is rising, which is concerning in the absence of data that this is safe (see chapter 10), though at least with legalization they are generally consuming a safer product.

We can all agree that no one has solved the problem of how to minimize the illicit market, except perhaps to avoid taxing the legal market to death, as for example they do in California.

Mini Ted Talk: I think making edibles into yummy treats that a small child or a pet would eat its way through is reckless and dangerous. I wrote a piece on this for Harvard Health, "Cannabis Is Medicine—Don't Make It Taste Good." A little kid, or a pet, wouldn't have any reason not to eat the whole bag of gummies. That's their job. The experience would be terrifying at best, and they might even become extremely ill and end up in the intensive care unit. At minimum, we need child-proof packaging and much better labeling. I was recently at a medical dispensary that had a chocolate bar with 1,100 milligrams of THC—this is insane and could really hurt someone! If a puff is about five milligrams, that would be the equivalent of 220 puffs. That is a dangerous weapon. People counter that with, "People should just be responsible" or "Medicine shouldn't have to taste bad." Being a primary care doctor for twenty-five years teaches you that all people aren't always responsible! I agree that medicine shouldn't taste bad, but that doesn't mean it should be put into candies that are particularly palatable to kids—surely there is a middle ground. End of Ted Talk.

I also wonder about the new concentrates that so readily expose users to such high doses of THC, up to 90 or so percent. This is not the plant we evolved with for thousands of years and know to be relatively safe. I don't think it matters if the flower is 10 or 20 percent THC; it's silly to try to legislate this type of cap. People titrate to their own level of comfort and generally do not enjoy the feeling of having taken too much. These types of limits just make medicine more expensive for medical patients and fuel the illicit market. The concentrates *are* really intense, and their use hasn't been studied. We don't know how safe they are, especially for younger users. People retort, "Hash has been around for thousands of years." The current market in concentrates has gone well beyond the hash of the past in strength and availability. Also, smoking hash that is 30 percent THC is quite different from dabbing crumble or wax that is 90 percent. My concern is balanced with the knowledge that making any of these things illegal merely drives the behaviors underground and provides huge incentives for people to use the illicit market, which is always more dangerous. Education ultimately works better than criminalization.

Stepping back a little and putting things in a historical context, Cannatopianism is now more hopeful and accepted than it has ever been. Legalization is spreading around the globe. The percentage of Americans who think cannabis should be fully legal continues to increase—69 percent at this writing, including more than 50 percent among every major political party.[15] More research on medical utility is being funded, both outside of the United States and, begrudgingly, despite the Schedule I status, within the United States. More data on medical benefits is flowing in, and we are expanding our understanding of what valid data is with real-world evidence (see chapter 7). Arrests and incarceration are trending down, statewide referendums are passing (or cannabis is being legalized by legislature), and more state governments are wholeheartedly supportive of legalization. Most believe it's a question of when, not if, cannabis will be legalized on the federal level as we clean up the past excesses and abuses of our criminal justice system. This is a story of regular citizens standing up to one of the most powerful propaganda and corporate juggernauts in the world and facing it down.

The two narratives, Reefer Pessimism and Cannatopianism, represent millions of people on both sides, with different persuasions and opinions. While there are some reasonable voices in the middle, which resonate with both sides, in general, the two narratives seem to reinforce and radicalize each other—like everything else in this country right now.

As legalization is impending, we must take what is helpful and what rings true from each of these narratives in order to fashion a unified and cohesive conception of this plant: its biology, its actual harms, and its medical and wellness potentials. As we develop a deeper understanding of how these stories split apart, what forces nurtured and influenced each of them, how they evolved, and what relevance each has to the modern realities of cannabis science and policy, we can cobble or bludgeon them back together into cannabis common ground.

## CHAPTER FOUR
# DOOBIE NO HARM
### Doctors and the War on Drugs

Why is it that when you go to your doctor to ask about, or for, medical cannabis, or tell them about your medical usage, hoping to integrate it into your care, they don't seem to know anything about it? Maybe they look embarrassed and try to change the conversation. They might mutter something dismissive like, "That's not a good idea," "That hasn't been proven yet," or "That's addictive," and then start prodding you about your undone colonoscopy or a cholesterol test that is needed. The sensible dictum to "tell your doctor about your medical cannabis use" collides with the grim reality that when you do, nothing helpful occurs.

It wasn't always so. Throughout the second half of the nineteenth century and right up until 1937, when cannabis became effectively prohibited in the United States by the Marihuana Tax Act, doctors routinely prescribed cannabis tinctures and considered it to be an effective, mainstream medicine. It wasn't controversial.

So how did American physicians go from being ardent proponents of, experts in, and defenders of cannabis medicine in the 1930s to their current black hole of knowledge about even the basics of medical cannabis? The passage of the Tax Act in 1937 made it virtually impossible thereafter to perform research or to treat patients with cannabis, so the accumulation of further lived experience treating patients with cannabis came to an end. Without lived experience, people are susceptible to manipulation and propaganda, which was provided in spades by the Federal Bureau of Narcotics. Many doctors were still in favor of cannabis, having used it successfully with their patients before the prohibition, but now this conflicted with political reality.

45

Harry Anslinger, the mercurial director of the Federal Bureau of Narcotics, waged a campaign to force doctors into allegiance with the government's position on cannabis. He was phenomenally successful. In 1967, just thirty years after the American Medical Association testified *against* criminalization, the AMA's position expressed in an editorial in the *Journal of the American Medical Association* was that "cannabis (marihuana) has no known use in medical practice in most countries of the world, including the United States." (We'll ignore the fact that this statement makes no sense; in what countries *does* it have medical use? And why would it be useful there and not in the United States if not for political reasons?) The AMA goes on to state,

> The use of marihuana among Puerto Ricans and both southern and northern Negroes is reputed to be quite high. In all likelihood, marihuana use among the poverty-stricken urbanite is concomitant with other dependence-inducing substances and a broad range of asocial and antisocial activity.[1]

This piece closes with a rousing call to action: "Marihuana is centuries old, but it represents a constant danger. The responsibilities of the citizen, including the physician, are clearly defined. The time to begin is now." The AMA hasn't really changed its position much in the subsequent fifty-five years, aside from hiding the racism of their cannabis policies better, by appearing to support more racially just policies. For example, in 2022 they decided to support expungements of cannabis-related offenses, yet they remain opposed to cannabis legalization (so there will continue to be more cannabis-related offenses that need to be expunged).[2] This also makes no sense! It is no wonder that only 15–18 percent of American doctors belong to the AMA,[3] down from 75 percent in the 1950s.

Why on earth did the doctors of the time go along with this mandated propaganda campaign? Were they cowards or wimpy sheep who allowed themselves to be the accoutrements of a broader influence campaign? Or did they just not have access to better information? (The information was clearly out there, as my dad was able to find it, albeit with concerted effort.) Perhaps it is difficult to understand, in retrospect, the political pressures these doctors were under. Maybe they felt that they could no longer make any money prescribing cannabis, so they cynically, or pragmatically, decided not to fight for it. Either way, by capitulating so easily to this model, where overzealous government officials could dictate what doctors believe, say, and do for their patients, they missed an invaluable opportunity to avoid repeating the mistakes of alcohol prohibition and to push back at the start against our War on Drugs that has been unraveling the fabric of our society since its inception.

As a new generation of doctors rose through the ranks; survived the indignities, foul odors, and bodily fluids of medical school; donned their white coats and recited the Hippocratic oath, a collective amnesia seemed to set in about the fact that doctors had, not so long ago, readily utilized and supported cannabis as a treatment. This amnesia was fostered by the menace of relentless political pressure, as well as the juicy lure of research dollars, which were strictly awarded to researchers investigating the harms of cannabis. Studies of benefit simply were not funded. Imagine if we had studied aspirin, or any medicine, only from the vantage of harm. We would have learned that it causes bleeding ulcers, but if we had stopped there, we wouldn't have the foggiest idea that it helps prevent heart attacks and strokes. There are millions of deaths and disabilities that we never would have prevented.

This sea change in medical practice was not initially driven by any legitimate or evidence-based discussions of health concerns, but by external forces to which the doctors succumbed: sociopolitical and corporate forces. The criminalization of cannabis was never based on anything medical or health related. Later on, doctors would come to parrot and amplify the U.S. government's harmful claims about cannabis, and these vastly exaggerated concerns eventually became integrated into the accepted belief system of modern medicine. If you repeat something enough times, it can start to become your truth. Then studies were funded, performed, and interpreted so as to reinforce and amplify these beliefs. This isn't to say that none of these concerns had merit or that there weren't new concerns that came up in response to clinical situations, but there was a very particular context in which these concerns first arose.

As the cultural dislocations of the 1960s hit full force, tensions across our society were boiling over. Cannabis became a powerful symbol, for both sides. For the counterculture, it meant freedom, creative thought, community, cultural liberation, and rebellion. For "straight" people, it became emblematic of moral decay, degeneration, and rejection of the establishment. Unfortunately, many physicians lent their skills and expertise to help club the young protestors with stereotypes about male cannabis users as brain-damaged, sperm-depleted, breast-growing, amotivational primitives who were shedding IQ points daily. Our nation's physicians almost exclusively marched with the establishment, even though it was not scientifically supported (with unbiased science) or socially beneficial.

All along, there were a minority of doctors who stood up for honesty about cannabis, or at least for not criminalizing the users of it. Generally doctors, ever-present authority figures, were firmly placing themselves on the wrong side of the War on Drugs. The end result—continuing to this day—was the evolution of a profound rift between the lived experience of patients who used medical cannabis and the accepted belief system of medical professionals.

The fact that science can be warped by cultural forces has been evidenced so many times throughout history, including by its widespread misuse in the War on Drugs. But as astronomer Carl Sagan often wrote, science is ultimately self-correcting. Eventually research started to catch up with the truth about cannabis. By the time I started medical school at the Boston University School of Medicine in 1993, scientists were making one breathtaking discovery after another about the endocannabinoid system, though studies on the clinical use of cannabis still lagged far behind. My father's then-new 1993 book *Marihuana, the Forbidden Medicine* was just coming out to great fanfare. In this book, my father explained,

> The largely undeserved reputation of cannabis as a harmful recreational drug and the resulting legal restrictions have made medical use and research difficult. As a result, the medical community has become ignorant about cannabis and has been both a victim and an agent in the spread of misinformation and frightening myths. What follows is largely a book of stories because most of the evidence on marihuana's medical properties is anecdotal. Someday the systematic neglect of the research community will be remedied and the authors of a book on the medical uses of marihuana will be able to review a large clinical literature.[4]

Every time I read these words, I feel like he's speaking to me from 1993. Just as he predicted, this current book, about a medicine that is now less forbidden—in no small part due to his tireless efforts—will be able to draw from a much deeper well of clinical research than my dad's book could have.

None of the advances in understanding the endocannabinoid system penetrated the hermetic medical school bubble I was in. It was like the Dr. Seuss story *Horton Hears a Who!* But in the opposite direction: no one inside this hermetic environment could hear any new ideas from outside about cannabis unless it was a very particular type of idea in a very specific language. Few of my peers seemed interested, except my roommate, and he was from Cyprus and wasn't brought up with (or didn't care about) the same antidrug messages. To me, this presented great cognitive dissonance. Not only had cannabis vastly alleviated the suffering of my brother Danny, but I knew that profoundly important and relevant things were happening scientifically and politically, developments that should have been of great interest to medical practitioners and instructors. Yet this all seemed to be happening in a reality that was utterly divorced from my experience at medical school.

My medical school education on the topic of cannabis was oddly abridged, given that tens of millions of Americans were using it and half of all Americans had tried it. It consisted of perhaps a few minutes in lectures on pharmacology and a few passing mentions in other contexts, such as under "drugs of abuse" or during the lecture by a forensic psychiatrist on some of the most gruesome cases of psychosis and violent crime (which, in retrospect, had little to do with cannabis and which did illustrate the seeping into medical education of deliberately constructed stereotypes).

To me, it felt as if our curriculum had arrived, unedited, from the federal government's official "This Is What We Want Doctors to Think about Cannabis" file. We learned about the "gateway theory" that pot use leads to harder drugs (it doesn't). We learned about the amotivational syndrome, in which you lose drive and motivation as a consequence of cannabis use (you don't). We learned that cannabis use lowers IQ, even though subsequent studies contradicted this once they remembered to factor in socioeconomic variables (privileged kids do better on standardized tests than poor kids do).

The medical benefits of cannabis were given some very scant lip service, as they couldn't entirely ignore that so many patients were using it, such as for chemotherapy symptom relief. No one was upset when I raised my hand in my pharmacology class and said, "But what about the fact that people with HIV are using it effectively for pain control and to prevent weight loss?" but no one seemed particularly interested either. The lack of curiosity or willingness to think outside the box within which our education was packaged seemed pervasive, only partially to be explained by how exhausted and beaten down we were.

This formalized and stereotyped education fully contradicted the experiences that, even back then, some of my first patients were relating to me about the notable benefits they were experiencing. The take-home message—throughout all four years of medical school—was that cannabis was a drug of abuse with little medical benefit and certainly not something worthy of much bandwidth in the curriculum. I begged to differ.

In the year 2000, my senior presentation during medical residency at Harvard's Brigham and Women's Hospital was on medical cannabis. I had hoped that Harvard would be more open-minded and accepting about cannabis than medical school at Boston University had been, but I should have factored in how conservative Harvard was. After all, this was the institution that—at that very moment—was retaliating against my dad for his cannabis advocacy, though I didn't realize at the time that this was still going on. The Harvard Medical School attitude now is somewhat more progressive on cannabis than it was back then, especially after some key donations, such as the multimillion-dollar donation in 2019 to Harvard and MIT from Charles Broderick for cannabinoid research.

My father, whose long-standing office at the Massachusetts Mental Health Center was just a few blocks away, came to my presentation. My classmates were young enough to be skeptical about the propaganda about cannabis that our profession was feeding us. Many of them had used it in college without harm, and certainly all of them had friends who had done so. They all had patients who were using it, with benefit, and mostly without harm. So I don't think that many of my colleagues were particularly anti-cannabis at that point. They all respected my clinical skills and intellect. What was lacking was a conviction that this would ever be a legitimate treatment. There was no context for my presentation because cannabis has always been discussed in light of substance misuse, not in terms of wellness. As such, I don't think my presentation penetrated very deeply. The sense in the room was, "This is the latest eccentric idea Peter is enthusiastically espousing. How quaint. Time to go back to real medicine." Decades later, some of these same colleagues now refer patients to me.

I have always integrated medical cannabis into my own primary care practice. With my patients, I often find cannabis to be effective for mild to moderate chronic pain and insomnia, though I've also had success with a wide variety of other conditions, including anxiety, spasticity, PTSD, fibromyalgia, and, coming full circle, chemotherapy-induced nausea and vomiting. I based my practice on a combination of whatever clinical research existed at that point in time—there's more every year—the past cases I've cared for, whatever "real-world evidence" there was, my patients' preferences, and my deep personal understanding of the effects of cannabis. I had a secret weapon: I could always call my dad or stop by his office and run cases by him.

As with other medications, cannabis doesn't always work for any particular person or condition, and it has side effects and toxicities to look out for. My rule of thumb is to ask, "Is this safer than the alternative I would be using?" If the alternative is something like opioids or benzodiazepines (e.g., Valium), cannabis is usually safer. Cannabis has worked often enough, and well enough, to make it an indispensable tool in my toolbox.

The irony is that, as a primary care doctor, having medical cannabis as an option to help my patients actually makes my work life a lot easier— and would do the same for other doctors if they took the time to learn about it. For example, we don't have an abundance of safe and effective medications for insomnia, assuming you've exhausted the nonmedical options. You start a patient on something that is supposedly relatively harmless like melatonin—though recently even this has been questioned. When that doesn't work, to me it seems obviously safer to offer a few drops of a gentle CBD-predominant cannabis tincture (mostly CBD with just a little bit of THC, maybe a 4:1 or 12:1 ratio), which will allow my patients to drift off to sleep in a mild, relaxed euphoria, than it would be to break out the heavy-duty tranquilizers such as Ambien or trazodone. Similarly, for chronic pain, why destroy the kidneys with daily NSAIDs if a modest dose of cannabis does the trick? What other medicine simultaneously alleviates four or five things at once to improve the symptoms of fibromyalgia (pain, insomnia, anxiety, quality of life)? There were reasons why doctors once used cannabis so widely and are starting to do so again—it works, and it is often a safer alternative.

Many doctors today, who tend to be overwhelmed and burned out, would rather not deal with cannabis at all. It is one more thing to be added to an already overly full plate. Life was simpler when they just had to read a few dismissive paragraphs of Reefer Pessimism in medical school and then, in response to patient inquiries, regurgitate the post-1937 party line that cannabis is addictive, harmful, and has no medical utility. The problem is, at first gradually and then in larger numbers, patients stopped buying this message. Currently 94 percent of Americans support legal access to medical cannabis. Doctors can no longer get away with shutting patients down with a pejorative, commanding, "You don't use marijuana, do you?" (Of course not, doctor!). It is difficult to think of anything else that 94 percent of Americans agree on.

Patients are hungering for high-quality information and are expecting their doctors to know enough about cannabis to have intelligent, helpful conversations about it. Cannabis-savvy patients aren't inclined to give doctors the benefit of the doubt, perhaps knowing that cannabis has been legalized despite the doctors who (with certain notable exceptions) have been firmly ensconced on the wrong side of the War on Drugs, with medical associations weighing in on the wrong side of virtually every cannabis-related state ballot initiative. Patients have led, doctors are following, and thus doctors are starting from a point of questionable credibility on this issue. That said, most polls show that people would prefer to get accurate information about cannabis from their doctors than from anyone else.

According to a 2017 study in the journal *Drug and Alcohol Dependence* titled, bluntly, "Physicians-in-Training Are Not Prepared to Prescribe Medical Marijuana," it was documented that only 9 percent of medical schools have medical cannabis in their curriculum and that "84.9% reported receiving no education in medical school or residency on medical marijuana."[5] Our "endocannabinoid system"—the vast network of neurotransmitters and receptors that controls a whole host of bodily functions and which also provides the mechanism by which cannabis acts—isn't taught at a majority of medical schools. This is astounding because this system is vitally important to virtually every internal system we have and mediates such essential functions as sleep, emotional processing, energy expenditure, appetite, and memory. Because of the War on Cannabis, research and teaching on it has been delayed and is lacking. According to a study by Dr. David Allen in 2013, only 21 of 157 schools—13 percent—mentioned the endocannabinoid system in even one course.[6]

If doctors haven't been taught the basics of medical cannabis, and if they haven't been taught the underlying physiology by which these basics would make sense, and if instead they have been subjected to a steady stream of misinformation, it is understandable that they wouldn't be particularly open-minded about, and welcoming of, this field.

What's stopping doctors from getting up to speed now? Aside from the holes and misconceptions in their education, which is fixable, some of the main obstacles are as follows:

- Modern medicine is used to working with medications that are single compounds, and cannabis is a plant that has five hundred or so compounds in it. For this reason, it is difficult to envision it being approved by the FDA, or patented either. Big Pharma is unlikely to sponsor any trials of whole cannabis, as patients can grow it on their own, so there is no profit incentive.

- Cannabis is a poor fit for evaluation by the same scientific means that have been the "gold standard" for Western medicine—the randomized, blinded, placebo-controlled trials. For example, you can't "blind" someone as to whether they are given cannabis or a placebo, as most people tend to notice if they are stoned or not. If you start craving Doritos or chocolate, or start *really* enjoying the music or waxing poetic about the meaning of life, that is an obvious tip-off. Cannabis often alleviates several symptoms at once—for example, pain, sleep, and anxiety. Conventional medical studies often measure just one metric at a time. We need a different lens altogether through which to view the efficacy of cannabis (see chapter 7 on real-world evidence).

  I should note here that some of the concerns my cannabis-averse colleagues have are quite legitimate. Even if you make the argument that the research has been unfairly suppressed for the last eighty years by the War on Drugs, there still *is* a relative lack of evidence into the clinical benefits of cannabis—at least the type of evidence we are used to—compared to many other treatments that we use, though this is changing (see chapter 7 on what counts as evidence). Doctors themselves have good reason to doubt treatments that have not been scientifically established. Patients present anecdotal evidence for all types of miracle cures and flaky treatments—magnets, mega-vitamins, homeopathy, herbal brews—which we feel perfectly comfortable dismissing in the absence of evidence, so why should we hold cannabis to a different standard? Why not stick to treatments that have been proven?

- The dosing can be extremely inconsistent, nonuniform, and rather foreign to many doctors. Take this Sour Diesel gummy and call me in the morning.

- Smoking a medicine is anathema to doctors, and anything that is smoked is hard to conceptualize as a medicine. While vaping cannabis with a dry herb vaporizer (which heats to a much lower temperature than combustion and has many fewer unhealthy particulates) is much safer than smoking, this idea hasn't been adopted or understood by most doctors. Though topicals, tinctures, inhalers, skin patches, suppositories, and edibles are all viable options, the stigma persists in the eyes of medical professionals, as many patients still do smoke it. An extremely bright and well-regarded psychiatrist friend of mine recently said to me, sort of in a huff, "How can inhaled burning plant material possibly be a medicine?" (As just explained, it doesn't have to be burning or inhaled.)

- Cannabis is quite enjoyable when used recreationally, causes a mild euphoria, and for many people can enhance the enjoyment of food, sex, music, nature, and art. Medicines aren't viewed as enjoyable—this makes them suspect. Due to the intrinsically puritanical nature of our society—and as a hangover from the War on Drugs—pleasurable substances aren't medicines, and medicines aren't meant to be enjoyed. (Think of the expression "Take your medicine.")

- Utilizing medical cannabis involves ceding quite a bit of control to patients. Doctors don't control the dose, strain, or delivery method beyond the ability to make suggestions (if they know enough about it to do so), which can then be modified by budtenders. Saying, "Try taking a sip of the strain Northern Lights from your vaporizer when you get nauseous," is very different from saying, "Take ten milligrams of Compazine." This exercise in doctors not being control freaks could actually be good for doctors and patients alike, as doctors could stand to relinquish some power in this relationship, and patients often thrive with more autonomy. However, even I get nervous when I hear stories of budtenders at dispensaries giving my patients advice like, "My cousin's sister-in-law had a headache five years ago at a Dead concert and said that Afghani Hash made it go away, so why don't you try some of our infused bubble hash for your migraines?" Certainly, the budtenders—all of whom seem quite well-intentioned—do need mandatory education and regulation if they are even tangentially going to be giving out medically related suggestions.

- Utilizing "real-world evidence" instead of only one type of evidence (e.g., randomized controlled trials, or RCTs) is a cognitive shift (see chapter 7).

- Doctors never asked to be the "gatekeepers" of cannabis and resent being thrust into this role.

So, what can doctors do to get on the same page as patients and be in the care loop? Be humble. Educate ourselves. Be open to learning things we don't know and to listening to the wisdom of other types of healers. Be comfortable saying, "I don't know—let me look it up," or sending patients to someone who does know. Don't bluff—that never turns out well. Don't add to the stigma. Most of all, don't shut down communication. There are many reasons why doctors and patients need to have open communication about cannabis, including side effects and potential drug-drug interactions.

That doesn't mean you can't express your opinion if you disagree; just do so respectfully in order to keep the channels of dialogue open.

The way in which doctors embrace cannabis will be, in essence, a personality test for the entire profession. Can we muster the humility to learn this new field, to undo our past mistakes, and to help move the yardstick forward on social justice?

Meanwhile, what can patients do? Many patients have as bad a pot problem as doctors do, with the internalized stigma that has come from decades of Drug War propaganda and a lack of helpful knowledge. The shame and self-doubting can be off the charts. I have had elderly patients slink into my office, check that the door is fully closed, look around as if to check that the shades are drawn, and then slyly whisper, "Doctor, I'm in pain, I can't sleep. I can't take Advil anymore because of my kidneys. Is it OK to . . . to try marijuana?"

Time slows. A dangerous pause. I wonder whether to wait for backup. I know my duty.

"That's it, Grandma, on the floor. Right now! Hands where I can see them. I'm calling the DEA!"

I use my stethoscope to bind up the miscreant, press the panic button in my exam room so security will arrive, and move on to the next patient.

OK, not really. But the stigma is real, and sadly many patients are unnecessarily conflicted and feel needless guilt and concern. Over time, this stigma will continue to die down as millions of Americans are having positive experiences themselves—or with loved ones—using medical cannabis.

Patients must not let their doctors off the hook. Educate yourselves. Expect us to know this subject. Push back when we say things that aren't true or that reek of paternalism, propaganda, or stigma. Bring us articles to read. Quiz us when you see us again. Remember—with this issue, you have been leading, and we have been following. We screwed this up. We got it wrong. Our lack of both courage and independent thinking perpetuated the War on Drugs, which destroyed so many families. Help us finally enter the twenty-first century on cannabis. While we are getting up to speed and trying to reform our conservative medical institutions on this issue, do your best to find safe, credible sources of information that you can share with us.

An increasing percentage of doctors, particularly younger ones, are with you on a quest to become better educated on this issue. This is evidenced by a 2018 piece in the medically related online magazine *STAT*, written by two Harvard medical students, "Med Schools Need to Get with the Times on Medical Marijuana, Chronic Pain, and More," which bemoans the current, shocking lack of education. According to this piece,

> the majority of physicians-in-training are not being prepared to have informed conversations with their patients about medical marijuana, let alone recommend it as a treatment. This mismatch is striking, reflecting a failure on the part of medical schools to adapt to changing laws and a changing culture around marijuana.[7]

In a study published last fall, researchers found that fewer than one in ten medical schools included medical marijuana in their curricula. Two-thirds of medical school deans reported that their graduates "were not at all prepared to prescribe medical marijuana," and a quarter reported that their graduates "were not at all prepared to answer questions about medical marijuana."[8]

Even more worrisome, the survey demonstrated that almost 90 percent of physicians in the final stages of their training—residents and fellows—felt they weren't at all prepared to prescribe medical marijuana, and more than one-third felt they were not able to accurately answer questions about it. Almost 85 percent reported receiving no education about medical marijuana during medical school or residency.

It turns out that most doctors truly do believe that cannabis is an important medicine, which makes it all the more tragic that we are so far behind on this issue and that the medical societies are so out of touch. According to a 2019 piece, "A Survey of the Attitudes, Beliefs and Knowledge about Medical Cannabis among Primary Care Providers," 58 percent of PCPs believe that medical cannabis is a legitimate medical therapy.[9] Yet "one-half of providers were not ready to or did not want to answer patient questions about medical cannabis, and the majority of providers wanted to learn more about it." These results are similar to a 2021 study, "A Systematic Review of Medical Students' and Professionals' Attitudes and Knowledge regarding Medical Cannabis," which showed that 77 percent of medical students and 65 percent of medical professionals believe that cannabis has therapeutic utility. Fifty-eight percent of students claimed to have an "adequate or better" understanding of medical cannabis, whereas only 33 percent of medical professionals thought their knowledge was adequate or better.[10] Another 2021 study showed that 68.9 percent of doctors believe that cannabis has medical use.[11] This number seems to grow every year.

All studies showed a large demand on the part of medical students and doctors for more and better education. This, of course, needs to be modern, quality education, not the same nonsense we've been given. A 2020 flagship continuing medical education course for primary care, put on by a very prestigious medical school that will remain unnamed, had an abysmal session on medical cannabis. It was worse than I could have imagined. I actually felt embarrassed for our field and for my institution. The speaker started the lecture stating that he didn't know anything about medical cannabis, and then quoted facts from a "textbook for doctors" that he clearly didn't realize was written by people who were making a polemical case that cannabis *wasn't* useful as medicine.

The introduction to this "textbook for doctors" was written by a retired drug warrior at the Hudson Institute, who concluded, "We can now count the costs of the spreading acceptance of legalized drug use as serving to damage not only public health and criminal justice, but national security as well."[12] No bias there. Duck and cover—legal weed is coming! The book curated which studies they cited to misleadingly paint a dismal picture of the harms and benefits of medical marijuana. The best part was in the section on palliative (or end-of-life) care. They felt it important to alert us that "eye redness, caused by dilation of blood vessels in the eye, is one of the most notorious side effects associated with cannabis use"—it is difficult not to satirize. In my own head, "God forbid if one of my dying patients who is suffering from metastatic cancer and crippling bone pain suffers from *eye redness*! Not that!! Oh no!!! The hall monitor might catch them . . . get some Visine stat!" The dedication reads, "Dedicated to those who have . . . lost loved ones to any substance of abuse and addiction, including marijuana." No one has ever died from consuming cannabis!

Using a book like this is like using a textbook written by creationists to teach evolution. I'll spare you the story of when I tried to give feedback to the course directors. It was like trying to change the trajectory of a slowly moving iceberg. Not successful. Doctors don't need more of the same stigmatizing anti-education. Doctors need actual, helpful, practical education so as to be able to work with patients and meet them where they are, or at least understand what they are saying. We need to unite, not divide.

There's a taboo on medical doctors using cannabis, or at least discussing their use publicly, because the medical boards are antiquated, undereducated, and reflexively punitive on this issue. Even using medical cannabis can get you into hot water. One can only wonder about the origins of a double standard where doctors are allowed to consume alcohol, sleeping pills, muscle relaxants, antihistamines, Valium, Neurontin/gabapentin— whatever intoxicating and debilitating "legal" substances they want, as long as it isn't the "evil weed." As cannabis is becoming legal and is increasingly confirmed to be less harmful than alcohol and many of the prescription drugs we so freely prescribe, it begs the question: why are the medical boards not evolving more rapidly on this issue?

I did have a recent chat with someone on the Massachusetts Medical Board, and he was quite supportive of medical cannabis for patients. However, we didn't specifically discuss use by physicians. Horror stories of harassment and excessive punishment abound. When I first started as an associate director of the Massachusetts Physician Health Service, in 2013, I couldn't believe that doctors were actually getting in trouble for using cannabis. The addiction doctors spoke about cases so suspiciously—"he said he just had a few puffs at a dinner party"—implying that the client must have been compulsively smoking cannabis since preschool. The way they spoke about it, taking a puff or two—in a legal state, enough to get slightly buzzed and have a nice time—sounded, as they discussed it, as if, intoxication-wise, it were on the same level as having injected several speedballs of cocaine and heroin. Again, lived experience is vital to accurately gauge these things.

According to a 2018 piece in the prestigious online physician magazine *KevinMD*, "Using Marijuana Two Times a Month Cost This Doctor His License," a doctor, in a state where cannabis was fully legal, took a routine preemployment drug test.[13] He had admitted to twice-a-month cannabis use because . . . why not? It's legal, generally harmless for most adults, and far safer than alcohol and many of the prescription meds doctors are allowed to use. He had no idea that there was a destructive stigma against doctors using cannabis. The drug test was positive for cannabis. He was forced to go to rehab and was diagnosed with "severe marijuana dependence" and "told that he needed to stay for 90 days of inpatient treatment, which they just happened to offer on-site, at a cost of over $50,000." He refused, and the board yanked his license. He has not practiced medicine since, in an age of severe impending physician shortages.

Currently, in some ways our medical system is in a slow-motion collapse. This is due to the "great resignation" of many doctors, particularly PCPs, who are suffering the ill effects of burnout and moral injury. Many are quitting or are cutting down their hours, while others are sleepwalking through decreasingly meaningful careers as doctors continue to become commodified and treated like cogs in someone else's machine. We are under relentless pressure from our hospitals to see more patients, for less money, and we are increasingly burdened with idiotic administrative tasks. Because we can't unionize, we are defenseless against this nonsense. I've seen the care get more dangerous every year. We are constantly undermined by the insurance companies in our attempts to procure the care that our patients desperately need. Many, if not most, people—doctors included—utilize some chemical to relax at night or on the weekends to "take the edge off." It would be great if society, and people, were such that none of us needed anything, but it isn't, and they aren't. Until now, the only (legal) choice for doctors has been alcohol, which is more dangerous and incapacitating than cannabis on every metric.

As cannabis becomes legal, there's absolutely no reason that doctors shouldn't be allowed to choose it instead of alcohol. The relaxation, insight, mindfulness, and fellowship that cannabis provides could help many doctors work through the burnout and depersonalization they are currently suffering from. For many, this could be exactly the type of wellness they need. Cannabis, if used modestly, doesn't give you a noticeable hangover compared to alcohol. Just as for pilots, there should be some guidelines in place about safe usage, such as perhaps a neurosurgeon not using it less than thirty-six hours before surgery (or whatever turns out to be evidence based, with unbiased studies).

If doctors can handle making life-or-death decisions for patients, they ought to be able to handle the recreational usage of legal cannabis. With one less punitive and senseless policy to contend with, maybe fewer of us would quit medicine.

A few words about my father's involvement with the cannabis issue. In the late 1960s, my dad, a psychiatrist at Harvard Medical, decided to look into the research on marijuana, to "see what all these foolish young people were doing to themselves." Never one to do things halfway, he started from a blank slate and spent countless hours in Harvard Medical's vastly resourced Countway Library, reviewing every bit of the current and past research on marijuana.

He was subject to conflicting cultural influences around cannabis. On the one hand, as an establishment Harvard staff psychiatrist, he was about as firmly ensconced in the school of Reefer Pessimism as one could be and was exclusively schooled in the contemporary psychiatric/governmental line about decreasing sperm rate, men growing breasts, plummeting IQ, amotivational syndrome, genetic damage, brain damage, etc. As my dad described it once he had escaped from the intellectual bubble, "the established belief views marijuana as an addicting drug that leads to personality deterioration and psychoses and to criminal behavior and sexual excess."

On the other hand, politically, he was a progressive, it was the late 1960s and early 1970s, and friends of his—including his best friend, the astronomer Carl Sagan—were using cannabis, without obvious negative impact. They were openly discussing the benefits, such as enhanced connection, creativity, spirituality, and sexuality. He was determined to get to the bottom of the issue.

What eventually resulted from this exploration was his landmark book, published in 1971, *Marihuana Reconsidered*, in which he reevaluated, from scratch, virtually everything that is known about this plant, from its ancient uses to the contemporary science. He completely undermined the rationale for the criminalization of marijuana even though that is not at all what he set out to do. The evenhanded, scholarly tone and the meticulous research enhanced the credibility of the book. *Marihuana Reconsidered* beautifully depicts the rich cultural history of cannabis use throughout the last several thousand years. It explores why certain brilliant historical figures such as Théophile Gautier, Charles Baudelaire, Allen Ginsberg, and Carl Sagan (who used the pen name "Mr. X" in the book, as he was still in the cannabis closet) used marijuana and what it did for them. It reviewed the known harms and weighed in on which of these were actually evidence based and which were mainly feverish creations of the U.S. government's War on Drugs. He concluded that criminalization was more damaging to the youth than the cannabis itself was:

> We must consider the enormous harm, both obvious and subtle, short range and long term, inflicted on the people, particularly the young, who constitute or will soon constitute the formative and critical members of our society by the present punitive, repressive approach to the use of marihuana. And we must consider the damage inflicted on legal and other institutions when young people react to what they see as a confirmation of their view that those institutions are hypocritical and inequitable. Indeed the greatest potential for social harm lies in the scarring of so many young people and the reactive, institutional damages that are direct products of present marihuana laws. If we are to avoid having this harm reach the proportion of a national disaster within the next decade, we must move to make the social use of marihuana legal.[14]

The dedication of *Marihuana Reconsidered* originally read, "To Danny: Children are the greatest high of all." The reprinted paperback said, "In Memory of Danny," as my brother succumbed to his leukemia in 1973. My dad's efforts earned a glowing front-page review in the *New York Times Book Review* under the title "The Best Dope on Pot So Far."

My dad's efforts didn't go unnoticed by the then drug warrior in chief, Richard Nixon. According to one of the daily presidential briefs obtained by star reporter Dan Adams of the *Boston Globe*, *Marihuana Reconsidered* was summarized for Nixon as follows (borrowing, we think, from a book review in the *Gaffney Ledger*),

> It's not easy for anxious parents to listen with an open mind to arguments for legalization of marijuana. They're apt to feel that only a wicked or foolish person would want to see pot more readily available to young people than it already is. Dr. Lester Grinspoon is neither wicked nor foolish. After long and careful study of all sides of the question, Grinspoon is convinced that present anti-marijuana laws are doing far more harm than good. He believes that "If we are to avoid having this harm reach the proportions of a real natural disaster [we need to reform the marijuana laws]." This conclusion, and an impressive array of arguments to support it, are presented in his new book, *Marihuana Reconsidered*. Grinspoon acknowledges that use of marijuana may under some circumstances be harmful to some people, particularly adolescent chil-

dren. But a detailed review of medical evidence leads him to this verdict: "The harm resulting from the use of marijuana is of a far lower order of magnitude than the harm caused by the abuse of narcotics, alcohol, and other drugs." There are equally reputable and conscientious medical scientists and law enforcement officials who vehemently disagree with Grinspoon's conclusions. This agonized issue is one on which every citizen has a responsibility to make up his own mind. Grinspoon's book is a cogent presentation of one of the possible viewpoints.[15]

The name Grinspoon is circled, and a note is written: "H—I'm sure I recall—this clown is far to the left." (H was presidential advisor Bob Haldeman.) This makes me fairly certain that another infamous Nixon quote—"You know, it's a funny thing, every one of the bastards that are out for legalizing marijuana are Jewish. What the Christ is the matter with the Jews, Bob? I suppose it is because most of them are psychiatrists"— was directed at my dad.

It might have confirmed Nixon's most paranoid fantasies about Jewish psychiatrists if he only knew that within a year or two, my parents would be buying pot illegally for my brother Danny, to help him as he was dying from leukemia.

My dad's book and advocacy did much more than ruffle the corrupt feathers of Tricky Dick. *Marihuana Reconsidered* provided much-needed intellectual credibility, leadership, and ammunition to the nascent legalization movement, which continued to gain momentum. His follow-up book, *Marihuana, the Forbidden Medicine* (*MTFM*) was a dynamic overview of the current state of medical cannabis research, supplemented by case studies. It presented an eloquent defense of anecdotal evidence in the presence of our government's effective restriction on funded research of the benefits of medical cannabis. Borrowing the nerdy locution of his friend astronomer Carl Sagan, he referred to anecdotal evidence as "the N of 1 study," meaning a study with only one subject. In *MTFM*, which came out in 1993, he notes that since 1967, more than ten million people had been arrested on cannabis charges. That number has doubled by now.

In 1971, *Marihuana Reconsidered* provided an initial bright light illuminating the path out of the first half century of cannabis darkness, which began with the Marihuana Tax Act in 1937 and which became much darker with Nixon's War on Cannabis. *MTFM* became a second beacon, and just in time. This 1993 book proved critical, along with the work of hundreds of exceptionally dedicated activists, when California voted by ballot measure to legalize medical pot in 1996. I have colleagues who told me that the book *MTFM* is what made them go into the field of medical cannabis.

Decades later, when my dad was eighty-nine years old, a piece written by the editorial staff of the *Harvard Crimson* titled "Grinspoon, Reconsidered" reviewed my dad's many unique accomplishments and discussed how Harvard Medical had retaliated against him for his work on cannabis and psychedelics by repeatedly denying his promotion to full professor. My dad's CV boasts a list of accomplishments and publications that would have qualified him ten times over—eleven books and over 180 scientific papers. The *Harvard Crimson* concluded:

> Given the circumstances surrounding his promotion, we believe these biases may well have had a significant effect on Grinspoon's attempt to become a full professor.
>
> The immense good Grinspoon's novel research has done for not only his discipline but for societal issues and law reform is difficult to dismiss and warrants recognition. It has been used to fight for the decriminalization of marijuana possession, which has disproportionately affected communities of color.
>
> In the future, we hope that researchers and members of the Harvard community make every effort to recognize novel contributions irrespective of societal trends.[16]

In response to this article, and to a similar one on the front page of the *Boston Globe*, Harvard Medical did . . . nothing.

Over a span of fifty years, through times of setbacks and disappointments, including the dark Reagan years and their long aftermath, my dad persevered. In 2016, long retired but still extremely active, he had the satisfaction of observing the legalization of cannabis in his home state of Massachusetts. There is a picture in the *Boston Globe* of him taking a huge hit while smoking with family friend and activist (for veteran access to medical cannabis) Stephen Mandile, who was given the honor of buying the first joint legally sold in Massachusetts. He wanted to share it with my dad. The strain was Jack Herer, named after another legendary activist. My dad called it a "dream-fulfilling event."

## CHAPTER FIVE
# COSTS OF CANNABIS CONFUSION
## The Cash Cows Are Mooing Loudly

Often when I consult with patients or families about medical canna-bis, they are bewildered because they have received conflicting and contradictory advice from several different providers. Of course it's not an uncommon experience for patients to receive differing advice—that's what happens when patients request second opinions, or just because physicians have varying practice styles. But rarely in medicine are patients put into the situation where there are such fundamental disagreements, and where there is, de facto, almost always a second, contradictory opinion.

Among most clinicians, there are a few areas of general consensus about cannabis, such as avoiding cannabis before driving, avoiding dur-ing pregnancy (except in special circumstances—see chapter 10), and not using during teenage years. Most of us would agree that smoking is the least healthy way to consume cannabis. However, even this may contradict the advice a patient receives from budtenders, shamans, herbalists, natu-ropaths, or whomever patients go to once they realize that they won't get much useful, specific, or nonjudgmental information from their doctors about how to utilize cannabis.

Even within the same hospital, patients can get starkly contradictory advice about cannabis or report that the advice I gave them was met with stern disapproval by other providers. "I saw Dr. Jones for my pain, but I don't think she's a big fan of medical marijuana." I usually qualify any advice I give with the contextualizing information that there are a broad range of opinions about cannabis, that many doctors aren't entirely in agreement with medical cannabis, and that no one has a monopoly on the truth. I emphasize that it is important to be open and to communicate with all providers for the sake of safety. Dr. Staci Gruber, an esteemed cannabis researcher, in her landmark 2016 study "Splendor in the Grass?" put it as follows:

> Despite the rapid changes in policy, many legislators, consumers, physicians, and the general public remain misinformed about marijuana.[1]

Many patients are diligently trying to educate themselves, but it's unclear where to go for unbiased, quality education.

Part of the problem is that we truly just don't have a definitive answer to some of the basic questions about cannabis, such as "what does it do to the teenage brain?" (see chapter 13), so people default to the scientific "truth" that conforms with their ideological views of cannabis. As Nietzsche said, "Convictions are more dangerous enemies of truth than lies." In other words, in the absence of truths that are "written in stone," one is free to pick studies that evidence a more Panglossian or a more Pessimistic narrative about cannabis. There are plenty of studies from which you can construct a truly scary view of what happens to the teenage brain, especially with heavy usage before the age of sixteen. There are plenty of other studies that don't show much, or any, effect on IQ once the playing field is leveled by factoring in things such as poverty and education.

To add to the confusion, the same study can produce vastly different interpretations and headlines depending on the editorial bent of the news outlet or advocacy group. For example, say cannabis use were to go down broadly after legalization in all adolescent age groups in a particular state, except for a modest bump in fifteen-year-olds. Some headlines will emphasize "teen cannabis use dangerously rising," while others might report, "teen cannabis use down overall." Sometimes a particular newspaper visibly shifts its editorial position. When the reactionary cannabis hater and casino billionaire Sheldon Adelson bought Nevada's largest newspaper, the *Las Vegas Review-Journal*, the editorial policy went from pro- to anti-legalization for the upcoming referendum.[2] The joys of capitalism!

The list of people impacted by this ongoing societal indecision and endless debate about the benefits and harms of cannabis certainly includes teens, who hear what they want to hear. Like the kids of divorced parents, if teens get two different answers to a question, they will naturally pick the answer that suits them best. The key is telling them the truth about cannabis, recognizing its appeal, explaining the harms, and understanding that they might experiment or have questions. Keep focused on the message "just say wait" until they are older and their brains are better developed, so they don't risk harming themselves. Just like it is better if divorced parents are able to speak with one voice for the sake of the kids, it would be better if we all spoke to teens with a unified message about cannabis. Most teens truly don't want to hurt their brains.

Next on the list is medical patients. Hopefully we are nearly done with the "cannabis isn't a medicine" nonsense from the Dark Ages, though some medical societies still put "medical cannabis" in quotation marks. It makes it much more challenging to treat patients in a safe and effective manner if they are getting contradictory information about what is safe and effective. The stigma makes all communication more difficult. Some elderly patients are clearly uncomfortable even asking about medical cannabis.

It's not helpful when, for example, the International Association for the Study of Pain concludes, in 2021,

> Due to the lack of high-quality clinical evidence, the International Association for the Study of Pain (IASP) does not currently endorse general use of cannabis and cannabinoids for pain relief.[3]

Millions of patients are using cannabis and other cannabinoids successfully for pain, and even the 2017 National Academies of Sciences, Engineering, and Medicine (NASEM) report concluded, after filtering through thousands of studies, that cannabis is effective for pain. Further, there is an avalanche of real-world evidence supporting this. The IASP might try treating *at least one* patient with cannabis before so categorically rejecting this treatment modality. One has to ask, why would a patient make up that their pain is well controlled? It's often the opposite scenario: "My pain goes to eleven, and the only medicine that works is one that I once had that starts with a P . . . Per . . . Perc . . . Percocet?"

To his credit, the chair of the IASP, Professor Andrew Rice, said,

> We do not wish to dismiss the lived experiences of people with pain who have found benefit from their use. This is not a door closing on the topic but rather a call for more rigorous and robust research to better understand any potential benefits and harms related to the possible use of medical cannabis.[4]

That is more compassionate, but the issue was widely reported as "pain society says cannabis doesn't work for pain," further muddying the issue.

Some specialties would lose business from legal cannabis, such as pain, addiction, and psychiatry, by virtue of people treating their own pain, anxiety, and depression with cannabis, or as the definition of cannabis "addiction" narrows so as not to include medical cannabis patients or court referrals (see chapter 9). It is such an odd coincidence that these are generally the same specialties that say they don't think it is effective or that it is too dangerous.

With contradictory messages and understandings about cannabis—how addictive, how dangerous, how helpful—how can we expect legislators to craft coherent laws or make a logical attempt to dismantle our racist and sadistically punitive Drug War–era laws? Other consequences of confusion are a hostile federal bureaucracy that interferes with and undermines state laws instead of working in concert with them to make them safer and more effective. Medical research is a mess, with too many restrictions and hurdles to overcome, and with most of the research having been done on the pitiful weed grown by NIDA, the Moldy Mush strain, which makes it difficult to prove anything.

Another outcome of our cannabis confusion, and from our society's Drug War mentality, is a fetishization of drug testing for cannabis. This results in countless, needless job losses due to failed drug tests for cannabis. A positive test for cannabis often just means that you have used it within the last several weeks; it by no means indicates that you are acutely intoxicated. It's quite possible to receive a positive test if you've never been high anywhere near your place of work. It could also mean that you used a nonintoxicating CBD product with a trace amount of THC in it. In 2022, as I was writing this, headlines appeared on this very subject: "Wells Fargo Analyst Says Federal Marijuana Testing Mandate to Blame for Trucker Shortages and Rising Costs."[5]

For many federal jobs, especially those that need security clearance, a history of cannabis use automatically prohibits candidates from even applying—this deprives our government of many of the best and the brightest.

Some people were pushing drug testing more than others. Dr. Robert DuPont, the drug czar under Nixon and Ford, the first head of NIDA, a lifetime fellow of the American Psychiatric Association and of the American Society of Addiction Medicine (ASAM), had a large role in sustaining our damaging obsession with drug testing, as he was an influential advocate for testing over a span of decades. As he was doing this, he was also making a fortune from a variety of drug-testing companies that he founded or was working for.

DuPont argued to test virtually everyone, and to vastly increase criminal penalties, such as for pregnant women. He published a policy paper that recommended "not only testing the adults on public assistance but also their children."[6] According to Google Books, he wrote three books, *Drug Testing in Treatment Settings*, *Drug Testing in Schools*, and *Drug Testing in Correctional Settings*, published by the Hazelden Foundation— which is part of the rehab industry and, as such, makes a huge amount of money from drug testing and the consequent referrals to rehab.

To learn more about DuPont's attempts to criminalize everyone and monetize the War on Drugs, read the article in the *Daily Beast* titled "Jeff Sessions' Marijuana Adviser Wants Doctors to Drug Test Everyone." According to this article,

> A national model bill he [DuPont] helped write in 2010 called on law enforcement to test anyone stopped for suspicion of driving under the influence for all controlled substances, and arresting them if any trace at all shows up in their system—regardless of the amount. While the bill includes an exemption for drivers who consumed a drug pursuant to a prescription, it would not apply to medicinal-marijuana users because doctors are not currently allowed to prescribe pot, only offer a recommendation for its use.

Further, it reads "Any person who provides a bodily fluid sample containing any amount of a chemical or controlled substance . . . commits an offense punishable in the same manner as if the person otherwise possessed that substance," adding in a footnote: "This provision is not a DUI specific law. Rather, it applies to any person who tests positive for chemical or controlled substances."

With no shame or irony,

> after leaving federal service, DuPont joined the former head of the Drug Enforcement Administration, Pete Bensinger, to cash in on urine testing.

The firm they founded, Bensinger, DuPont & Associates, provided drug testing services to some of America's largest corporations.[7]

There are numerous other financial entanglements, with different drug-testing companies, that DuPont worked with and received payment for. Tragically (in my opinion), DuPont was the chair of the American Society of Addiction Medicine's Drug Testing White Paper Writing Committee and—due to his active outspokenness about cannabis, perpetuating stigmatizing notions like the "amotivational syndrome"—is partially responsible for ASAM's historical hostility and ingrained bias against medical cannabis. I feel that their newsletter, which I read weekly, curates their articles about cannabis to feature the harms and ignore most of the benefits. This is a disservice to their members and fuels the gap between addiction specialist and patient on this issue. How can one understand why a patient uses cannabis if they don't learn something substantial about its benefits?

Reefer Pessimists would say that the costs of having such confusion around cannabis include a missed opportunity to put in restrictions on the cannabis industry before this industry does what the tobacco and alcohol companies did: advertise to teens and get a ton of people hooked. One recent Pessimist lashed out on Twitter,

> The cannabis industry is no more interested in social equity than is the tobacco industry—it's just a convenient argument to persuade leftists that allowing corporations to sell addictive products is good.

This obviously oversimplifies the situation (not to mention that weed is less addictive than nicotine), yet I understand the concern. I believe the cannabis industry is a "big tent" with lots of different people in it, many with benevolent agendas, others fueled by greed. If instead of fighting over legalization, both sides could work together to figure out how to legalize safely, we would be much more effective at regulating and steering this industry in the right direction.

Other important problems are plodding toward eventual solution, such as how to better put equity and social justice at the forefront of legalization, how to make cannabis banking legal so that all transactions don't have to

COSTS OF CANNABIS CONFUSION

be done in cash, or how to get medical cannabis covered by health insurance so it is affordable for the less well-to-do. It is difficult to work toward all of this when you are still fighting just to keep people out of prison in states where cannabis is still illegal.

Where I live, in Massachusetts, cannabis is legal both medically and for adult use. The contradictions inherent in it being legal on the state but not on the federal level are endless. Even though it is also legal in Maine and Vermont, it is illegal to drive with it over the border between two legal states. This "interstate drug trafficking" is a major federal offense—though it would be fairly difficult to get caught unless you were calling unwonted attention to yourself.

Medical cards in some states are not necessarily respected or protective in other states. This seems to be particularly true if you are Black and are traveling in the Deep South, as was the case for Sean Worsley. Worsley, a veteran who had a valid medical marijuana card from Arizona, was just passing through Alabama. When filling up his car with gas, a local police officer noticed that he was playing music and "laughing and joking around." The fuzz told him he was violating the town's "noise ordinance." Worsley turned the music down immediately, but the cop had by then smelled some cannabis from within the car. Worsley tried to show him his medical marijuana card but was greeted with, "Alabama does not have medical marijuana," handcuffs, felony charges, homelessness, and eventually a five-year prison sentence.[8] He served our country and now he's serving time—all because our laws are contradictory and incoherent, with some good old-fashioned racism thrown in.

The craziness even goes down to the molecular level. According to federal law, CBD is legal if it comes from the hemp plant, but it is illegal if it comes from cannabis, even though it is the same molecule. You can't make up anything this ridiculous.

Is it clear yet why everyone is confused?

Like the truths obscured by all the cannabis smoke in a Plato-like hotboxed cave, many of the different stakeholders in the cannabis discussion are chained to the limits of their vantage points, and their interests. Their knowledge is formulated in the shadows of their training, experiences, educational exposures, ideological biases, and, sadly, disproportionately, their livelihoods. With both cannabis and the prohibition of cannabis, the quote from

Upton Sinclair has never been more apt: "It is difficult to get a man to understand something when his salary depends on his not understanding it."[9]

How does one reconcile the different voices that are brought to the cannabis conversation? Recognizing them is a good first step. I've already discussed the Reefer Pessimists and the Cannatopians, but what other voices are out there contributing to the cacophony?

- The cannabis industry, which believes in its products and its mission, publishes educational materials that tilt toward the optimistic. Rules for advertising vary from state to state. The fear of the Reefer Pessimists is that this industry will follow the path of Big Tobacco and Big Alcohol and target teens as well as problematic users (who buy a lot of cannabis).

- The tobacco and alcohol companies. They seem be transitioning from resisting legalization to adopting a "you can't beat, so join 'em" attitude and are investing in cannabis-related products. It is thought that some of the pro-cannabis lobbying groups are "front" groups for Big Tobacco and, to a lesser extent, Big Alcohol. According to attorney Shaleen Title, who is a former cannabis control commissioner in Massachusetts, a fierce and effective advocate for social equity, and the CEO and cofounder of the Parabola Center[10] think tank, which fights for "cannabis policy for people, not corporations,"[11] "tobacco behemoths are pouring billions of dollars into the new legal marijuana industry, seemingly determined to target marijuana consumers and patients as their next prey."[12]

- The traditional recovery community, such as Alcoholics Anonymous members, and the rehab industry, who feel, or are taught, that "a drug is a drug is a drug." They often espouse a strict abstinence-based recovery paradigm (excluding tobacco and caffeine . . .) and have been very unaccepting of cannabis use in recovery (or the use of lifesaving medications such as Suboxone and methadone for that matter). These prejudices are starting to change, though at a glacial pace (see chapter 9).

- Law enforcement has every incentive to exaggerate the harms of cannabis as they make a fortune from Drug War budgets and asset forfeiture. Many times, I haven't found their data to be particularly credible, be it the DEA, the Office of Homeland Security, local police stations (who keep saying they found fentanyl in cannabis and then retracting, "Whoops, we were wrong!"), or particularly government-sponsored groups such as the High Intensity Drug Trafficking Areas (HIDTA) program.

- The U.S. government is still putting out exaggerated nonsense about cannabis, but this has moderated a bit in tone, and their funding is slowly starting to expand beyond merely seeking to just find harms. It is going to take a long time for the U.S. government to regain trust on this issue.

- I discussed the role, and the voices, of the medical profession in chapter 4.

In short, it's like the Tower of Babel out there! How do we get all of these people, with their conflicting agendas and biases, speaking the same language?

One thing that further adds to the confusion is the process of ballot initiatives on whether to legalize. This process engenders contentious public campaigns, with money pouring in on both sides. Cannatopians and Reefer Pessimists alike feel that they are outfunded, outspent, and outgunned. Rather than working to find patches of common ground, they succumb to pressure to brandish their more extreme arguments, which then assault the airwaves and the earlobes. In some ways, both sides have pulled further away from an invisible point in the center where the objective truth about the plant must lie. The sides radicalize and reinforce each other.

With each new state ballot initiative about legalization, millions of dollars pour into each media market to promulgate these two largely incompatible versions of reality, neither of which is exactly accurate. Advertising isn't helpful, as the issues are always more nuanced than can be portrayed in sound bites, and ads obviously come with an agenda. They are not public service announcements. The corporations and the wealthy are increasingly dominating the debate, taking it partly out of the hands of the grassroots. We've discussed the industries that have supported the Reefer Pessimists in chapter 2. At key times the Cannatopians have had some major help from a small number of billionaire philanthropists, including George Soros, Peter Lewis (the CEO of Progressive Insurance), and John Sperling (founder of the University of Phoenix).

The situation is further complicated by the fact that almost everyone has a strong gut reaction to the cannabis issue. Many different ingredients go into these filters: lived experience of the effects of cannabis on yourself or on loved ones, education (or propaganda), familial attitudes, political leanings, community beliefs, and financial incentives.

Sometimes people can and do change their opinions, however fervent, on cannabis in the face of new information, or new incentives. This often happens when a friend, family member, or acquaintance discovers the benefits of medical cannabis—such as in the context of a new cancer diagnosis—and starts sharing their experience. People reevaluate what they have been taught of harms and benefits in light of experience that contextualizes (or even disqualifies) much of what they've been told.

Some people shift the other way, such as if their teen or young adult has engaged in problematic cannabis use or, worse, experienced a psychotic episode in which cannabis was involved—not an uncommon scenario. In these cases, they tend to regret, or have at least modified, their previously liberal, permissive views on cannabis.

These cognitive/emotional biases that virtually all people have toward cannabis are profoundly unhelpful. They immediately affect how any new data is perceived and interpreted. Just as a vaccine skeptic might summarily dismiss a new study about the safety of vaccines, whereas the medical and scientific community would be inclined to accept it at face value, new facts and studies about cannabis are received and evaluated very differently. I see this on social media every day as each new study comes out. I usually know who is going to heap praise on it and who is going to savage it, regardless of the soundness of its methodology or whether it even makes any sense. This is as unhealthy as a scientific and social dialogue can get—the science is prejudged by the results.

I have to be careful to watch my own cognitive biases, having grown up in a cannabis-accepting environment and having had almost entirely positive lived experiences with cannabis as a provider, patient, and consumer. I try hard not to fall into cognitive traps by recognizing that it *is* an emotional issue for me: it helped my dying brother; it was the life work of

74

my dad, who is one of the people I admire most in the world; it helped me get off opioids; and it's given me a phenomenal tool to help many of my patients who are suffering. But these facts, or my feelings about the drug, ought not to have any effect on my assessment of the accuracy or validity of the scientific literature.

In reality, none of us are Mr. Spock–like and able to entirely divorce ourselves from our emotions. One technique I use is that I try to pretend that I'm reading something practical and apolitical, like something to do with my day job, such as a medical review article on hypertension or insomnia, or an article about different techniques and outcomes for removing earwax in a primary care population. Snore. This takes much of the emotion out of it.

These filters further polarize all of us and blind us to the true harms and potentials of cannabis. In addition to understanding, admitting, and factoring in our own biases, we need to dial down the polarization so a more reasonable and respectful dialogue can ensue. There's no reason to include vitriol in your tweets.

What can be done to bring the two sides back together? To a certain extent, the fighting will die down as federal legalization becomes a fait accompli—both sides can at that point stop brandishing their most aggressive arguments. The younger people are, the more in favor of legalization they tend to be, so, demographically, the future is bright for legalization. Public support for legalization is rising in all other demographics. As of this writing, Republicans are introducing cannabis legalization bills in the U.S. House to compete with those of the Democrats, though support generally is higher among Democrats and Independents. If both sides of the aisle are trying to legalize, it is just a matter of time and hammering out the details. Further, as more high-quality, neutral research comes out, our knowledge of harms and benefits will greatly improve, which will lead to more incontrovertible cannabis common ground.

Maybe it's time to try to circle back around, share a (metaphorical) peace pipe, and see what we can hammer out in common.

Before moving on to a discussion of the currently known harms and benefits, it is important not to shy away from the consequences that the War on Cannabis has had on our citizens and to the fabric of our society.

## CHAPTER SIX

# BLUNT TRUTHS
## The Harms of the War on Cannabis Users

What have been the harms of criminalizing cannabis users? The damage, when added up, is staggering and includes about twenty *million* arrests in this country over the last fifty years. According to the ACLU, of the 8.2 million marijuana arrests between 2001 and 2010, 88 percent were for simple possession of marijuana.[1] This has led to lifelong criminal records and in some cases imprisonment. It also resulted in vast amounts of collateral damage such as student loans denied, housing forfeited, voting rights revoked, and families broken. The cycle of poverty created can last for generations, and it disproportionately affects communities of color.

An increasing awareness of these injustices, along with a pervasive yet growing sense that we've all been sold a bill of goods about cannabis by our government and many of our experts, combine to explain the astounding groundswell of public opinion in favor of legalization. As legalization spreads across the United States and across the globe, one might be tempted to think that arrests for simple cannabis possession have gone away. Unfortunately, that is not the case. In 2019, more than half a million Americans were arrested for cannabis-related charges, the vast majority of which (91.7 percent), as usual, were for simple possession.[2] In 2020, it was better, but there still were 350,000 arrests, with most of these arrests serving no purpose whatsoever. There shouldn't be *any* arrests for simple cannabis possession. I believe that we should be focusing on expunging these harmful criminal records and on restitutions to people and communities that have been harmed, not on perpetuating greater harm.

Further, even though arrests are trending down, according to the paper "Racial Disparities in the Wake of Cannabis Legalization: Documenting

Persistence and Change," "substantial racial disparities persist following legalization." A common saying is that the War on Drugs is nothing more than a war on (certain groups of) people.[3] This is particularly true for the War on Cannabis. This chapter will attempt to give a flavor of what transpired during our government's half-century war on cannabis users, in which all cannabis users—including medical users—were hounded and persecuted by the U.S. government. It may give some insight into why the Cannatopians are so passionate about their cause and why they are so skeptical of any studies, warnings, or official pronouncements from any department of the U.S. government about cannabis.

## The Social Construction of Drug Epidemics

According to integrative medicine pioneer and best-selling author Dr. Andrew Weil, "the ubiquity of drug use is so striking that it must represent a basic human appetite."[4] Writer Michael Pollan echoes this thought when he cites the paucity of cultures and civilizations that have existed without the use of any psychoactive substances. The difference between heroin, which will promptly get you arrested, and codeine, morphine, or oxycodone, which we frequently prescribe in clinics, is merely a few atoms. We freely accept the deadliest of drugs by the score—tobacco and alcohol, along with dozens of addictive, intoxicating prescription drugs—yet we have demonized much less dangerous drugs, including most psychedelic drugs, just because of their cultural or racial associations. Our drug control regime is incoherent and deadly.

Why are we waging war on cannabis users? I discussed how cannabis changed from being an accepted medicine eighty years ago to a prohibited medicine in previous chapters. The effects this switch had, and the zeal with which the U.S. government enforced its misguided cannabis policy, is discussed here.

Does this "war" fit any type of pattern?

In the book *Drugs and Drug Policy: The Control of Consciousness Alteration*, authors Clayton Mosher and Scott Akins discuss the demonization of illegal drugs and the "social construction of drug epidemics." The main points they make are that:

1. "The drug warrior industry, which includes both the private sector and a massive government bureaucracy devoted to 'enforcement,' has an enormous economic incentive to keep the war raging." (This is part of why criminalization fit so well in the 1930s—alcohol prohibition had just ended, and there was a huge bureaucracy to support and justify.)

2. "Government officials need drugs in order to create heroes and villains and, in many cases, to divert attention away from the issues which have caused the drug use in the first place." (Such as homelessness, limited access to medical care, unemployment, racism, and inequitable economic opportunity.)

Therefore,

3. "As a result of these needs . . . government and criminal justice officials in the United States, frequently assisted by the popular media, have engaged in a concerted campaign to demonize certain drugs in order to justify their prohibition."[5]

According to Mosher and Akins, common techniques include blaming the commission of crime on these drugs (whether or not they actually are responsible); associating these drugs with bizarre or deviant actions such as uncontrollable sexual urges or violent acts ("voodoo pharmacology," where the drug takes over); and, finally, asserting that the particular drug in question is "consumed primarily by members of underrepresented groups" and that the substances are "distributed primarily by evil foreign traffickers."

Hmm . . . sound familiar?

Mosher and Akins go on to discuss several fluffed-up "epidemics" that fall into this pattern of governmental demonization. Every single aspect of it is true for cannabis, from blaming it on the Mexicans, to associating cannabis with sexually deviant and violent behavior, with the users at a complete loss to control themselves. As an example of this, in the movie *Reefer Madness*, people try to rape and shoot each other after using cannabis.

I have to again cite a 1967 quote from an official position piece in the *Journal of the American Medical Association*:

The use of marihuana among Puerto Ricans and both southern and northern Negroes is reputed to be quite high. In all likelihood, marihuana use among the poverty-stricken urbanite is concomitant with . . . a broad range of asocial and antisocial activity.[6]

One could argue, fairly effortlessly, that the AMA were playing the part of "useful idiots" in laying the groundwork for Nixon's upcoming War on Drugs.

As a cannabis user, it was easy to get arrested for cannabis, and I had many close calls. For example, next to the main lawn of Swarthmore College, I was enjoying a smoke with a few friends on a beautiful spring evening. Suddenly, out of nowhere, the fuzz appeared, sirens blaring. The officer physically cornered us with his squad car, jumped out, got right into our stoned faces, and barked at us.

"Do you have any cigarettes in your pocket?"

"Um . . . no, officer, of course not. Smoking is bad for you."

"Then what were you just smoking? Empty your pockets."

I handed him my beautiful hand-carved wooden pipe and, sadly, my entire stash of high-end weed. One of my friends, a fellow philosophy major, started to argue with him about how morally bankrupt his entire position was and the ethical and racial abyss in which the officer was placing himself by accosting us. This wasn't helping the prospects for getting us off the hook. Once we were able to shut my friend up and the officer could get a word in edgewise, he threatened to arrest us but instead settled for giving us a vicious tongue lashing.

How would being arrested for harmlessly and innocently smoking a little weed with friends on the Swarthmore College campus have helped anything? It is easy to come up with a long list of things it might have harmed. I doubt left-wing, Quaker-themed, drug-accepting Swarthmore would have kicked me out, but it would have precluded medical school, as admission committees don't particularly approve of things like criminal records or drugs.

If I weren't a middle-class white college student, I likely would have been arrested and charged—this infraction would have truly compromised all of my future prospects.

Had we been arrested, we would likely have all dealt with something similar to the ordeal my friend and roommate went through a few years later. Brian was a successful consultant with the U.S. government who specialized in mitigating contaminants. We shared an apartment in Washington, DC, during the time when I was working at Greenpeace's national headquarters. Our apartment was right near the National Zoo, and when we hung out on our back porch on summer evenings, we would hear the lions roaring as well as many of the other animals. It sounded like we were on safari.

Brian was talented at brewing beer, but the only thing that truly quieted his constant anxious rumination was cannabis, which he would use at night. You could see a full-body unclenching with just one puff. Then he'd be happily socializing rather than just worrying neurotically about hypothetical problematical scenarios.

One afternoon, I was down at the Washington Mall with a friend—the same friend that gave the stoned sermon on morality to the cop at Swarthmore five years earlier. We were enjoying the splendid summer weather tossing a Frisbee when we received a panicked phone call: "This is Brian. I've been arrested for weed. This is my one call. They took my glasses, belt, and shoelaces. I can't see anything, and I'm sitting in a freezing cell with nothing to do. I'm going to lose my job. I'm freaking out. You have to bail me out."

"Hang on, Brian, we'll be there. This will be OK."

What did he get arrested for? A nickel bag of pot, which is five dollars' worth. It comes in a tiny bag and is probably about enough to consume in six modest puffs. It was late 1980s cannabis, with a lower THC content than today's weed. It was barely enough to get one person high, once. He was buying it from a street dealer in Meridian Hill Park, which was right down the street from where we lived. He had no other source, as this was in the dark days before the advent of legal weed. Unbeknownst to him, the entire transaction was being watched by law enforcement, who materialized and pounced just after the deal was consummated. Brian said they had difficulty locating the five bag—and almost had to let him go—because they had him shoved up so hard against the police car that they couldn't access the inner pocket he had hidden it in.

They threw the book at Brian because they were trying to move up the chain to implicate a drug dealer of some significance, which was bad luck and bad news for Brian.

Brian's plight was as good as you could get for a cannabis arrest. It was in DC, not in Georgia or Alabama, where the laws were draconian, leading to years in prison. Most importantly, and unfairly, he was a white professional whom the criminal justice system would greatly favor if he acted a certain way, choreographed by his expensive attorney. Being a professional, he could afford a specialized attorney (whom my dad hooked him up with). With all of these advantages, he still suffered from several years of immense anxiety over this, thousands in legal fees, repeated court appearances, mandatory drug testing, and lots of uncertainty. He was barely able to hang on to his job and had to contend with this blemish on his record. He didn't have cannabis to help him relax anymore, so he started drinking much more heavily. It is mind-boggling that he went through all of this grief and punishment—and that our society wasted all of these resources—for the crime of self-treating his anxiety with a tiny bag of weak cannabis.

Black people have had it far worse. They use cannabis at the same rate as whites do, yet they are arrested at almost four times the rate of white people.[7] The smell of cannabis is considered "probable cause" in many states, particularly in southern states, and this allows the policeperson to snoop around and look for things to bust them for. Blacks are much more likely to end up in prison for the same infractions and to suffer far more severe consequences from the same criminal records. This impacts jobs, finances, housing, and education. Families are broken up.

It is no wonder that, at my twin brother's wedding, when my older brother and I snuck outside with some family friends to smoke a joint, they were much more concerned about concealment than we were. I was totally insensitive. We were in a slightly darkened alleyway, and I said, "We can just smoke here; no one will care." One friend gave me a pointed look and said, "Not if you look like us." We found a much more secluded place to spark up.

I doubt Brian would still be working for the government if he had dark skin, and he may well have ended up behind bars. In 1989, there were four hundred thousand other cannabis arrests in the United States, all equally as useless and destructive.

A seminal event in the history of the persecution of cannabis users was the institution of mandatory minimum criminal sentences. While most egregiously utilized to incarcerate millions of Black Americans during the "crack epidemic," mandatory minimums have also ensnared hundreds of thousands of cannabis users. The Last Prisoner Project is a highly worthy nonprofit that works to get all remaining cannabis prisoners released. One of their founders, entrepreneur and dogged cannabis rights advocate Steve DeAngelo, sent me an article about Allen Russell, who is a Black man serving a life sentence for cannabis possession.

In 2017, Russell was caught with forty grams of cannabis—several hundred dollars' worth. According to the Equal Justice Initiative, Mr. Russell was arrested in his apartment in November 2017 wearing only a white tank top and his underwear after Hattiesburg police breached the windows of his apartment and exploded a flash-bang grenade by his front door, then entered the apartment and threw a chemical agent to force Mr. Russell out.

After arresting Mr. Russell, police seized a pair of jeans from the apartment. They found bags in the jeans that were tested and found to contain 43.710 grams of marijuana. Mr. Russell was convicted of possession of marijuana in an amount greater than 30 grams but less than 250 grams—an offense punishable under Mississippi law by a $3,000 fine, up to three years in prison, or both.[8]

Unfortunately, in Mississippi, if you are a "habitual violent offender," defined as having committed other crimes, involving violence, you get life in prison, even just for cannabis. Mr. Russell did have some prior charges, some home burglaries *when he was a teenager* and one charge of possession of a firearm (which, even in Mississippi, felons aren't allowed to possess). Despite the fact that all of his convictions were clearly nonviolent, without any physical altercations or confrontations, they were treated as if they were violent crimes because a 2014 law defined burglary of a residence as a "per se crime of violence." As such, he is stuck in prison *for life* for the same cannabis that, in many other states, you can openly walk in and buy, or have delivered to your home, grow, or make a good living selling. His appeal of his conviction was turned down in 2021.[9]

Is Mr. Russell entirely blameless? No. Should he have known the local laws and culture? That would have helped. Did he take a huge risk? Yes. Does he deserve life in prison (or any time in prison) for forty grams of weed? Of course not. To say that this is an unproductive use of the criminal justice system, as well as a waste of a human life, is a huge understatement. He needs job training, not lifelong imprisonment. Hopefully the Last Prisoner Project, with their dogged efforts, will get him set free.

A dramatic escalation of the War on Drug Users occurred under Reagan's watch with changes in the Posse Comitatus Act. The Posse What Act? The Posse Comitatus Act is a federal law signed by President Hayes in 1878 that limits the role of federal troops in domestic law enforcement. This prevents the president from using the army as a police force—it is why the United States isn't (yet) a banana republic. In 1981, as part of Reagan's War on Drugs, the Military Cooperation with Civilian Law Enforcement Agencies Act was passed, which essentially suspended the Posse Comitatus Act in certain scenarios, such as suspected drug smuggling.

If you contrive a big enough moral panic, I guess you need to call in the army to quell it. Or, one way to make a moral panic look like an urgent, perilous moral panic is to infuse images of militarized police forces into the nightly news.

This suspension of a law that was put in place to protect civilians unsurprisingly resulted in the trampling of the civil rights of millions of Americans. It allowed Reagan to attack drug growers and users with the full force of our military. It militarized the police across the country. The "War on Drugs" was transformed from a metaphorical war into an actual war, with warlike weapons and gear, against our own citizens.

Once the military has entered a realm of civil society, it is extremely difficult to get it out. This is one of the ways in which the War on Drugs will be a gift that keeps on giving (or, more accurately, the grift that keeps on grifting). The police forces never demilitarized.

Just when Nancy Reagan was promoting the scientifically nonsensical strategy of "just say no" and whipping up the "parents' movement" into a frenzy about drug use, newly beefed-up police units were barreling into neighborhoods, and arrests for nonviolent cannabis crimes went up to almost one million arrests per year. This "war" was sold by industry-supported advocacy groups such as the Partnership for a Drug-Free America. The partnership endured a scandal when it came out that they were being funded, at least in part, by the tobacco and alcohol companies.

It sounds so cynical and dystopian: the two most deadly drug industries, tobacco and alcohol, financially supporting a broad-based propaganda campaign, wrapped in the trappings of patriotism and public health, to support a militarized war against other drugs—all based on capitalism and racism—to ensure a continuing stream of revenue to these two highly deadly industries.

One program that I remember hearing about at the time, which I thought was extremely repressive, was Operation Green Merchant, conducted under the first Bush administration. Cannabis cultivation had largely been chased indoors by the helicopter raids of the Reagan administration. In response, the feds began targeting indoor hydroponic growers. They did this by having Congress pass laws that made legal objects, such as grow lights, illegal if used for an illegal purpose. (So a baseball bat is illegal if I use it to brain someone? It seems that the action not the object is what is problematic in these cases. And why weren't thousands of guns then illegal? Hypocrisy abounds.)

These laws allowed the government to subpoena records from hydroponics stores, secure wiretaps, and subpoena shipping records from UPS. They concentrated on the businesses that advertised in the magazines *High Times* and *Sinsemilla Tips*. According to a 2020 article from *High Times*, "Operation Green Merchant and H. W. Bush's War on Drugs,"

> on October 26, 1989, now known to the hydroponic equipment and marijuana industries as Black Thursday, the DEA raided garden stores in 46 states, seizing assets and arresting 119 people. Over the next two years $17.5 million in assets were seized and 1,262 arrests were made. Agents dismantled 977 grows and 57,000 plants were destroyed. Even though stores were becoming more and more careful about separating themselves from the cannabis market, the narcs were relentless. They entrapped store owners and workers by "offer[ing] us women, guns, and money if we'd show them how to grow pot and sell them gear," as one hydroponics retailer put it, and would pose as hippies or medical patients to try and solicit information about growing ganja.[10]

The DEA posed as veterans in pain who needed medical marijuana in order to manipulate the heartstrings of the workers at hydroponics stores, to encourage them to disclose enough information about how to grow medicinal cannabis to allow them to be arrested. One might wonder how pretending to be a sick veteran who needs help in order to arrest the person generous enough to offer that help is in any way ethical or productive. Further, asset forfeiture is a profound conflict of interest—it allows law enforcement members to enrich their departments as they arrest people suspected of drug dealing. There is no requirement for legal proof, no warrants—just the ability to take and keep property. It can be extremely difficult, if not impossible, to get your property back, even if you prove your innocence.

Operation Green Merchant came to an end after facing growing backlash from many people, including those whom the feds mistakenly targeted for no-knock arrests, people who had nothing to do with cannabis. There was also backlash to its obvious overreach, air of entrapment, and senseless and excessive cruelty. With stunts like this, the DEA was offering a lot of PR assistance to the legalization movement.

We weren't just terrorizing cannabis users in the United States. In 1946, Anslinger, the head of the Federal Bureau of Narcotics, was appointed to the United Nations to represent and export U.S. drug policy. Tragically, the United States began to use its economic might to coerce other countries into adopting similarly punitive cannabis laws around the world. This process culminated in 1961 in the Single Convention on Narcotic Drugs, which placed strict restrictions on the cultivation of cannabis and other drugs. For example, cannabis now had the same restrictions on it that opium cultivation did. These restrictions on cultivation are what resulted in NIDA taking control of our country's supply of research weed and thus generating the Moldy Mush strain that made it more difficult for researchers to demonstrate anything about cannabis. It wasn't until December 2020 that cannabis was removed from Schedule IV of the 1961 UN Single Convention on Narcotic Drugs.

We also poisoned a lot of people, foreign and domestic, with paraquat, a defoliant that the U.S. State Department aided, funded, and encouraged the Mexican government to spray on cannabis crops to eradicate them. Paraquat is a powerful herbicide but also a poison that can gravely damage lung tissue. Unfortunately, if you harvest the cannabis right after it has been sprayed, you can still sell it, and it is indistinguishable from nonpoisoned cannabis. According to a 1978 article in the *New York Times*, "Poisonous Fallout from the War on Marijuana,"

Because of the distribution patterns of Mexican marijuana, paraquat-sprayed marijuana is sold mostly on the West Coast to teen-agers, on the East Coast in ghettos, and, across the nation, to the estimated 200,000 Armed Forces enlisted personnel who smoke.[11]

We were now destroying the lungs of teens, disadvantaged city dwellers, and our military. NORML filed suit to stop the use of paraquat, but this legal action was preempted when Senator Charles Percy filed an amendment that blocked funds for this toxic program, thus relegating it to the dustbin of history as another failed attempt to exterminate marijuana use (and, to a certain extent, users) no matter what the cost.

The War on Cannabis isn't over. At the time of this writing, a person in one part of the United States can make millions selling weed where another could end up in prison for selling the same product. One is still far more likely to get arrested for cannabis if you have dark skin. We still have hundreds of thousands of arrests for simple cannabis possession every year.

Beyond legalization, we have tremendous work still to do in terms of expungements of criminal records and reparations to communities of color devastated by the War on Cannabis. If you expunge someone's criminal record, at least they can start over, though many will be starting from scratch. We need to make sure that those who have been disproportionately impacted by prohibition are preferentially offered involvement in the new cannabis industry. This is essential so that they have an opportunity to generate back the wealth that was siphoned off, forfeited (i.e., stolen by law enforcement), or lost while behind bars during the last fifty years of targeted enforcement of drug laws.

Due to the diligent and courageous work of tens of thousands of activists over half a century, we are finally heading in the right direction, toward an end to the "prohibition for profit" industries, at least with respect to cannabis. As with all aspects of cannabis reform, this won't continue to move forward without a continued, concerted effort. There is plenty of prohibitionist pushback. The cash cows are mooing loudly in outrage. No matter what physical or mental harms cannabis may cause, they pale in comparison to the physical and mental harms inflicted upon all of us by our ugly War on Cannabis.

# Part II

# HOW HARMFUL? A MEASURED APPROACH

## CHAPTER SEVEN

# WHAT COUNTS AS EVIDENCE?

What do we actually know about cannabis? What are the harms, what are the medical benefits, and what are the quasi-medical or extramedical benefits? In representing what both sides argue are the most feared harms and the most appreciated benefits, and by critically analyzing these positions and the data that supports them, if it does, I'm hoping to come up with a sensible "middle ground" that most can agree on, or at least live with.

I intend to derive a gestalt viewpoint, grounded of course upon whatever science we have. This science absolutely has to be understood within the context of the social history in which it was performed. Any diligent student of the philosophy of science can tell you that (most) science isn't done by robots in a vacuum in the middle of space, and that people's biases and agendas can greatly impact what we look at, what we find, and how we interpret the results. If *ever* there was an issue that required the science to be understood through the lens of the social agenda through which it was funded and interpreted, it is cannabis.

I don't represent myself as having all the answers. By profession, I'm not an epidemiologist, cultural historian, neuroscientist, or primary researcher. On some issues, I will straightforwardly conclude that our evidence base is lacking and will point to the research that still needs to be done or the questions that remain to be answered. I've studied this plant my entire life, have treated thousands of patients with it, and I've usually been comfortably welcomed, or at times equally criticized, by both "camps."

If, at a bare minimum, we can facilitate communication between doctors and patients—the lack of which is incredibly dangerous—this will be a win. If we can open up civil discussion between Utopians and Pessimists, even better. Then, at least on this one cultural sticking point, the world will be a slightly less polarized place, perhaps providing a road map for solving some of our other intractable issues.

To start, let's evaluate what does and doesn't count as "evidence."

Doctors currently attempt to rely on "randomized controlled trials" (RCTs) to determine what is or isn't true or valid in medical care, though certainly there was plenty of medical care—thousands of years' worth—that occurred before RCTs were invented. We routinely utilize many treatment modalities that haven't been proven to be effective by RCTs, such as much of the care for pregnant patients—whom it isn't ethical to experiment on. There are other, important types of evidence that get nudged out of the way by the current climate of preferentially, and somewhat selectively, elevating RCTs über alles. When it comes to cannabis, there is a relative shortage of RCTs due to our government curating the research for the last fifty years, and this is often mistakenly (or opportunistically) conflated with "there is no evidence that cannabis works" for one or another particular indication.

RCTs include two critical principles. First, they are "double-blinded," so the biases of the researcher as well as the test subjects cannot factor in—neither group knows what treatment, if any, a particular participant is receiving. Studies have shown that bias can come from either source: the participants can "expect" to get better if they know they are getting an active treatment, and researchers subtly treat them differently due to the knowledge of the treatment they have received. Hence, they are "double-blinded"—the patients and the researchers are both blinded. Secondly, the studies are "placebo controlled" so that one can differentiate a treatment response from the placebo effect, which can be quite high, up to 30 percent for some pain medications.

RCTs are considered to be the most rigorous type of evidence to prove or disprove the efficacy of certain treatments and are commonly referred to as the "gold standard." RCTs showing benefit are usually needed as part of the package of evidence required by the U.S. FDA to approve a medication and for insurance companies or Medicare to reimburse for their use. It isn't at all clear how a botanical medicine like cannabis, comprised of five hundred different ingredients, would make it through this process.

We absolutely need standards of evidence. Otherwise, anyone can claim anything and everything, which is an open invitation to snake oil salespeople. For example, as I drive to my primary care clinic, I listen to the local AM Spanish-language radio stations to improve my Spanish. These stations are almost exclusively Evangelical, which explains why, after I spend months throwing every tool I have into healing a patient, some of my patients then raise their hands and announce, "Thank the Lord that I am healed." (I guess, in that worldview, it's true that the Lord created doctors, hospitals, medications, and primary care doctors such as myself, though it does seem like an unfair misattribution of credit! If they do well, the Lord gets credit, but if they do poorly, we can get sued. Unfortunately, the Lord also created malpractice attorneys.)

One infomercial that I frequently hear consists of two actors chatting, one as a doctor and one as a patient. The (fake) doctor explains how the special vitamins for sale can clean out your prostate or can rejuvenate your liver. When my patients ask me about this, I can explain to them that there is absolutely no evidence that these things work in this way. You can't "clean" or "rejuvenate" internal organs with vitamins. At best, they are a waste of money, if not, as an unregulated supplement, downright poisonous to the liver and the kidney. This is something that most doctors would agree with (unless they are the ones selling the vitamins . . . you would be surprised, but places like the Cleveland Clinic, which has blanketly prohibited their doctors from recommending medical cannabis, sell all kinds of unproven vitamin and supplement preparations online under the guise of "wellness").

It is important not to underestimate the power of the placebo effect, which is why researchers go so far out of their way to separate out this effect—a main advantage of RCTs. Using placebos used to be an accepted medical practice, though it is no longer allowed, as it conflicts with the "informed consent" component of the patients' rights movement. Decades ago, when my family was on vacation, the query was made, "Is there a doctor on the flight?" My dad dutifully stood up. A young woman was having a massive anxiety attack. They asked my dad to evaluate her and let them know whether to turn the plane back to its airport of departure. My dad chatted with her in his calming psychiatric voice, gave her a sedative, and told her, "This will calm you right down in twenty or so minutes but might make you sleepy," and he sat down next to her for the remainder of the flight as the pilots had requested. She calmed down in about twenty minutes as the pill kicked in and actually fell asleep because she perceived the pill as quite sedating. She, the captain, the crew, the airline, and the other passengers were profoundly grateful to my dad for treating her anxiety and allowing the flight to continue. All my dad had given her was a sugar pill.

Many of the mainstream, corporate medical institutions, such as the American Psychiatric Association and the American Medical Association, are currently saying there isn't enough "evidence"—specifically referring to RCTs—for cannabis to be considered a safe and effective medicine. This is in contradistinction to the millions of people who are visibly and undeniably using it as a safe and effective medication. In effect, the lack of RCTs has become a club used by conservative medical institutions and prohibitionists to fight (quite unsuccessfully so far) against legalization of medical cannabis. It is important to emphasize that most doctors themselves are in favor of legalized access to medical cannabis—it is just the professional societies that supposedly represent them, and which wield a certain (dwindling) amount of societal influence, that are against this. It is up for discussion whether this institutionalized resistance to medical cannabis is due to the lingering influence of Big Pharma, whether it results from the perceived need to zealously guard a moat around the professional territory of some physicians, or whether it is just the dreaded old fart syndrome (OFS).

All of this begs the following questions: are RCTs the only type of evidence there is? Are RCTs foolproof? Is the rest of medical practice strictly dictated by RCTs, or are they employing a double standard for cannabis? Are there other types of evidence appropriate and acceptable?

Controlled experiments were not needed to recognize the therapeutic potential of chloral hydrate, barbiturates, aspirin, curare, insulin, lithium, or penicillin—pharmaceuticals introduced before the double-blind controlled study was invented. It is somewhat of a myth that all modern medicine is entirely based on RCTs and is completely "evidence based." Much of what I do as a PCP isn't based on RCTs. I would bet that we have never "proven" with an RCT that people hear better when you remove their earwax, but this is a helpful procedure that lessens isolation and improves cognition—it is self-evidently helpful. You can witness the results.

At the same time, the use of anecdotes can be misleading. As my dad wrote in a blog,

> Anecdotes present a problem that has always haunted medicine: the anecdotal fallacy or the fallacy of enumeration of favorable circumstances (counting the hits and ignoring the misses). If many people suffering from, say, muscle spasms caused by multiple sclerosis take marijuana and only a few get much better relief than they could get from conventional drugs, those few patients would stand out and come to our attention. They and their physicians would understandably be enthusiastic about marijuana and might proselytize for it. These people are not dishonest, but they are not dispassionate observers. Therefore, some may regard it as irresponsible to suggest on the basis of anecdotes that cannabis may help people with a variety of disorders.[1]

So, are there any categories of evidence besides RCTs and anecdotes? Are RCTs really as bulletproof as they are portrayed as being?

Dr. Tom Frieden was the head of the Centers for Disease Control (CDC) from 2009 to 2017. In 2017 he wrote a compelling piece in the *New England Journal of Medicine* called "Evidence for Health Decision Making—Beyond Randomized, Controlled Trials." In this piece, he describes some of the limitations of our "gold standard" and makes RCTs sound perhaps more gold plated than gold standard. Frieden points out that RCTs don't always apply to people outside of the carefully selected study population. For example, if you study a high-risk group, the results might not apply to larger populations that don't share those particular risks. RCTs usually don't last long enough and aren't large enough to capture rare or delayed side effects, such as, say, the heart valve problems that resulted from the diet drug fen-phen. Because RCTs are so expensive and are under time limitations, they often rely on surrogate markers (e.g., numerical estimates of level of pain), not what truly matters clinically (e.g., quality of life). They can become clinically outdated because they take years to plan and execute. Finally, "RCTs are also limited in their ability to assess the individualized effect of treatment, as can result from differences in surgical techniques, and are generally impractical for rare diseases."[2]

Frieden goes on to mention,

Many other data sources can provide valid evidence for clinical and public health action. Observational studies, including assessments of results from the implementation of new programs and policies, remain the foremost source, but other examples include analysis of aggregate clinical or epidemiologic data.[3]

Frieden goes on to evidence this claim with examples including such varied issues as the harms of tobacco and the causes of infant death syndrome. He concludes that "current evidence-grading systems are biased toward RCTs, which may lead to inadequate consideration of non-RCT data."[4]

One of the many challenges in conducting RCTs with cannabis is its complex pharmacology. Cannabis has hundreds of molecules in it. Different strains or "chemovars" of cannabis have different effects—some are uplifting and creativity generating, while others make you sleepy, relaxed, horny, and hungry. RCTs usually test one isolated substance at a time. With cannabis, an RCT would most practically assess one "strain" at a time, so any given result wouldn't necessarily apply to a person using a different one of the eight hundred or so different types of cannabis. My experience with the energizing sativa Durban Poison would likely be different from your experience with the soporific indica Northern Lights.

Further, there are many different ways to consume cannabis (smoke, vape, edible, tincture, suppository, topical, skin patch, inhaler, etc.), and the consumption method dramatically impacts the effect, clinically and phenomenologically. An RCT tests just one of these, so the results wouldn't necessarily be generalizable to the way someone else might be using the cannabis. My inhaled Durban Poison experience would absolutely be different from what you go through after eating brownies made from Northern Lights! I might spend a few hours happily writing, organizing things, cleaning my house, or exercising, whereas you might spend six to eight hours lounging on the couch, watching *Rick and Morty*, eating the best chips you've ever tasted, or listening to the Grateful Dead. These two strains/consumption methods obviously would not have the same medicinal effects.

Further, with cannabis, blinding is a big problem. You can't fool people with placebos. Why? Because most people who are paying the slightest bit of attention to their surroundings would likely notice if they are stoned. It's not a state secret that THC is psychoactive. This is why people have gone to so much trouble throughout history, risking arrest, to use cannabis in the first place—it changes your consciousness (it expands), how your muscles feel (as if they've been massaged), how you experience time (very slowly), and how you perceive the world (full of mystery and enchantment or, if you take too big a dose, very menacing). As such, it is extremely difficult to blind.

Some investigators tried to get around this obstacle by using Benadryl (diphenhydramine) or Lorazepam (a benzodiazepine, like Valium) to fool people. Now, as someone who has smoked plenty of cannabis in my past, I can tell you that no one who has *ever* experienced cannabis would be fooled by this. It's as if a researcher were trying to pawn off Sudafed mixed in muddy water as a large cup of coffee—good luck with that. This is one place where it might save some time, money, and effort if more cannabis researchers had tried cannabis and had a better lived understanding of the actual effects of cannabis. While it's true that cannabis, Benadryl, and Lorazepam all can make you drowsy, the quality of the experience is entirely different. Benadryl makes you feel groggy, drugged, and as if you are brain dead, and Lorazepam makes you sleepy and relaxed—perhaps it is possible to confuse these two if you have never taken either one of them. But cannabis makes you euphoric, thoughtful, and enhances all of your senses, starting with your vision perception—things are seen in high relief (no pun intended) and in much more vivid detail. It would be extraordinarily difficult, even to the least observant person on the planet, to confuse this cannabis experience with that of either Lorazepam or Benadryl.

You could try using cannabis-naive patients; they might be fooled by such a substitution. However, then you are giving one group Benadryl and Lorazepam, which might have a clinical impact on whatever you are studying, and you aren't comparing it to a placebo. It becomes an entirely different type of study, a comparison or "non-inferiority" study between cannabis and Benadryl/Lorazepam instead of an RCT.

A 2021 paper, coming from several of the leading medical cannabis experts in the UK, called "Real World Evidence in Medical Cannabis Research," reiterates many of these themes and drills down on some of the specific difficulties there are in conducting standard research on cannabis and cannabis-based medicines. They define real-world evidence (RWE)

as "evidence derived from health data sourced from non-interventional studies, registries, electronic health records and insurance data."[5]

The authors list a treasure trove of RWE supporting the medicinal use of cannabis, including national survey studies and analyses of government records, clinical/dispensary data, registries, and databases. For example, one of the cited studies is from Germany, and it follows people for twelve weeks and demonstrates, by analyzing data from a large pain registry, that an under-the-tongue preparation of THC and CBD is highly successful for severe chronic pain, especially neuropathic pain. Other examples of RWE studies include studies that demonstrate the effectiveness of cannabis to treat the symptoms of fibromyalgia and a study from the New Mexico Medical Cannabis Program (MCP) that shows "clinically and statistically significant evidence of an association between MCP enrollment and opioid prescription cessation and reductions and improved quality of life."[6] They also reference a wide range of large, ongoing studies, mostly in Europe and Canada, that are utilizing RWE to determine exactly what cannabis can and cannot help with.

The authors also have helpful suggestions as to how to make RWE more accurate and relevant:

> It is important that studies standardize their methodology according to those set out by regulatory authorities to ensure research has the greatest impact. Moreover, they should seek to directly address questions set out by governing bodies as areas where there is insufficient research.[7]

Instead of everyone going off in a different direction with different measures, let's figure out what the insurance companies and governmental bodies feel they need so that the bar of evidence has been reached to approve and pay for medical cannabis.

No one is suggesting that we get rid of RCTs. Rather, we ought to broaden the definition of "evidence" to include those studies that more fully incorporate the actual lived experience and voices of patients. RCTs and RWE can truly complement each other. There are some ways in which RWE can answer questions that RCTs can't. For example, per the UK paper, "RWE has broader inclusion criteria, accounting for factors like non-standard dosing, and is not limited by scope of disease, thereby improving ecological validity."[8] Also, because RWE often includes longer-term data with longer follow-up, these studies can capture rare or delayed side effects of treatments.

It's important to note that there are also some serious limitations to RWE studies, which is why RWE studies haven't traditionally been considered to be the gold standard. A big difficulty can be determining causation from associations that are seen. As discussed previously, association does not equate to causation. For example, all the people who are reading this book were born. Being born is clearly associated with reading this book. But being born didn't cause people to read this book, and reading this book didn't cause people to be born. One of the authors of the above paper, Dr. Mikael Sodergren, suggested some other ways to help maximize the value of RWE in cannabis:

1. Universal terminology of medications to allow comparisons across practices and between different countries. Our acetaminophen is your paracetamol—this is confusing!

2. A minimally acceptable clinical data set or standard.

3. Global collaboration with support from governments and regulators to incentivize transparent data collection and publication.[9]

These intelligent suggestions would increase the clarity, coherence, and applicability of RWE.

Dr. Kevin Boehnke is a cannabis researcher at the University of Michigan who, in a 2019 piece, "National Trends in Qualifying Conditions for Medical Cannabis," echoes many of the above suggestions. He cites the ongoing Schedule I status of cannabis in the Controlled Substance Act as a huge barrier to harnessing more RWE. According to Boehnke,

> We could develop a rigorous observational data collection process for individuals using medical cannabis. These data would complement and inform the slower but more rigorous clinical trials. . . . If cannabis were rescheduled, the legal ramifications of collecting these data would be reduced, and patients with a medical cannabis license could opt into a patient registry that tracks use patterns, changes in symptoms, products

SEEING THROUGH THE SMOKE

used, changes in other medications, and safety issues. If collected effectively, these naturalistic use data could act as an incredible resource to investigate outcomes of real-world dosing regimens for various reasons (eg, cannabis as a substitute for opioids) and also examine population-level trends for adverse effects. . . . . These data could be used for drug development by aligning cannabis product composition with symptom relief in specific conditions, leading to clinical trials that are more targeted than those in the current scientific literature.[10]

There is no reason why this shouldn't take place, except our government's stubborn maintenance of cannabis in Schedule I (the legal category that applies to substances with no medical utility and high abuse potential). Change is starting to happen organically, at least in other places. In December 2021, the Medicines and Healthcare Products Regulatory Agency in the UK issued a press release in which they announced new guidelines created to incorporate RWE into their process "to support clinical trials which could get medicines to patients sooner." They said,

When used in this innovative way, real-world data has the potential to make a huge difference when it comes to bringing medicines through clinical trials to patients. . . . Real world data could make it more feasible for trial sponsors to repurpose existing medicines for new conditions. Because of this, and the growing need to find more cost-effective ways of conducting clinical trials, our new series of guidelines focuses on how to use real-world evidence to aid regulatory approval, helping to bring medicines to the patients who need them, sooner.[11]

I suspect other governments and institutions will be doing the same and that this type of evidence is going to become much more accepted and widespread. Gathering this type of RWE is much more feasible and effective now than in past years because of improvements in Big Data and machine learning, which allows this kind of information to be harvested and analyzed from multiple databases. Why not apply this rapidly improving technology to help improve people's lives with medical cannabis?

This expansion of the definition of "evidence" will make it more difficult for the sclerotic medical societies in the United States to continue to ignore RWE in general, and particularly as it relates to cannabis. It might also encourage the U.S. FDA to accept a broader definition of "evidence" as well when deciding which drugs to approve.

In considering the near blanket dismissal of RWE by professional medical organizations when it comes to cannabis, several preliminary thoughts come to mind. This might be a valuable clue as to why there is such a gulf between many doctors and their patients in terms of perceptions of the efficacy of medical cannabis. Maybe the two groups have been accepting and relying upon different types of evidence all along. From the old guard medical establishment's perspective, there aren't RCTs—regardless of the politics of the past—so there's just not enough evidence to responsibly get on board. Add this to the stigma, the federal illegality, the controversy, the lack of standardization, and the lack of knowledge—it's easier to just say no and to pass the patient off with a general caveat that it's not safe and there isn't enough evidence.

From many patients' perspectives, you know cannabis is working for you. This is your experience. You don't need an RCT to know that it helps you to relax and to get a good night's sleep. It beggars belief that your doctor still has his or her head in the sand on this issue. It's been down there for decades! (How do they breathe?) After all of the official lies from the government, to be told that there's no "evidence" from your doctor feels like the George Orwell quote, "The Party told you to reject the evidence of your eyes and ears. It was their final, most essential command." Of course medical cannabis works! Who are these people? I'm telling them my pain is gone! First, they didn't believe me when I said it wasn't gone, and they thought I was looking for opioids, and now they don't believe me that it is gone. I can't win.

Ironically, RWE has been deemed of sufficient quality and strength by detractors to fuel their claims that cannabis is harmful. Most of the studies that purport to show that cannabis causes addiction, induces heart attacks, lowers IQ, causes psychosis, etc. are based not on RCTs but on RWE, mostly observational studies. We don't give people who have cardiac risk factors cannabis in order to see if it causes heart attacks; that would be unethical. "Go smoke this and call me back tomorrow if you are still alive." So, we are stuck with RWE in a lot of these cases. Yet, this begs the question, why is RWE adequate to demonstrate the harms of cannabis but not to support its benefits?

Some are concerned that certain of the current indications for medical cannabis, in states where it has been legalized, have leapfrogged ahead of the science. It is true that we wasted so much time and energy fighting over *whether* medical cannabis should be legal that its eventual legalization has often occurred in a piecemeal and disjointed fashion. There are complicated issues involved in deciding what should be an indication for medical cannabis. Where do we set the bar for evidence? What types of evidence do we consider? Should patients be allowed to try cannabis for their condition if they believe in it, even if the evidence base isn't robust? (And if this is the case, should insurance companies have to pay?) To me it makes sense to give fairly wide latitude to the doctors and their patients, as they would know best what helps them and how to integrate cannabis into their care.

Sometimes, when I read the lists of approved uses for cannabis in some of the states, I wonder, for example, "how could cannabis possibly help with decompensated liver cirrhosis? Or the flu?" Of course, it is true that cannabis can make a patient with decompensated cirrhosis feel more comfortable by helping with symptoms such as nausea, pain, insomnia, anorexia, and anxiety. This is particularly helpful, as there are many other medications, which one ordinarily might use (NSAIDs, Tylenol), that you can't take when your liver is not healthy. In this case, cannabis is a treatment for symptoms when you can't take anything else. Seems reasonable. Is this "evidence based"? Again, it depends on your definition of evidence.

I'm all in favor of judiciously and sensibly incorporating RWE into the assessments of the benefits and efficacy of medical cannabis. However, it seems to me that some clinical situations would require a higher degree or quality of evidence than others. If I am alleviating a problem that is uncomfortable but not dangerous, such as a migraine, I'm willing to attempt this with less evidence. The worst-case scenario with the migraine is that the cannabis doesn't work and we try something else. Lots of medications do and don't work for migraines, and we learn this through trial and error.

On the other hand, if we wish to use cannabis to treat a progressive disease like a growing cancer—this is just an example—we would need a *much* higher standard of evidence. First of all, the risk of failure—pain, death, and disfigurement—is unacceptably high. Secondly, if patients are using cannabis with the belief that it is curative, they are more likely not to use something that has been proven to work, such as chemotherapy. In that case, we are actually harming the patient, as cannabis, by itself, isn't known to cure cancer. In such a situation, I would opt for a much higher bar of evidence and would prefer to have some RCTs confirming my therapeutic choices.

So maybe, as we incorporate RWE, we could keep in mind what the clinical scenario is and what the consequences are. Not all illnesses and potential treatment failures are of equal import. Treating symptoms is very different from attempting to impact the trajectory of disease.

## CHAPTER EIGHT

# DOES CANNABIS CAUSE PSYCHOSIS?
## Chicken Meets Egg

Cannabis use and psychotic disorders such as schizophrenia are strongly associated—no one argues against this fact. This means either that cannabis causes psychosis (including disorders like schizophrenia), that people with psychosis are particularly avid for cannabis as a form of self-treatment, or that the same factors, such as specific genes, push certain people toward both excessive cannabis use and psychosis. These explanations are not mutually exclusive. The dictates of the War on Drugs historically caused our government and many of the researchers it funds to emphasize the first explanation, that cannabis causes psychosis. Let's see what the evidence shows.

Cannabis, along with alcohol, amphetamines, steroids, psychedelics, and other drugs, can cause a transient "substance-induced psychotic disorder." Cannabis is the most likely substance to do this. For the most part, this is an agreed-upon side effect of cannabis. Further, people who develop one of these transient psychotic disorders are more likely to progress to schizophrenia if the disorder was caused by cannabis (as opposed to being caused by amphetamines or steroids, etc.). Does this prove that cannabis "causes" schizophrenia? No.

The fact that worldwide rates of cannabis use have skyrocketed over the last sixty years, going from very few cannabis users across the globe in the late 1950s to hundreds of millions of users currently, *while rates of schizophrenia have remained rock stable worldwide* (around 1 percent of the population), is an unassailable argument that cannabis is *not* contributing to an overall increase in schizophrenia.

Some die-hard Pessimists are scraping to show an increase, somewhere, anywhere, in the rates of schizophrenia so they can blame it on cannabis. How about in Denmark between 2000 and 2012? A recent study arguing that, yes, cannabis does cause schizophrenia referred to this as evidence of rising rates of schizophrenia, but what the article they were citing actually said is,

> The increased incidence of schizophrenia could partly be explained by better implementation of the diagnostic criteria for schizophrenia in child and adolescent psychiatry and improved access to early intervention services, but a true increase in incidence of schizophrenia *cannot be excluded*.[1] (emphasis added)

"Cannot be excluded" is quite different from "the rates are rising," and if this is the most compelling evidence of increasing cases of schizophrenia worldwide, you can rest assured that there hasn't truly been an increase.

Is cannabis innocent of all charges? Absolutely not. Schizophrenia is caused by a complex interplay between genetic risk and environmental factors. Cannabis is thought to act as one of several environmental factors that can trigger schizophrenia *in people who are already predisposed toward psychosis by virtue of their genetic makeup*. If there is no genetic tendency toward schizophrenia, cannabis does not increase the risk.

What this means is that while cannabis doesn't "cause" schizophrenia per se, cannabis might precipitate an earlier presentation of schizophrenia in vulnerable people, that is, people with a family history showing vulnerability to this disease. An earlier age of onset of schizophrenia is associated with worse outcomes because, among other reasons, you have less of a chance to establish adult life skills before the psychosis hits and undermines your progress.

On a practical level, this means that people who are considering using medical cannabis ought to be carefully screened for a family history of schizophrenia in order to assess their risk. Such a family history doesn't absolutely mean they can't use medicinal cannabis (though that would certainly be a safe, reasonable choice), but that they have to be extraordinarily careful, as their risk is higher. People don't always know their full family history, especially for mental illness and other stigmatized diseases that might not have been freely discussed. If any type of psychosis is diagnosed, cannabis use should cease immediately, as ongoing cannabis use might also worsen its course. CBD doesn't have to be stopped, as CBD is thought to act in an antipsychotic manner in conjunction with other treatments (see chapter 20).

The following are some ways to minimize risk:

- If you have a personal history of substance-induced psychosis, any type of psychotic disorder, or schizophrenia, it is recommended that you avoid cannabis use, as it may trigger or aggravate your condition or interfere with your recovery.

- If you have a family history of schizophrenia or other psychotic disorders, it is far riskier for you to use cannabis than for someone without such a family history. You ought to strongly consider avoiding usage unless there is a compelling medical reason to use.

- Instead of super-high THC levels, which are currently fashionable in the United States and Europe, it is safer and healthier to go lower on the THC and to always blend in some CBD, which is thought to be protective against both psychosis and many of the other detrimental effects of THC (see chapter 20).

- Always attempt to inform your health care professionals about your cannabis use, no matter how dismissive they may seem, in case you run into difficulties with it. It is critical that your care team know all the drugs and medicines you are on, even if they don't approve (though, ideally, they have the bedside manner not to shame patients away from important disclosures).

Psychosis is defined as "a severe mental disorder in which thoughts and emotions are so impaired that contact can be lost with external reality." Many of us feel that way until our first sip of morning coffee, but this refers to something much deeper and more pervasive. There are different flavors of psychosis, ranging from experiencing transient psychotic symptoms, to psychosis triggered by substances, to first-episode psychosis that can last for weeks or months. Finally, there are much longer-lasting psychotic diseases such as schizophrenia, which is a lifelong diagnosis without a definitive cure.

Psychosis is not anxiety, tension, depression, uncooperativeness, or several other items in the laboratory rubric that researchers use to categorize (pathologize) cannabis users, called the Positive and Negative Symptoms Scale (PANSS). This scale is what some researchers have used to measure "psychosis" after exposing research subjects to THC. Being high is not psychosis either. If you define psychosis to overlap with the effects that cannabis can frequently cause, such as being "spaced out and seeming separated or detached from the test environment, has said or done something bizarre or needed redirection," you can prove that cannabis causes "psychosis," but it isn't particularly helpful or convincing.

There are several factors that complexify the search for clarity on the relationship between cannabis and psychosis. The first is pressure that has been exerted on the scientific community by the War on Drugs over the last half century. A central tenet of the War on Drugs, pushed by the apparatus of antidrug leaders from Anslinger, to Nixon, to Reagan and beyond is that "cannabis causes insanity." A young researcher in the 1980s, for example, whose thesis was that cannabis was unlikely to cause psychosis, would have had an extremely difficult time being funded by NIDA and would have moved on to study a different topic. For someone interested in proving that cannabis does lead to schizophrenia, or any harm for that matter, the funding spigot was wide open, and these studies have proliferated. This has created a profound bias in our scientific canon over the last half century—making cannabis seem more harmful and less beneficial—and it is unclear how we can best deal with this.

It is also critical to remember that correlation isn't causation. Ice cream consumption and drownings both rise at the beach in the summer—they are correlated. But the ice cream use doesn't *cause* the drownings, unless maybe you feel guilty about breaking your diet and try to swim across the English Channel to burn off the extra calories.

It can certainly *appear* as if cannabis is causing, or helping to cause, the psychosis. In many cases, teenagers or college students experience heavy cannabis use weeks or months before their psychotic break. I don't think anyone would argue that the cannabis is helping the situation, or that the cannabis is a good idea in these scenarios, but did the cannabis *cause* the problem?

There are generally (at least) four different ways of looking at this:

1. Teens and young adults who use cannabis at a young age increase their chances of developing schizophrenia and other psychotic disorders later. This is because the use of cannabis directly causes or contributes to psychosis.

2. Intensive self-treatment with cannabis, often along with other substances such as tobacco and alcohol, is a prodromal (i.e., before the main symptoms come out) component of schizophrenia and other psychotic disorders. Cannabis may be particularly effective for people attempting to self-treat the disquieting feelings that precede overt psychosis, which is why "pre-psychotic" people are so forcefully drawn toward cannabis. (The psychosis is causing the heavy cannabis use.)

3. Specific genes cause both the psychosis and the excessive cannabis use. That is, the same genes that code for heavy cannabis use also code for schizophrenia—there is "shared liability." A variety of this is that the "genetic predisposition to schizophrenia makes cannabis users especially liable to psychotic experiences." This was the conclusion of a 2021 study, "Cannabis, Schizophrenia Genetic Risk, and Psychotic Experiences: A Cross-Sectional Study of 109,308 Participants from the UK Biobank." They conclude, "Thus, cannabis use was disproportionately highly correlated with psychotic experiences among individuals at high genetic risk of schizophrenia."[2]

4. A fourth hypothesis, as articulated by Harvard Medical's star cannabis researcher Dr. Staci Gruber (and colleagues), who is clearly one of the brightest, most evenhanded and non–agenda driven researchers in the cannabis space, is that "the association between cannabis use and psychosis would not be observed if confounding variables were properly controlled for." Generally, according to Dr. Gruber and colleagues, "mounting research suggests that cannabis use alone is not sufficient to cause psychotic disorders."[3]

One study that received huge amounts of uncritical press on this sub-ject—despite about a dozen crippling flaws (detailed below)—was a 2019 study by lead author Marta Di Forti, "The Contribution of Cannabis Use to Variation in the Incidence of Psychotic Disorder across Europe (EU-GEI): A Multicenter Case-Control Study." In this study, researchers assessed rates of psychosis in multiple cities with stronger cannabis versus rates of psychosis in cities with weaker cannabis. The strength of the can-nabis was binary, broadly based on whether the average potency of the cannabis confiscated by the police in that particular city was greater or less than 10 percent THC. Di Forti's researchers reiterated the already known association between cannabis and psychosis: "The strongest independent predictors of whether any given individual would have a psychotic disor-der or not were daily use of cannabis and use of high-potency cannabis."[4] This study is often taken as gospel, including in a recent 2022 *New York Times* piece, which quoted a researcher who said, "We definitely know that there's a dose-dependent relationship between THC and psychosis," and went on to explain,

> One rigorous study found that the risk of having a psychotic disorder
> was five times higher among daily high-potency cannabis users in Eu-
> rope and Brazil than those who had never used it.[5]

What was unique about this study was that Di Forti's researchers went further and concluded that the higher rates of psychosis seen in the high-THC cities are *caused by* the stronger weed. In other words, citizens in London and Amsterdam had higher rates of psychosis than did citizens in Palermo, and this is because the average cannabis, citywide, had THC lev-els greater than 10 percent, as opposed to less than 10 percent in Palermo.[6]

Further, by "assuming causality," they went on to predict how many cases of psychosis could have been prevented if "high-potency cannabis were no longer available." For example, "if high-potency cannabis were no longer available, 12.2% of cases of first-episode psychosis could be prevented across the 11 sites, rising to 30.3% in London and 50.3% in Amsterdam." They are claiming to have proven that the average THC in cannabis used by cannabis users was higher than 10 percent in some places and lower than 10 percent in others, and that *this difference alone* caused far more individuals to develop psychosis in those cities where the average THC level was higher than 10 percent. Consequently, a large number of cases of psychosis could be prevented by restricting access to this high-potency cannabis. They suggest that half the cases of psychosis in Amsterdam could have been prevented by shutting down the coffee shops and by restricting access to high-potency weed.

This study was manna to the Reefer Pessimists because, despite its beginning-to-end flaws, it *appeared* to be an extremely meticulous epidemiological study attempting to *causally* link cannabis use to psychosis. This study involved plenty of patients, so it had statistical power, and multiple different cities, so it was generalizable. They claimed that the mechanism and timing of cannabis causing psychosis were biologically plausible and that this study was consistent with and built upon previous studies that have come to similar conclusions (beware of this maneuver, which is highly circular—discussed below in point 9). Further, it appeared to show a link between strength of cannabis and rates of psychosis—as cited so confidently by the expert in the above *New York Times* piece. The press, including the medical press, dutifully reported on it without any critical thought or skepticism.

There were a few critical issues with this study that didn't get much attention:

1. How does this study determine chicken versus egg? It doesn't; that's why they have to "assume causality," which is dubious. Pre-psychotic persons could be drawn to places with stronger cannabis and more cannabis culture, just as plausibly as the stronger cannabis could be making people sick (if it even does make people sick). People could have gravitated to cultural centers with stronger cannabis that would more effectively "self-treat" their "pre-psychotic" conditions. The directionality here is quite problematic.

2. Just because an average citywide THC level in those samples (that happened to be confiscated by the police—even this isn't necessarily representative) is above or below 10 percent THC, that doesn't account for what any particular individual was using. If I live in Boston and the average THC level is 11 percent, that doesn't by any means prove or suggest that I, as

an individual, use cannabis that has that potency. I could be using some mellow 4 percent cannabis with CBD in it, or I could be using a strain as high as 30 percent.

3. As if to prove the above points, they say in the "limitations" section, "Data on cannabis use are not validated by biological measures, such as urine, blood, or hair samples." So, they don't truly know much of anything about the cannabis-related behavior of *any* of the subjects they counted as evidence.

4. They didn't test any individuals for CBD levels or other cannabinoids. Cannabis is comprised of hundreds of different compounds that work together. CBD is thought to be medicinal in general and specifically protective against some of the harms of THC, *especially psychosis*. It makes no sense to not test, ask about, or include CBD, as the lack (or presence) of CBD (and other cannabinoids) could likely be impacting the results. (One could plausibly argue that the level of CBD is almost as important as the level of THC with regard to psychosis.)

5. There are lots of other "confounding" factors (factors that influence the results that they couldn't account for) that they didn't or couldn't factor in and which could have provided an alternative explanation for these findings. For example, in their samples, *the cannabis users also smoked more cigarettes and used more other drugs than the nonusers*, so how do they know it was the cannabis causing the problems and not the other drugs? (They don't.) What about alcohol? Or trauma? Or maybe life is more stressful in those cities, which could trigger both cannabis use and psychosis.

6. They "assumed causality to prove causality." I'd flunk out of my Introduction to Logic course at Swarthmore College within the first week if I tried this. I can't imagine what my professor would say to me if I did this. He once bellowed at a classmate, "If my grandmother had wheels, she'd be a bus," for committing a much more minor logical transgression.

7. It's not clear by what mechanism "high-potency" cannabis would cause more psychosis than "low potency." People tend to titrate their dose to their comfort level. Instead of smoking three puffs of 7 percent THC cannabis they smoke one puff of 20 percent (which, ironically, is better for the lungs). Higher-potency cannabis doesn't mean bigger dose, and dose, ultimately, is the variable that matters.

8. They also bring in "biological plausibility" to bolster their claims. Many things in medicine that have biological plausibility don't actually turn out to be true when studied. Hormone replacement therapy was plausibly supposed to be healthy for postmenopausal women until we learned that it caused net harm and lower survival. "Plausibility" just means you can create a realistic mechanism, not that it is true.

9. As a general point, many of these studies on the "causation" of cannabis harms reference each other for validation. In this study, they mention, "Our findings confirm previous evidence of the harmful effect on mental health of daily use of cannabis, especially of high-potency types." Yet other studies reciprocally refer to this study for confirmation and essentially say, "We don't really prove causation, but our conclusion of causation is confirmed by the Di Forti study." If you understand all of these studies to be as inconclusive as they truly are, it's sort of a shell game for these researchers to refer to each other to bolster their credibility. They are trying to create a self-fulfilling illusion of more scientific certainty than the individual studies actually warrant.

10. The PAF (population attributable fraction) stuff is highly speculative (see below), bordering on BS—they truly have no idea if *any* of the cases of psychosis were caused by cannabis, let alone a specific number.[7]

For an eleventh point, and elaboration on some of the others, I'll defer to the official rebuttal in the *Lancet*,

Marta Di Forti and colleagues conclude that removing one environmental factor—daily high-potency cannabis use—would reduce the incidence of all psychotic disorders in Amsterdam, the Netherlands, by 50%. . . . We think that this is very unlikely given that Sullivan and colleagues confirmed the heritability of schizophrenia to be about 80%. Therefore, attributing this complex multifactorial brain disorder to one environmental factor such as high-potency cannabis use seems counterintuitive, especially given that 33.6% of the patients assessed by Di Forti and colleagues had never used cannabis.[8]

Ouch. It goes on,

The reported 50% population attributable fraction (PAF) for cannabis use in Amsterdam becomes even more questionable with a recent two-sample bidirectional Mendelian randomization study showing that *the causal direction was from schizophrenia to cannabis use and not vice versa. Indeed, high-potency cannabis use can lead to drug-induced psychosis and high-potency cannabis use might trigger earlier onset of psychosis in genetically vulnerable individuals who would have developed psychosis anyway. But these conclusions are all very different from stating that high-potency cannabis use is responsible for 50% of incident psychosis cases in Amsterdam.*[9] (emphasis added)

Unfortunately, the media, as demonstrated by the above-cited *New York Times* article, have been conditioned to take the bait when it's a study of the harms of cannabis. The BBC reported this study with this headline, "Potent Cannabis Increases Risk of Serious Mental Illness," and they go on to report, "They estimate around one in 10 new cases of psychosis may be associated with strong cannabis, based on their study of European cities and towns. In London and Amsterdam, where most of the cannabis that is sold is very strong, the risk could be much more."

Now, as you can see from the objections I've raised, this study doesn't show that "potent cannabis increases the risk of serious mental illness." This is journalistic laziness and scientific illiteracy raised to a rarified art form.

Or, as Dr. Carl Hart, the brilliant director of the Psychology Department at Columbia, bluntly summarizes: "Those studies are poor and crappy—they're correlation studies." Hart continues, "What they're calling strong correlations are about the same correlations when you look at cat ownership in childhood and likelihood to go on and have a psychiatric illness."[10]

Amen to that, though if you ask me—a dog person—cats *are* pretty annoying and can definitely drive you crazy. (I had to say at least one controversial thing somewhere in this book.)

As mentioned, virtually all recreational drugs and many medicines can cause a disorder called "substance-induced psychosis," which usually resolves within weeks to months but is quite dangerous and can at least temporarily derail your life. This is one of the risks of using drugs and medicines, whether its alcohol, amphetamines or other stimulants, cannabis, sedatives, steroids, or one of the hallucinogens. Some people who develop substance-induced psychosis go on to develop lifelong schizophrenia (seemingly if they are genetically presupposed to it). It is critical to determine who these people are so that we can prevent these negative outcomes.

In a 2019 study called "Transition of Substance-Induced, Brief, and Atypical Psychoses to Schizophrenia: A Systematic Review and Meta-analysis," researchers studied people who went from substance-induced psychosis to schizophrenia to see which drugs were the most common culprits. The average rate of transition for all comers was 25 percent (i.e., one-quarter of all people with substance-induced psychosis when on to develop schizophrenia). Yet a higher percentage of cannabis-induced psychosis went on to schizophrenia at thirty-four percent. Therefore, those who developed substance-induced psychosis—by no means a rare disorder—from using cannabis were more likely to develop schizophrenia.[11]

But what about the familial risk scores? Kendler's team noted that the familial risk scores for psychosis were twice as high as in the population at large. This strongly suggested that the cannabis was interacting with other risk factors, in this case a genetic predisposition, to increase the risk of developing schizophrenia in vulnerable individuals. Again, the cannabis doesn't, on its own, cause the schizophrenia (though it may help trigger it or precipitate it earlier).

Kendler and colleagues, in a 2019 paper titled "Prediction of Onset of Substance-Induced Psychotic Disorder and Its Progression to Schizophrenia in a Swedish National Sample," first examined who gets substance-induced psychosis in the first place and noted that "individuals with substance-induced psychotic disorder had, on average, one-third of a standard deviation higher familial risk score for . . . psychosis than the general population—a highly significant difference." People with a family history of psychosis tended to get substance-induced psychosis. They conclude, "Focusing first on substance-induced psychotic disorder, we could confidently reject the hypothesis that the disorder arises solely from the psychotogenic effects of the substances of abuse."[12]

Take a pause. Deep breath. This stuff is difficult! Bear with me.

Finally, and critically, looking in the other direction, at a population of patients with schizophrenia, Kendler found that, among all cases of schizophrenia, *the family risk score for psychosis was the same whether or not your schizophrenia was or wasn't preceded by a substance-induced psychotic disorder.* As they say,

> with respect to familial risk for psychosis, patients with substance-induced psychotic disorder who develop schizophrenia are indistinguishable from patients with schizophrenia without a history of substance-induced psychotic disorder.[13]

This is absolutely critical: if cannabis (or the other substances) were *causing* the schizophrenia, the cases of schizophrenia from substance-induced psychosis should have had *lower* familial risk than the other cases of schizophrenia—*because cannabis should have accounted for some of the risk.* In other words, some of the risk should have been from the cannabis and some should have been genetic, and, as such, the familial risk ought to be lower in these cases if cannabis was contributing to/causing the psychosis. If the genetic risk is the same, per Kendler,

> these results support the hypothesis that in substance-induced psychotic disorder, drugs of abuse may precipitate the development of schizophrenia but do not typically have a strong causal role in the emergence of the chronic psychosis.[14]

In Kendler's words, "Schizophrenia following substance-induced psychosis is likely a drug-precipitated disorder in highly vulnerable individuals, not a syndrome predominantly caused by drug exposure."

In summary, despite the Drug War–inspired claims of the last fifty years, cannabis does *not* cause schizophrenia.

I had a bird's-eye view of the cannabis–psychosis connection during a visit from a college-age friend of my family. Ron was on break from college where he studied engineering at one of the most prestigious university programs in the world. I had known this kid since he was ten years old. I was aware that he had used cannabis, at least casually, during high school, which I didn't approve of. He was bright, together, and successful, and I didn't give the cannabis much thought, except to express, in response to his open discussion of the issue with me, why I absolutely wouldn't use cannabis at his age because of concerns about brain development. If I had said, "STOP SMOKING MARIJUANA RIGHT NOW," he would have tuned out and stopped listening after the word "marijuana"—another clueless adult lecturing about weed. We have better success if we meet people where they are and focus on harm reduction. They might not do what we want them to, but at least it's open for discussion, which gives you a chance and maintains your credibility in their eyes. It also leaves open vital avenues of communication.

His family had moved away from Boston, and it wasn't until much later that I learned he had been having trouble in his new high school, likely related to his cannabis use. During a period when he was using heavily, he started to believe his entire high school was ganging up on him in a coordinated plot. This resolved with cessation of cannabis and some therapy. Lesson learned (hopefully). His entrance scores to his elite graduate program were some of the highest the school had ever seen. The future was full of promise.

When he stayed at our home over a break after his first year at university, I was shocked to see that he seemed solely interested in getting stoned from the moment he arrived. Not sociably high, a puff or two to relax—he was getting stoned to oblivion at every possible opportunity. He was using no other drugs and no alcohol, but cannabis to extreme excess. I've never seen someone so avid for cannabis. It was the only thing he wanted to do with his friends, or alone, with all of his free time.

This didn't seem like "cannabis addiction" per se—this went far beyond. It was as if an inner robot were instructing him to seek and consume cannabis above all else. Cannabis addiction doesn't usually present like that. It's more like people can't stop using it, and it has begun to crowd out the other things in their lives. With his monomaniacal compulsion to use, he was acting as if he were heavily addicted to something far more

114

rewarding, like meth or opioids. Nothing was going to stop Ron from getting high. His whole visit was oriented around this; we, the hosts, were incidental.

The old Ron shone through at moments. Even though the conversation kept reverting, one way or another, back to cannabis, he had absolutely no symptoms suggestive of psychosis. He was just very high most of the time, and refractory to my efforts to impact his use.

I was highly alarmed by his behavior, and I had several frank discussions with him about my concerns. On various occasions, I was on the verge of calling his parents, even though he was well over twenty years old and legally an adult. His parents were overseas, but they knew me and would have flown in and gotten him help. He pleaded with me not to, claiming that they would cut off tuition and make him move home, which was in a different country from all his friends and his school program. It would ruin his life. He gave me the deepest assurances that he would get it under control.

As he returned to school overseas, he was stable for three or four months, and then he started feeling increasingly stressed, lonely, and alienated. He felt like he wasn't connecting well with the other kids. He wondered if this prestigious program was truly a fit for him after all, despite his Herculean efforts to get accepted. The other students were exclusively interested in making money, and this seemed empty to him.

To deal with his distress and uncertainty, he started smoking cannabis, at first with friends and then every day for a period of three weeks. No other drugs were involved, and minimal alcohol. He has no known family history of psychosis or schizophrenia. He started to develop a more severe paranoia that went beyond what he had experienced in high school. He was having disturbing thoughts that he couldn't shake. He was a Nazi. He had raped a girl—this is what his psychotic mind was telling him. He'd be sent to prison, which was merged in his mind with the hospital, where he could have received help. At other times, he believed that all of these disturbing occurrences were all just a prank being pulled on him by the headmaster—an idea that was even more confusing than the other thoughts.

Fortunately, his family was able to swoop in, get him hospitalized, and keep him safe. I spoke to him several times in the immediate aftermath, and it was heartbreaking, speaking to this incredibly gifted kid who was now struggling just to get words out due to the heavy-duty antipsychotic medications he was on. Months later, he was rapidly heading back to baseline and was back in school, at a less stressful and competitive institution. He has committed not to use cannabis again. I explained to him that it could retrigger everything, and this truly is the last thing he wanted.

In his opinion, he thinks that his crash and burn was at least in part because of the cannabis, but he's not quite sure how it contributed. He says it's tough to dissect what happened because he was in such rough shape. About the cannabis, "It didn't help."

He concluded, "Cannabis was the spark that set the fire off."

To say that "cannabis was the spark that set the fire off" is a great way to put it and intuitively synthesizes much of the research cited above. Cannabis can precipitate psychosis if the conditions are in place. But if there wasn't anything there for the spark to set on fire—a large pile of pre-psychotic, psychologically flammable wood—then there would be no fire. Cannabis is a component of a complex multifactorial web. It doesn't cause lasting psychosis by itself in someone who is not prone to it.

The problem is, how do you determine who is at risk? Even if you know that someone is at risk, what do you do about it? If these behaviors are coming from a magnetic genetic attraction to cannabis, it isn't easy to get the person to abstain. Abundant research shows that people already predisposed to schizophrenia are more driven to use cannabis. Consider a 2014 study, "Genetic Predisposition to Schizophrenia Associated with Increased Use of Cannabis":

> In a sample of 2082 healthy individuals, we show an association between an individual's burden of schizophrenia risk alleles and use of cannabis. . . . These findings suggest that part of the association between schizophrenia and cannabis is due to a shared genetic etiology.[15]

In other words, those with gene variants linked to increased schizophrenia risk were more likely to use cannabis, and to use more of it than others. The same genes are causing the schizophrenia and the cannabis use. Perhaps a component of Ron's intense compulsion to use cannabis when visiting was genetically mediated (though he has not been diagnosed with schizophrenia).

If a person is over eighteen and you don't have any parental or legal control, or other leverage, how do you stop them from lighting up? Keeping cannabis illegal makes things worse—it makes the cannabis more dangerous as it isn't regulated, it makes it harder for people to ask for and to receive help due to stigma, and it gives people criminal records—all without impacting the amount of cannabis used. Do you threaten to kick your relative or friend out of the house? Then they are at risk of more dangerous addictions, homelessness, and poor mental health outcomes. "Tough love" can kill people.

There's a lot of grandstanding, but I'm not sure anyone has the answer to this.

According to the Di Forti study discussed above, there's a 50 percent chance that Ron's psychosis was "caused" by the fact that the average potency of the cannabis confiscated by the police in Paris, where Ron was going to school, was greater than 10 percent. By now, you should see that this is nonsensical. If there was no limit to his access to cannabis and to the dosage he consumes of THC, how does the strength matter? Unless you want to posit something like the stronger cannabis got him high faster, more efficiently, or more dangerously. You'd have to argue, "Because it took only three minutes to smoke half a joint (of stronger weed), instead of taking him six minutes to smoke a full joint of weaker weed, he has a higher risk of psychosis." That's like saying you're more likely to become an alcoholic, or to develop psychosis from using alcohol, if you drink port rather than wine, because it is twice as strong.

As Dr. Carl Hart points out, most of the studies showing that cannabis "causes" psychosis are hobbled by the fact that they are observational in nature—they view disease at one fixed point in time, making it impossible to judge cause (chicken) and effect (egg). A recent study that was longitudinal, meaning it followed people over time—a much more valid way to understand cause and effect—has come out addressing this very issue. Impressively, they followed fifteen hundred twin pairs. This study, "Adolescent Cannabis Use and Adult Psychoticism: A Longitudinal Co-twin Control Analysis Using Data from Two Cohorts," followed these twins from adolescence into adulthood, testing their genetics and their "psychoticism" in relation to cannabis use:

We found no evidence of an effect of cannabis on psychoticism or any of its facets in co-twin control models that compared the greater-cannabis-using twin to the lesser-using co-twin. We also observed no evidence of a differential effect of cannabis on psychoticism by polygenic risk of schizophrenia. Although cannabis use and disorder are consistently associated with increased risk of psychosis, the present results suggest this association is likely attributable to familial confounds rather than a causal effect of cannabis exposure.[16]

Their conclusions strongly support the "it's explained by familial confounds" hypothesis over the "cannabis causes psychosis" one.

To be conservative, acknowledging the ongoing uncertainties and debate over this issue, I would advise that cannabis users (and providers) do the following:

1. Keep the dosages of THC as low as possible, whether using for medical or adult use. For medical, use the minimal effective dose. For adult use, consider getting pleasantly high, not wasted, and don't mix cannabis with other drugs.

2. Use strains high in CBD, which is protective against psychosis (as well as other side effects of cannabis, such as memory impairment—see chapter 20), or supplement your cannabis use with CBD.

3. If possible, know your family medical history and share this with your doctor. If you have a risky family history, such as a large streak of schizophrenia, skip the cannabis or proceed with great caution.

4. If, after using cannabis, you notice strange and unpleasant thoughts that don't mesh with your usual beliefs or your peers' reality, stop the cannabis use. I would also get professional help.

5. Avoid the "concentrates" such as wax, shatter, crumble, etc.— good old-fashioned cannabis flower should be strong enough, especially given how much stronger it has become in recent decades. According to one 2020 study, concentrates don't

necessarily get you "higher"; they just cause your THC levels to spike.[17]

6. Take periodic tolerance breaks (stop using for two to four weeks) to lower your tolerance and, consequently, lower the total dose of THC. By doing this, you can get the same effects from the cannabis, whether recreational or medical, save lots of money, and it's healthier.

It is critical to remember that all drugs and medicines have their harms. There is no free lunch, including with cannabis. We must rely on education and common sense, not on criminalization, in order to encourage people to maintain a healthy, measured relationship to this plant, which isn't going anywhere.

## CHAPTER NINE

# PEOPLE GET ADDICTED TO WEED?

C annabis can be addictive, but it is debatable how addictive it truly is. The psychiatric and addiction communities have very different ideas about the addictiveness of cannabis than the cannabis community does.

According to the field of addiction psychiatry, cannabis use disorder (CUD), a term often used synonymously with cannabis addiction, is diagnosed quite objectively when patients fulfill a certain number of criteria over time that have been carefully validated. Some of these include tolerance, withdrawal, cravings, inability to control use, use in hazardous circumstances, and continued use despite negative consequences. The consequences of having CUD range but can be quite severe, especially in teens and young adults who are particularly susceptible. CUD is associated with lower happiness, an unsatisfying social life, lack of career success, lower socioeconomic status, car crashes, emergency room visits, cognitive decline, problems with other drugs, other psychiatric diagnoses, suicide, and low motivation. The use of cannabis should generally be discouraged, except in cases of, as they term it, quote, unquote, "medical" use.

Mainstream addiction psychiatrists believe that CUD is common, and some studies purport to show that CUD afflicts up to a quarter to a third of adult cannabis users. It ranges from mild, to moderate, to severe depending on how many of the criteria are met. According to the American Society of Addiction Medicine (ASAM), "between 9.3% and 30.6% of American adults who use cannabis have CUD."[1] The fact that this range is gigantic—more than a factor of three—foreshadows a discussion of whether the criteria are somewhat, or possibly vastly, overinclusive and whether they are sensibly applicable to typical cannabis users or medical cannabis patients. To confuse things further, the definition of "cannabis addiction" and the diagnostic criteria for CUD have evolved and have changed with each iteration of the psychiatric diagnostic codebook, which makes it more difficult to track and compare rates over time.

Many addiction specialists feel that, while perhaps not as life threatening as opioid use disorder or alcohol use disorder, CUD is dangerously dismissed and underappreciated. It knocks many lives off track, especially teens and young adults. As perceptions of the harms of cannabis decline, and as legalization progresses, more people are attempting to self-treat psychiatric disorders such as anxiety, depression, and PTSD with cannabis. The psychiatrists (who, coincidentally, make their living by prescribing psychiatric medications) feel that psychiatric disorders are best treated by psychiatrists with bona fide psychiatric meds, not with cannabis, which can potentially make these conditions worse. They feel that we are putting a large swath of our population at risk for an increase in rates of addiction. As a society, we are experimenting on ourselves.

Many people in the cannabis community don't believe that cannabis is addictive—they think it is just another bogus U.S. government propaganda point. A common story is, "I used it for twenty years and then I was able to stop on a dime without any problems. How can it be addictive?" Others think it can be mildly or infrequently addicting, with an occasional person who goes off the rails. They wonder who these one-quarter to one-third of adult cannabis users are who supposedly become addicted. Few in the cannabis community appear to have much direct experience with cannabis addiction despite knowing hundreds, if not thousands, of people who seem to use cannabis without problems. They cite the versatile wellness benefits of cannabis and note how at odds this is with the negative attention one must muster in order to focus in on the small minority of people who run into difficulty. The disconnect between their own experiences and observations and the extreme rhetoric from some addiction specialists causes them to deny, reject, and ignore most, if not all, information and advice from the addiction community.

Cannabis proponents point out that the majority of studies of its addictiveness have been funded and conducted under the auspices of the War on Drugs, where there was, and still is, massive institutional pressure and financial incentive to demonstrate harm. In essence, the community says, "Cannabis is about well-being, not addiction. Go focus on alcohol or something that is actually destructive. We didn't ask for your 'help' and don't believe your rigged studies. Leave us alone." They feel that needlessly pathologizing so many cannabis users harms people and fuels the vast "prohibition for profit" industry that has callously ruined so many lives.

These are two vastly different sets of assumptions that we need to reconcile. It brings up an interesting question: who *does* know more about cannabis and cannabinoids? Is it the cannabis users, who have long-standing, lived experience with the drug, many of whom work in this field as researchers, health care providers, entrepreneurs, or budtenders? Or is it the addiction psychiatrists, many of whom have never used it themselves, have never actually treated patients with cannabis for anything (only for "cannabis addiction"), and who almost exclusively are exposed to information about the downsides because they have been steeped in an anti-cannabis milieu for decades? Both groups are, to a certain extent, subjected to their own echo chambers of curated information. It is likely that they both have different pieces of the truth to contribute, the Pessimists telling us about what could go wrong, and the Utopians telling us what could go right. In my experience, it is the moderate, balanced cannabis clinicians who know the most about cannabis, as they treat patients, read *both* sides of the literature, and often have lived experience with the drug and with all of the people they have treated.

Part of this comes down to a fundamental conflict in a priori assumptions, one of harm, the other of benefit. This informs what people study, remember, internalize, emphasize, and focus on—the cognitive biases that help us filter an overwhelming amount of information every day.

My own sense is that many of the studies and assumptions of cannabis addiction are plagued by overly broad inclusion criteria for what constitutes CUD. Arguably, the disorder itself is inadequately conceived and doesn't reflect the current reality of cannabis use (this is discussed below). Further, many people use cannabis either for medical purposes or more generally for health and wellness purposes—categories that aren't even recognized, included, or asked about by the psychiatric community, who have anointed themselves as the ones to define the rates of addiction. The concept of "cannabis addiction" was formed during a time when our society had a very different view of cannabis, under major pressure from the War on Drugs, before medical marijuana use was widely recognized.

Just because there are positives to its use isn't to say that you can't get addicted to it; rather, it just demonstrates that it has been looked at with a distorted lens since its criminalization, and we may need to redefine these things in a more neutral and helpful way.

Another shortfall is that in many studies, the rates of addiction are determined by epidemiologists, not clinicians. To determine these rates, they utilize survey data harvested by laypeople, or even computer-assisted interviews, over the phone. Addiction is ideally supposed to be diagnosed through a structured clinical interview. The rates that come from number-crunching these broad surveys range from 9 to 30 percent. The wide range is likely because of how the questions are asked, which questions are asked, and how the answers are transformed into a diagnosis of CUD. The methodologies of these surveys, like the NESARC (National Epidemiologic Survey on Alcohol and Related Conditions) and the NSDUH (National Survey on Drug Use and Health), change over time as the government is forced to make concessions to reality (e.g., "legal trouble" is only because of criminalization, so it shouldn't be a criterion for being addicted—they had to remove this), making comparisons from previous times difficult.

According to a 2017 article in *Vox*, citing alcohol researcher Richard Grucza,

> The problem with NESARC, Grucza said, is it underwent major methodological changes between the 2001–2002 and 2012–2013 waves. Here are a few, originally noted by the Substance Abuse and Mental Health Services Administration (SAMHSA), which conducts NSDUH, and verified by the National Institute on Alcohol Abuse and Alcoholism (NIAAA), which conducted NESARC:
>
> • The NESARC changed some questions from wave to wave, which could lead survey takers to respond differently.
>
> • In the 2001–2002 wave, NESARC respondents were not given monetary rewards. In the 2012–2013 wave, they were. That could have incentivized different people to respond.
>
> • No biological samples were collected in the first wave, while saliva samples were collected in the second. What's more, respondents were notified of this at the start of the survey—which could have

led them to respond differently, since they knew they'd be tested for their drug use.

- Census Bureau workers were used for the 2001–2002 survey, but private workers were used for the 2012–2013 survey. That could lead to big differences: As Grucza told me, "Some researchers speculate that using government employees might suppress reporting of socially undesirable behaviors."

There is plenty of research out there that suggests even one of these tweaks could have significant impacts on survey responses. But to have all of these at once makes the two waves of NESARC difficult, if not impossible, to seriously compare. Researchers from SAMHSA told me that they would caution against trying to use the different waves of NESARC to gauge trends.[2]

Also, of course, the legality of cannabis is rapidly changing, which affects how people answer questions about their usage. These points are rarely mentioned in the news articles that report on this, whether they are sensationalizing a rise or a drop in cannabis addiction. The changes in the definition of CUD over time (see below) aren't included either.

When some cannabis addiction researchers claim that 30 percent of adult cannabis users have CUD, this begs the question, who exactly are these people? I can only scratch my head at these purported rates of CUD. There clearly exists a nontrivial group of predominantly younger people who *do* get into serious trouble with cannabis, but it is a smaller fraction, not one-third of adult users. I don't think we know the number, as our definitions are broken.

My own experiences might be subject to selection bias, as I grew up with extremely high-functioning cannabis users, but I've also interacted with thousands of people battling all types of addictions, to all types of drugs, from all walks of life, both as a person in recovery and as a treatment provider. I've treated doctors, nurses, and other patients, for a diversity of addictions, including to cannabis. I've dealt with many thousands of people, both professionally and personally, who utilize cannabis.

With a few dozen or so exceptions, the people I used cannabis with in high school, in college, during my five years working at Greenpeace, during medical school at Boston University, during my internship and residency at Harvard Medical, and further into adulthood, as well as people I interact with as a cannabis specialist under all kinds of circumstances—doctors, nurses, lawyers, professors, activists, academics, writers, laborers, you name it—most of them seem to have a healthy relationship with cannabis. Certainly not all of them, but it is a minority who get into trouble.

As a primary care doctor in an inner-city clinic, I see plenty of people who struggle in various ways, with cannabis sometimes being a component of this struggle. It is often difficult to say whether the cannabis is helping them walk through their disadvantaged circumstances with less misery or whether it is an unhelpful crutch that is increasing the hardship. But addicted? It's a question of definitions. My favorite definition is "continued use despite negative consequences." (This avoids the rabbit holes of "what do we even mean by addiction?" A learning disorder? A brain disease? How does addiction differ from psychological dependence, physiological dependence, habit, or strong attraction to something?)

What is the answer to the conundrum of the discrepancy between the 9 percent estimate and the 30 percent estimate? What about the perceived rarity of widespread addiction in the cannabis community? Are a significant proportion of cannabis users faring much more poorly than they appear to be? Do they just admit their troubles to anonymous (or computerized) callers on national surveys of drug use, but keep it hidden from their doctors, their families, and everyone else? Are they motivated and successful in public but then, the second they get home, they amotivationally plant themselves on their sofas and disengage from society (except to answer survey questions over the phone about their cannabis addiction)? Is there a separate pool of cannabis users, cut off from the main cannabis community, that is afflicted with all of the ills of CUD that we don't know about but that accounts for this troubled 9–30 percent of users? Are they all living under a bridge somewhere in Colorado, amotivationally unable to migrate due to cannabis legalization? Maybe they went there when it first legalized cannabis and smoked away their gumption to leave.

All satire aside, the numbers don't seem to add up. Though I bet that from a different vantage point, such as if you work as a pediatric addiction specialist who deals with the young people who do go off the rails, these numbers might seem plausible, even understated, because that's much of what you would see and treat every day.

Perhaps it's a question of definitions *and* vantage point.

125

About ten years ago, a few days after my monthly meeting with my psychiatrist, I was reading through my medical record out of morbid curiosity. His note was full of things like "well groomed" and "speech linear and coherent," which I thought gave me more credit than I deserved given how little caffeine I had imbibed at the early hour of our visit. I learned from my first visit with him to conceal my coffee or I'd get a stern lecture about the (valid) connection between my overconsumption of caffeine and my chronic insomnia. Even when I'm sipping on a watery Diet Coke during our visit, the note says, "Patient was actively consuming caffeine," as if I had freebased caffeine powder and was injecting it into both arms at once, while also snorting it and using a caffeine suppository.

All of a sudden my jaw dropped as I saw in my chart, "diagnoses of opioid and marijuana addiction." I checked to see if this was the correct chart. Where on earth did the marijuana addiction come from?

There is no argument that I am sixteen years into recovery from a vicious opioid addiction that had almost killed me several times over. This was public knowledge—I've written a memoir about it (*Free Refills*) and speak openly about my struggles with opioids. Where did the diagnosis of marijuana addiction come from?

There are eleven criteria for CUD. A patient needs to have two out of the eleven of these criteria for at least a year to qualify as "addicted" to cannabis, accompanied by "significant impairment of functioning and distress."[3] If you use cannabis, you can test yourself as we go along. Keep in mind that if you meet two or three criteria you have mild CUD, if you meet four or five you have moderate CUD, and six or more means severe CUD. Note: if you do in fact meet most or all of these criteria, depending on your thoughts about this particular definition of cannabis addiction by the end of the chapter, you might want to speak with your physician!

According to the DSM-5 (*Diagnostic and Statistical Manual of Mental Disorders*, 5th edition), the criteria for CUD are as follows:[4]

1. Use of cannabis for at least a one-year period, with the presence of at least two of the following symptoms, accompanied by significant impairment of functioning and distress.

Clearly I'd used it for at least a one-year period (or, by then, three decades . . .), but no one has ever claimed cannabis-related impairment of functioning. Cannabis had always been integral to helping me manage distress and maintain balance. Given the miserable (abusive) marriage I had been in and the stressful, exploitative career I was (am) trying to hold on to (primary care doctor), who knows how well I would have fared without it. (Answer: I stopped using cannabis for at least five years as I was drug-tested by the medical board for my opioid monitoring, without a thought, craving, problem, or difficulty. I didn't cheat once in five years. It didn't occur to me to cheat. All my tests were negative. I didn't miss it much, and I was fine without it, though my creative tank felt a little bit empty.)

2. Difficulty containing use of cannabis—the drug is used in larger amounts and over a longer period than intended.

I've had a lifelong pattern of taking just a puff or two; I've never liked taking more. (Most people self-titrate to their desired effect.)

3. Repeated failed efforts to discontinue or reduce the amount of cannabis that is used.

I'd had no failed attempts to discontinue or reduce; I've always been able to stop and start abruptly when need be, such as for international travel or drug testing.

4. An inordinate amount of time is occupied acquiring, using, or recovering from the effects of cannabis.

Aside from times spent in the past waiting for unreliable weed dealers, in the times before legalization: no, no, and no. There is minimal hangover or recovery if one uses modestly, and indeed even a night of heavy use results in significantly fewer effects than a comparable alcohol-induced hangover.

5. Cravings or desires to use cannabis. This can include intrusive thoughts and images, and dreams about cannabis, or olfactory perceptions of the smell of cannabis, due to preoccupation with cannabis.

Never experienced. It sounds more like what you'd get with opioid addiction, which I sometimes wonder if people partially conflate with cannabis addiction. I have had intense cravings for yummy food after consuming cannabis, but that's different. Also, why is this even a criterion? We have cravings for lots of different medicines and substances that we aren't considered addicted to. I can crave a beer on a hot summer day, but I am about as far from an alcoholic as you can get.

6. Continued use of cannabis despite adverse consequences from its use, such as criminal charges, ultimatums of abandonment from spouse/partner/friends, and poor productivity.

Poor productivity? In some ways, it was the key to my productivity at many times in the past. For example, in medical school. I used it every night to relax after studying for the medical boards—which enabled me to study harder during the day as I was well rested—and scored quite high (ninety-seventh percentile). Cannabis helped reset my brain for the next day's labors—I'm not saying this works for everyone. It also helps my writing—there's no paper I've written under the influence of cannabis that didn't receive a grade of an A or "Honors." But people have very variable levels of success (or failure) with this. Also, "criminal charges" are an artifact of the War on Cannabis and shouldn't be part of the criteria for "addicted."

7. Other important activities in life, such as work, school, hygiene, and responsibility to family and friends, are superseded by the desire to use cannabis.

No. Opioids used to utterly supersede these things, but cannabis—never. With opioids, I'd isolate from others and focus on the euphoria I felt; I'd take lots of naps where I'd be able to commune with my dopamine receptors in solitude. With cannabis, I'd engage all the more and remember to check in on people.

8. Cannabis is used in contexts that are potentially dangerous, such as operating a motor vehicle.

This would be very stressful and dangerous; I always made sure someone else was driving if I were to consume.

9. Use of cannabis continues despite awareness of physical or psychological problems attributed to use—e.g., anergia, amotivation, chronic cough.

It always motivated me and gave me energy. There is some stigma baked (no pun intended) into this question, like chronic marijuana users have no motivation or energy—this isn't evidence based. I have asthma, but it never seemed to make it worse, except one of those rare times at college when you take too big of a bong hit and are coughing and gasping for ten minutes. The use (of a bong) didn't continue.

10. Tolerance to cannabis, as defined by progressively larger amounts of cannabis needed to obtain the psychoactive effect experienced when use first commenced, or noticeably reduced effect of use of the same amount of cannabis.

Not really. My usual dose has been the same for four decades: one or two puffs (more toward one puff, as it has gotten stronger).

11. Withdrawal, defined as the typical withdrawal syndrome associated with cannabis, or cannabis or a similar substance is used to prevent withdrawal symptoms.

A few times, in my twenties, I experienced some very trivial symptoms that resolved in a day or two—far easier than stopping caffeine or opioids! Nothing like stopping benzodiazepines, which gave me a year and a half of misery. There *is* a withdrawal syndrome with cannabis, but that's true for many other medications we use, which aren't considered addictive (e.g., SSRIs).

As it turns out, I didn't even meet the low-hanging bar of two criteria that one needs to qualify for CUD. I didn't actually meet any of the criteria in any meaningful way. The one I came closest to meeting was withdrawal (though it wasn't within the last year, as required to be to be included), which, as we will see, shouldn't even be one of the criteria.

Why would this unfailingly kind and brilliant psychiatrist so automatically label me as addicted to cannabis? I suspect that my psychiatrist couldn't imagine me using cannabis over such a long time period without being addicted to it, especially in light of having had another addiction. I also suspect that this is a common occurrence, and it is because doctors, including psychiatrists, don't have a broad-based and long-standing scientific foundation about the endocannabinoid system—the set of receptors and neurotransmitters by which cannabis affects us. The way they've been taught about cannabis has been almost exclusively from the point of view of pathology. They have been fed, by the professional societies and the medical schools, unilaterally negative information about cannabis—until very recently, when the sheer force of public opinion has translated into pressure to lighten up and be more balanced.

Many doctors tend to equate all recreational drug use with misuse, especially if the drug is illegal and has been stigmatized. I feel this is medically misguided and needlessly judgmental. This stance also can be hypocritical if they consume alcohol or caffeine, as most doctors do. To justify this dual standard, one would have to invoke the fairly unconvincing standard of morality that "what is legal is just." This is the lowest of Kohlberg's six layers of moral development. This way of thinking was target practice in my moral philosophy seminar at Swarthmore College. (Further, psychiatrists increasingly don't seem to mind the fact that psychedelics are illegal, so that would be yet another double standard.)

Even though the majority—possibly the vast majority—of people who use cannabis use it without problems, and with at least some benefit, I suspect its use is still judged as fundamentally pathological by many doctors, particularly psychiatrists.

Fortunately, many doctors are slowly and steadily evolving their views on cannabis. It can be difficult to know if this is a sincere change, like CNN's Dr. Sanjay Gupta experienced as he realized that most of the studies were artifactually focused on harm and he started to read more of the international literature, which is more sensible. Some of these "hallelujah moments" seem like opportunistic ploys—to stay near the "center" and thus to stay relevant. If you don't acknowledge medical marijuana at this point in history, even in quotation marks, no one is going to take you seriously. As society swings in favor of cannabis, the reefer madness stuff doesn't play as well. As such, some people—who don't appear to be the slightest bit convinced that cannabis is anything less than the devil's lettuce—are begrudgingly modifying their public positions so as to remain part of the conversation.

Even Dr. Nora Volkow, the head of NIDA, one of the most historically cannabis-demonizing organizations ever, said in November 2021 in an interview with FiveThirtyEight, "There's no evidence to my knowledge that occasional [adult] marijuana use has harmful effects. I don't know of any scientific evidence of that."[5]

Another irony of my diagnosis was that I was given a scary-sounding diagnosis of cannabis addiction at a time when I was finding cannabis to be a helpful aid to my process of quitting the opioids. It helped more than any other treatment with the agonizing withdrawal symptoms, especially the nausea, muscle aches, abdominal cramping, insomnia, restlessness, and anxiety. More crucially, it helped give me the insight to understand that, no matter how bleak things seemed, I could and in fact *needed* to do this, for myself, my kids, my job, and my family. It helped me persevere. I have not encountered anything in life that generates more helpful personal insight than cannabis does (except possibly psilocybin).

Diagnoses have consequences, and stigma begets more stigma. Imagine if the Massachusetts Medical Board, which has been about as enlightened about cannabis as Fred Flintstone might be about climate change, found out about a diagnosis of cannabis addiction in a practicing physician. Go straight to rehab; do not pass go. My God, what a nightmare! In chapter 4, I discussed a case of a doctor losing his license for responsible, transparent medical cannabis use. Hopefully the medical boards are evolving on this issue.

Moreover, an erroneous diagnosis of a substance use disorder could affect health insurance status as a "preexisting condition," or it could undermine the treatment a patient gets from the next doctor who cares for them. What if they needed a sedative or painkiller? The next doctor might think, "Druggie cannabis user. I can't be giving him any sleeping pills or painkillers. He'll probably sell them to get more weed." Doctors can harm people when they erroneously assign them pathologies that they don't have, especially ones associated with stigma.

In the 2021 article "Drug Dependence Is Not Addiction—and It Matters," the authors, two of my heroes in the world of drug policy, my MGH colleague Dr. Sarah Wakeman and journalist Maia Szalavitz, point out the harms of incorrectly saddling a patient with a diagnosis of a drug use disorder,

> In the United States, misdiagnoses of addictive disorders can lead to a cascade of negative outcomes, including stigma, discontinuation of needed medications, undue scrutiny of both patients and physicians, and even criminal consequences. Misdiagnosis might also result in treatment that is inappropriate or harmful to a patient.[6]

I do think that propensity to get addicted to a particular substance varies from person to person. At one physician recovery group meeting, a doctor said, "I had my first drink at age fourteen and never stopped since." This is difficult for me to relate to, as I've never been able to drink more than one drink without falling asleep. In contrast, at a book talk for my memoir *Free Refills*, a woman in the audience said, "I took Vicodin after my C-section, and I didn't feel any euphoria. How did you *possibly* get addicted to that stuff?" Some of susceptibility to addiction seems to be luck of the draw: how our brains interact with a certain drug. Part of this has to do with genetics, part with past trauma, and part with our current mental health and life circumstances. With this in mind, I can imagine that a certain subset of people might experience cannabis in a way that is much more rewarding than most other people, especially at a vulnerable time in their lives. As a consequence, they could find themselves susceptible to getting addicted to it.

My personal opinion is that cannabis is about as addicting as caffeine. People get extremely dependent on caffeine to manage and enjoy their lives, not unlike cannabis. Caffeine usually isn't particularly disruptive, unless you develop palpitations, heartburn, anxiety, or insomnia. Heavy, regular users of either cannabis or caffeine are susceptible to symptoms of cravings, tolerance, and withdrawal symptoms.

Some very heavy cannabis users find the cannabis withdrawal symptoms to be all but intolerable. The withdrawal symptoms have been shown to make remaining abstinent from cannabis exceedingly difficult in these cases. These patients can have extreme difficulty sleeping and eating, as well as restlessness, boredom, and anxiety. The intolerability of these withdrawal symptoms can be a cause of relapse back onto cannabis in people who are trying to quit. They have learned, in effect, that using cannabis lowers their distress, and not using it raises their distress. This can be a setup for addiction.

I have experienced some mild cannabis withdrawal symptoms in the past during the times in my life—like when I worked at Greenpeace in my mid-twenties—when I was a heavier cannabis user. I frequently had to travel internationally and, depending on my destination, there might not be any cannabis where I was, such as when I went to Kiev to help open up a Greenpeace office in 1991. The withdrawal symptoms were not particularly enjoyable, especially the grumpiness and the insomnia, which lasted just a few days. It is child's play compared to opioid withdrawal, which I am also, unfortunately, quite familiar with, which is an incapacitating living hell that lasts for weeks. It's sort of like the difference between badly stubbing your toe and breaking five ribs. Both are unpleasant, but one is much worse and longer lasting than the other.

The addiction to opioids itself, beyond withdrawal, is generally more severe and life dominating as well. People who are addicted to cannabis don't tend to rob dispensaries to obtain cannabis as one might rob a pharmacy to acquire Oxycontin. They don't feign pain syndromes, forge prescriptions, or injure themselves to acquire cannabis. It's not that all or most people with opioid use disorder might do these things by any means, but they are common stories at NA meetings, which I've been to hundreds of. It is difficult to imagine, for example, a nurse or doctor addicted to cannabis being so far gone as to divert fentanyl from a patient who needs it, as we occasionally read about, sadly, with opioids and health care providers. A minority of patients do get majorly addicted to cannabis, and it certainly can wreak havoc on their lives.

Cannabis does cause a mild euphoria, but the experience of using it isn't *that* rewarding to our dopamine systems, as other drugs are such as heroin or meth. And the amount consumed is often limited by side effects such as anxiety, which is protective. It does seem to be more rewarding in teens, who are more susceptible to addiction. The head of NIDA, Dr. Nora Volkow, describes it well:

It's a learning process when you become addicted. . . . It's a type of memory that gets hard-wired into your brain. That occurs much faster in an adolescent brain.[7]

This didn't happen to me as an adolescent because I was extremely engaged in school, as well as my role as the loud but somewhat tone deaf bass player for our band, the Shades, but I can understand the temptation, particularly if you are bored and unhappy. This may be especially true with today's youth who have all these existential threats, such as climate change, hanging over their heads and who feel as if they are facing an uncertain future, financially, politically, and existentially. We all have to fight against the insidious "fuck it, why bother?" attitude.

I strongly suspect that many people with "cannabis addiction" or "CUD" in their charts end up with them there as much due to physician error (like my case), shortcuts, or thoughtlessness as to any actual problem with cannabis. As I was writing this chapter, I saw "cannabis abuse" in the chart of a patient who has been using cannabis to calm down and to focus since I started as his PCP fourteen years ago. He is a major success story, a primary care masterpiece, having transitioned from heroin to Suboxone without any relapses. He has his kids back living with him, and he's working again, living independently, and supporting himself. Over the last fourteen years, over forty or so visits, I've seen nothing that is damaging or harmful in his usage of cannabis. On the contrary, it helps him with his emotional equilibrium, with his "intermittent explosive disorder," much more than any of the psychiatric drugs have. Just like me, despite his previous struggles with opioid addiction, he wouldn't fulfill the criteria for CUD.

This patient's newly acquired psychiatrist reflexively checked off the "cannabis abuse" box in the electronic medical record after their first meeting. There was a brief mention about "chronic cannabis use" in the note. My patient said they hardly discussed it—he had just answered one question. There was no assessment of the eleven criteria that are supposed to define CUD or any discussion of harms or benefits. I suspect this practice is widespread due to the misconception that cannabis use must mean cannabis misuse, especially in people who look like him, with his tattoos and jewelry, who have struggled with addiction.

Part of the problem is that, until recently, there was no way to document cannabis use in our electronic medical records without in some way denoting that you are "addicted" or "abusing" it. For decades, all cannabis use, no matter how benign, has been denoted as "abuse," "dependence," or "addiction." The rates of "addiction" gathered by the researchers who comb charts will obviously be inflated if there's no other way to write that a patient uses cannabis beyond "abuse," "dependence," "addiction," or "CUD." Recently, there have been upgrades to our computer system so that one can now document cannabis use in the electronic medical record in a neutral way, such as "medical cannabis patient" or "cannabis user." I don't know why this critical fact isn't highlighted in the "limitations" section of more published studies, as it undermines the results of so many of the studies that are being done, particularly those trying to emphasize a particular harm of cannabis.

A more cynical reason that CUD might be overrepresented in the charts is that generally doctors get paid more if there's more "medical complexity." For example, I have received numerous trainings on how to make things look more medically complex on the record by clicking certain diagnoses so that my hospital gets paid more for the same amount of work. As a consequence, I suspect that many of the CUD diagnoses that have been added on are just fluffing up the complexity of, say, an ED visit that is for something entirely unrelated, where cannabis use was mentioned during the medical history taken by the medical students, who practice by asking about everything.

Other researchers, epidemiologist types, take these diagnoses of CUD—many if not most of which are almost certainly erroneous, as I discuss above—and do research based on massive data crunching of hundreds of thousands of charts. They treat all of these CUD diagnoses as valid and relevant. Then they conclude, from crunching the numbers, things like, "Increasing Trend of Cannabis Use Disorder among Young Patients Admitted Due to Acute Myocardial Infarction." To look at the methodology used in this study,

> She and her colleagues analyzed medical records of 819,354 people from a large public database of hospital stays. They identified people 18 to 49 who had been hospitalized for a heart attack *and whose records showed a previous diagnosis of cannabis use disorder.*[8] (emphasis added)

They conclude, "Our study highlights the increasing trend of AMI [acute myocardial infarction] hospitalizations with concurrent CUD."[9]

The press then runs with it. Per CNN, "Young adult cannabis consumers nearly twice as likely to suffer from a heart attack, research shows."[10] (That's not what the study showed! It was an association in an observational study, which can't show causation.) Note the evolution from "increasing trend [of association]" to CNN's "twice as likely to suffer." Then the anti-marijuana groups typically further exaggerate the claims, which have the appearance of being grounded in research (however fluffy). This entire vein of inquiry is quite disconcerting if you take a moment to question the obvious invalidity of many, if not most, of the CUD diagnoses in the chart.

As an aside, I don't mean to trivialize the content of this particular example, as there *are* some legitimate cardiac concerns with cannabis. It can act as a central nervous system stimulant and raise heart rate (especially if the user is anxious from too high a dosage), and therefore it could be implicated in potential arrhythmias and possibly heart attacks.

As we'll see, the diagnosis of CUD is even less coherent in medical patients.

Cannabis researcher Dr. Staci Gruber, along with her brilliant colleagues at the Marijuana Investigations for Neuroscientific Discovery (MIND) program at Harvard's McLean Hospital, raises the question of how accurate the measuring sticks for cannabis addiction are in medical cannabis patients. I've been questioning this for years, but Dr. Gruber is an actual neuroscience researcher. She is unbiased and equally in demand from both "sides." In previous, groundbreaking work, Dr. Gruber demonstrated that the cognitive effects of using cannabis were profoundly different in medical patients, where the cannabis seemed to improve cognition, than they were in recreational cannabis users, where tests of cognition were worse (see chapter 12).

In a 2021 paper, "Assessing Cannabis Use Disorder in Medical Cannabis Patients: Interim Analyses from an Observational, Longitudinal Study," Gruber's team started by noting the wide range of estimates of CUD in the general population from the epidemiological survey studies, with one study giving us a rate of 11–15 percent and another study giving us a rate of 30 percent.[11] All of these patients were unquestioningly assumed to be recreational users. There wasn't any consideration of the possibility that some (a significant amount?) of the symptomatology and use patterns that count toward CUD criteria could have been explained by legitimate medicinal use. Until very recently, most researchers put medical and recreational users in the same basket, with little to no consideration of the medical uses or benefits, as part of the institutionalized anti-cannabis bias.

Dr. Gruber's questions were whether the rates for CUD have been studied in medical cannabis patients (they haven't) and whether the traditional tools that we use to assess CUD are adequate to assess this (they aren't).

For her study, Dr. Gruber assessed a common screening test for CUD called the CUDIT-R, which provides a numerical rating to the frequency of things like, "How often do you use cannabis?" "How many hours were you stoned on a typical day that you used cannabis?" and so on, including issues like trouble stopping cannabis; failing to do what was normally expected of you due to cannabis; spending a great deal of time getting, using, or recovering from cannabis; having problems with memory or concentration after using cannabis; and using cannabis in hazardous situations like driving or caring for children. (There is obviously a gigantic chicken/egg problem with many of these questions—people might use cannabis because they can't concentrate.) Many of the questions employed by this briefer screening test overlap the formal diagnostic criteria for CUD.

Dr. Gruber's hypothesis was that medical cannabis "patients would exhibit increased frequency of use relative to baseline, but endorse few problems associated with MC use given their primary motivation for use is symptom alleviation."[12] For example, the use would go up, especially if they are just starting medical cannabis. In fact, they can get four points on the CUDIT-R just from transitioning from not using any to using it four times a week. You only need eight points total to qualify for "hazardous cannabis use" or, in other words, an addiction. Just starting to use medical cannabis every other day gets you halfway to an addiction according to this widely implemented metric. For this and a host of other reasons, they concluded that the CUDIT-R isn't a reliable way to assess CUD in medical cannabis patients. We need to transition to a measure that accepts and reflects the actual reality of cannabis use.

Gruber also points out that "definitive diagnosis of CUD can only be made using a diagnostic interview such as the Structured Clinical Interview for DSM (SCID)."[13] As someone who has experienced and recovered from addiction, and who has treated thousands of patients for problematic opioids, cannabis, alcohol, etc., I am quite convinced that one cannot diagnose something as complex and nuanced as "is this person addicted?" by analyzing the results of survey questions obtained over the phone. I am truly mystified as to why everyone ignores this point. Did I miss a memo? Addiction is a *clinical* diagnosis. If a stranger had called me with a survey about addiction, my opioid-addicted self, fifteen years ago, wouldn't have taken the call. I'd be worried it was the police or the medical board. To truly diagnose addiction, you need eye contact, a longitudinal relationship, possibly some drug testing, and a comprehensive medical and psychological exam. It isn't just plugging responses into a "one-size-fits-all" checklist.

Finally, Dr. Gruber then steals my thunder, as I've been saying this practically since I could first talk,

> As in the case of opioid use disorder, for example, tolerance and withdrawal criteria are not considered for individuals who are using opioids under appropriate medical supervision. With regard to cannabis, similar exclusions from DSM-5 criteria may need to be applied.[14]

I'd get rid of the "may" part. In fact, in a 2013 paper, "DSM-5 Criteria for Substance Use Disorders: Recommendations and Rationale," author Deborah Hasin, who has authored several of these studies implicating 30 percent of adult cannabis users as addicted, argues,

> An important exception to making a diagnosis of DSM-5 substance use disorder with two criteria pertains to the supervised use of psychoactive substances for medical purposes, including stimulants, cocaine, opioids, nitrous oxide, sedative-hypnotic/anxiolytic drugs, and *cannabis in some jurisdictions*. These substances can produce tolerance and withdrawal as normal physiological adaptations when used appropriately for supervised medical purposes. With a threshold of two or more criteria, these criteria could lead to invalid substance use disorder diagnoses even with no other criteria met. *Under these conditions, tolerance and withdrawal in the absence of other criteria do not indicate substance use disorders and should not be diagnosed as such.*[15] (emphasis added)

If the patient is using benzodiazepines, opioids, or cannabis for legitimate medical purposes, we ought to completely ditch the criteria of tolerance or withdrawal, as these are intrinsic parts of many medicines that we routinely use. And what does "in some jurisdictions" have to do with anything? Either cannabis is or isn't a medicine—it's a pharmacological thing, not something decided by the legislature or voters in Mississippi or Vermont. If a policeman is chasing me and I make it over the border from Idaho into Oregon, are my tolerance and withdrawal suddenly valid and noncontributory to a diagnosis of addiction?

For all the reasons cited above, Dr. Gruber concludes that

> CUD is likely a unique construct among those using cannabis medically, and existing tools developed for use in recreational consumers do not appear to be reliable, valid measures for assessing CUD in medical cannabis patients.

I believe that estimates of CUD have been wildly inflated by roping in millions who use cannabis medically. The dangers of overpathologizing have been discussed above. I would abandon the concept of CUD altogether and start from scratch. We need to create an untainted measure of cannabis addiction that accommodates the current realities of the drug so as to better target (and not mistarget) treatment.

What are the legitimate concerns about the consequences of having CUD? What does it do to your life, to your relationships, to your livelihood? Is it on par with other addictions, such as alcohol, meth, or opioids? Or is it more trivial, along the lines of our ubiquitous caffeine addictions? Is it somewhere in between? Does it vary? Or, like so many issues related to cannabis, is it in the category of "has only been dealt with under the auspices and funding of the War on Drugs, with the cannabis product used being mostly illegal and unregulated during the time, taken without the guidance of cannabis specialists, and under the strong self-reinforcing presumption of serious harm, etc.," so we don't really know?

A 2015 paper that has received a lot of attention in this area is "Prevalence of Marijuana Use Disorders in the United States between 2001–2002 and 2012–2013." This is where the "nearly three out of ten adult marijuana users manifested a marijuana use disorder in 2012–2013" comes from.

Once again, we see this published in *JAMA Psychiatry*, a publication that has had a mixed and sometimes one-sided history on cannabis research. The author sets the tone for the grave import of the study early on by describing the consequences of CUD and of use of marijuana in general:

> Studies have shown that use or early use of marijuana is associated with increased risk for many outcomes, including cognitive decline, psychosocial impairments, vehicle crashes, emergency department visits, psychiatric symptoms, poor quality of life, use of other drugs, cannabis-withdrawal syndrome and addiction risk.[16]

When you read something like this at face value, it is a wonder that any of us who have liberally partaken are still alive and able to function at all! It makes smoking a joint sound more dangerous than mainlining PCP.

Moving beyond the "associated" nonsense, which we've discussed above, does "use or early use of cannabis" truly result in a "poor quality of life"? We all have heard manufactured horror stories of "your brains on drugs," but I'd ask my readers, are most of the people you know who use cannabis experiencing a "poor quality of life"? And if they are, such as with teens or young adults who get into difficulty due to cannabis, or people living in poverty, is the cannabis a cause of this poor quality of life or an attempt to find some transient relief from the unhappy cards they've been dealt? If cannabis triggers psychosis, that is a definite harm and is of course "a poor quality of life," but this is truly the exception (i.e., it primarily occurs in people prone to psychosis), not the rule. Isn't a "poor quality of life" more commonly associated with excessive alcohol consumption with its attendant liver problems and violence? The above conclusions seem steeped in exaggeration, innuendo, and bias. If you follow the actual references, you uncover some pretty fluffy studies, or a lot of studies that don't actually evidence the point they are being referenced for.

For example, I followed the reference that was provided as evidence to support this particular statement about "poor quality of life" because improvements in quality of life are so frequently seen in studies of medical cannabis patients. It was an earlier study called "Gender Differences in Health-Related Quality of Life among Cannabis Users: Results from the National Epidemiologic Survey on Alcohol and Related Conditions," where they assessed "health related quality of life" with a twelve-item health survey, the SF-12, and then supposedly parsed out the contribution of cannabis use and CUD from all the innumerable other things that could be affecting quality of life. Their results were as follows:

Mean SF-12 mental summary scores were significantly lower (indicating a lower quality of life) among female and male cannabis users compared to non-users (by 0.6 standard deviations (SD) and 0.3 SD, respectively), and among females and males with CUD compared to those without CUD (by 0.9 SD and 0.4 SD, respectively). Controlling for sociodemographic variables and mental illness, each joint smoked daily was associated with a greater decrease in mental quality of life summary scores in females (0.1 SD) compared to males (0.03 SD).[17]

Mini-pontification: *This* is the study that demonstrates cannabis users, in general, across the world, across all time, have a "poor quality of life"? God help me! The differences were tiny—less than one standard deviation. Each time a male smoked a joint, his quality-of-life score, measured by a questionnaire, decreased by 0.03 standard deviations? This is science? This is math? And what about "reverse causation"? Couldn't people with a "poor quality of life" try to ease the misery or find some joy with cannabis? And what about confounding variables? Yet, *this* is the proof cited in an academic study printed in *JAMA Psychiatry* and widely cited by the press. End of pontification.

If things with cannabis really were so dire, why would they have to stretch things so hard to make it look bad, or rely on such thin fodder? I could come up with dozens of studies that show an *improved* quality of life with medical cannabis because, as people's pain and insomnia are better controlled, their quality of life improves. In dozens, if not hundreds, of "real-world evidence" medical studies (see chapter 7), improved quality of life is an extremely common outcome measure. For example, at my home institution, a recent NIDA-funded paper, "Effect of Medical Marijuana Card Ownership on Pain, Insomnia, and Affective Disorder Symptoms in Adults," showed (if you excavated deeply enough; they showcased the negative findings) that those who had more immediate access to medical cannabis "had greater score improvement in mental well-being on the SF-12."[18] The witnessed improvements in quality of life were larger than in the above-cited study "showing" worse quality of life with cannabis use.

This positive finding never made it into this study's "Results" or "Conclusions" sections of the study—again, you had to dig.

Unfortunately, due to its polemicized history, cannabis is not in the category of regular science, where you give the benefit of the doubt and just trust that everything is kosher. With cannabis, you *always* have to look beyond the headlines, read the entire study, check on the references, try to discern the (perhaps unconscious) agenda of the researchers, and take note of the social context in which the research is being performed, as well as its funding source and the affiliations of the authors.

As for the idea that cannabis use and CUD are "associated with substance use disorders," a major propaganda piece of the War on Drugs has been the idea that cannabis was a "gateway" to "harder" drugs. These claims haven't withstood the test of time. First of all, association is not causation, so that component of it has deliberately been misleading from the start. Further, most people start with alcohol or tobacco, not cannabis. As early as 1999, the Institute of Medicine of the National Academy of Sciences rejected the "gateway theory":

> Patterns in progression of drug use from adolescence to adulthood are strikingly regular. Because it is the most widely used illicit drug, marijuana is predictably the first illicit drug most people encounter. Not surprisingly, most users of other illicit drugs have used marijuana first. In fact, most drug users begin with alcohol and nicotine before marijuana— usually before they are of legal age.
>
> In the sense that marijuana use typically precedes rather than follows initiation of other illicit drug use, it is indeed a "gateway" drug. But because underage smoking and alcohol use typically precede marijuana use, marijuana is not the most common, and is rarely the first, "gateway" to illicit drug use. *There is no conclusive evidence that the drug effects of marijuana are causally linked to the subsequent abuse of other illicit drugs.*[19] (emphasis added)

Why people still bring up the "gateway theory" in scientific studies or news articles is beyond me. Ironically, cannabis is increasingly being seen as a gateway *out of* chronic pain, opioid dependence, and opioid addiction (see chapter 15). As for cannabis being "associated" with mental illness, we will discuss whether it improves or worsens the various mental illnesses in chapter 19.

In my experience treating CUD, these cases range in severity and consequence. Some people don't want to quit and don't think they have CUD—they were just getting frog-marched into treatment by concerned or controlling family members or a significant other, or they flunked a preemployment drug test. Without intrinsic motivation and a belief that you have a problem, it is difficult to make progress. Others need to quit because they had a change in circumstances—a trip overseas, a new job with drug testing, impending parenthood—that made ongoing use of cannabis impossible for them. This group is more motivated and usually can stop, at least for the time period required. It's easier to stop if achieving your goals depends on stopping. Other patients, usually males in their twenties in my experience, never stopped their heavy use from their college days, while their friends were all able to cut down as they transitioned into more adult roles. These people tend to be more heavily addicted, as cannabis tends to be a big part of how they cope with any kind of distress. People who are clearly addicted in the eyes of everyone around them, yet who have convinced themselves that their use is medical and vitally important to their well-being, are a challenge to treat. Also, there are many cases in which things aren't black and white: the cannabis is helping in some ways while harming in other ways.

I've seen plenty of cases that fit my definition of addiction, which is "continued use despite negative consequences." A good example might be a patient who frequently ends up overnight in the hospital for severe vomiting. Is this "cannabis hyperemesis syndrome" (CHS)? The only way to distinguish CHS from a similar problem called "cyclic vomiting syndrome" is to stop cannabis for three to six months and see if the vomiting resolves. Some patients can't do this. To me, if you can't stop using cannabis for three months to help diagnose a medical condition that is utterly screwing up your quality of life, causing you to barf like crazy and requiring several overnights in the hospital per month, that qualifies as "continued use despite negative consequences," or cannabis addiction.

Some cases can be extraordinarily upsetting and disruptive to parents, with a young adult essentially barricaded in their basement, jobless, socially isolated, and no longer developing social or life skills. They are content to smoke weed all day. Though, even in these cases, it can be difficult to know to what extent cannabis is the true cause of the problem, versus an effect of some other mental illness or trauma that they are self-treating. Often some of both is at play. The thing that finally got a few of these patients out of the basement, interacting with others and working, was a job in the cannabis industry. This transition, from slacking to working, greatly improved conditions and family morale. The parents were pleased that their young adult finally found something they took an interest in and that was motivating them to transition into an adult role. (This only works if they have an established ability to control their cannabis use.)

In my experience with the addiction recovery community, very few people take cannabis addiction seriously, for a variety of reasons. A majority of people have been in rehab for cannabis through the court system as opposed to being there due to an actual addiction. This has been inflating the numbers of cannabis addiction for decades. According to one study, 50.7 percent of rehab admissions in 2015 were mandated by a court or juvenile justice referral.[20] What happens is a judge gives the parents a choice for their kid: rehab or juvie. Any sane parent would pick rehab so as not to further damage their kid's future. The facility diagnoses and, more importantly, bills it as "cannabis addiction."

The unfortunate teen, stuck in rehab for up to ninety days, has to go through the motions of being treated for marijuana addiction. They have to repeat all the platitudinous twelve-step mantras day after day. "I admit that I am powerless over cannabis and I turn my life and will over to God to cure me." Blech. This nonsense is potentially as brain damaging as cannabis use if you ask me, having been through it for opioids. I truly respect that some people find it helpful. Yet, these patients are forced to pretend they had been addicted to weed and were getting into recovery, either by a judge or, for many professionals, by the medical or nursing boards. That's not addiction, even if it looks like it on paper. It is avoiding a criminal record or professional consequences because cannabis was still illegal.

At least the court to rehab conveyer belt seems to be slowing, as cannabis treatment admissions decreased by 26 percent from 2002 to 2015.[21] Our society is slowly coming to its senses about the futility of punishment as a response to substance use. The rehab industry will not let their cash cow wander off without a fight and invariably side against legalization when state ballot initiatives come up.

In the cases where a person is *truly* in rehab for an addiction to marijuana, other patients (myself included, at the time) are genuinely astonished. A commonly overheard, amalgamated conversation would be, in an incredulous voice, "I overdosed on Oxy and coke, had to be resuscitated twice, had a seizure, developed pneumonia and heart problems, got a skin infection, was in the hospital for three months, went bankrupt due to the medical costs, am dealing with criminal charges in several states, had my dealer beat the shit out of me, was dumped by my wife, lost my job, and my car, and my kids, and my dog; I went bankrupt and have hepatitis C, and you're here for . . . *weed*?" Substitute meth, crack, or what have you— it is difficult for many people to comprehend.

What I've ultimately come to understand over time is that suffering is suffering. In many cases, the exact drug is irrelevant. People can get addicted to many different substances and behaviors. If someone is addicted and dysregulated, they need sympathy, compassion, and treatment, no matter which chemical it is they are misusing. I've seen cannabis addiction throw some very solid-seeming life trajectories off track.

For those who *are* addicted to cannabis, we certainly could use better drugs and treatments for CUD. According to a 2018 paper, "The Current State of Pharmacological Treatments for Cannabis Use Disorder and Withdrawal," "research into pharmacotherapy for CUD has steadily grown from the late 1990s and early 2000s to the present. . . . Despite these efforts, to date, there are no FDA-approved medication treatments for CUD."[22] The best current treatments we have for CUD are behavioral therapies, piecemeal treatments for each of the withdrawal symptoms such as anxiety and insomnia, and treatment of the underlying conditions that are contributing to the overuse of cannabis. CBD is a promising new treatment possibility, as are molecules called FAAH inhibitors, which inhibit the breakdown of our natural levels of endocannabinoids, such as anandamide, and thus increase their levels.

Given that some people clearly do get into trouble with cannabis, but it almost certainly isn't nearly as high as a quarter to a third of adult users, how can we adjust the sensitivity of the definition of CUD so it better reflects reality? I would start by eliminating the categories of withdrawal and tolerance. This makes sense given how many useful and commonplace medications have tolerance and withdrawal as common features of their use, such as opioids, benzodiazepines, and antidepressants. This change would help avoid ensnaring the many patients who are using cannabis for medical reasons, or for reasons of wellness and enhancement, into an unhelpful category of "addicted." In the 2020 study "Probability and Correlates of Transition from Cannabis Use to DSM-5 Cannabis Use Disorder: Results from a Large-Scale Nationally Representative Study," the authors argue, "Depending on a substance to avoid physical withdrawal symptoms is neither necessary nor sufficient to define addiction."[23] This is also consistent with Dr. Gruber's article cited above which shows that CUD isn't accurately diagnosed in medical cannabis patients, in part because of the inappropriate inclusion of tolerance and withdrawal.

Next, I would go back to the widely accepted tradition that addiction is a clinically diagnosed disease. We should get rid of this habit of diagnosing millions of people by computer-assisted telephone interviews, which creates a moral panic, yet with cannabis just appears to create this hypothetically addicted body of people who don't seem to materially exist. If you give all these people a diagnosis of CUD, but very few of them act like they have CUD, think they have CUD, or are even aware that they might have CUD, how is this helpful? In the 30 percent study, the author complains that "only 13.2% with lifetime CUD participated in 12-step programs or professional treatment."[24] That's perhaps less of a failure of the treatment system and more a consequence of the fact that many of these people aren't actually addicted to cannabis. Of the 13.2 percent, a large portion were likely mandated to rehab by the courts, so the true number is probably even lower.

Next, I would increase the number of criteria one needs to qualify for CUD. There is evidence to suggest that a higher number of criteria results in a more accurate diagnosis. The more criteria you require, the more cases you might miss, but the more diagnostic certainty you have for the cases you have diagnosed. Given that we appear to be overdiagnosing cannabis addiction, this seems like a good trade-off, as it would help us to be more certain about the cases we diagnose. It would also help the patients take the diagnosis seriously.

If you got rid of tolerance and withdrawal (so there are now nine not eleven criteria) and made it so that you needed four out of nine to qualify (instead of the current two out of eleven), this would be much more accurate. If we did this, a more reasonable number of people given a diagnosis of CUD would *actually* have a clinically meaningful CUD.

In fact, some recent studies have shown that it is almost entirely "severe CUD," meaning six or more criteria met (of the eleven), that is associated with psychosocial problems. In my schema (without withdrawal or tolerance), that would equate to needing to meet four out of nine criteria. The main difference is that if we tightened this up, we wouldn't needlessly be diagnosing, pathologizing, stigmatizing, and as a consequence harming so many people who are using cannabis without problems and with benefit.

I would search for a way to incorporate the positives of cannabis use into our diagnostic considerations, to get a more nuanced view of why someone is using cannabis. I understand that this isn't a common feature of diagnosing an addiction, but it is the only way to make our approach to cannabis—which is a medicine as well as a drug of potential misuse, and which can have positives and negatives at the same time—remotely coherent.

What does it mean to be in recovery? As someone in recovery from opioid addiction, it breaks my heart to hear about people on methadone or Suboxone hassled at Narcotics Anonymous meetings: "You're not really in recovery because you're on a replacement drug." This is completely against the current science and the ethos of addiction treatment. It fully internalizes and weaponizes the stigma that we all should be fighting against together. This attitude goes back, in my opinion, to the religious, moralistic, and abstinence-only roots of Alcoholics Anonymous. People on medication for opioid use disorder (MOUD) are *absolutely* in recovery—health care providers are prescribing these meds; they are regulating known chemical deficiencies and allowing people to return to their normal lives. According to Dr. Sarah Wakeman, an addiction specialist at Man's Greatest Hospital (MGH),

> Taking these medications to function normally is not an addiction any more than taking insulin for diabetes or an antidepressant for depression is. . . . This myth amplifies stigma and represents an outdated view of addiction and treatment.[25]

Along the same lines, many people have used cannabis to overcome addictions to other more dangerous drugs such as heroin or booze, or downers. This tends to be done more by patients themselves than within the medical system, as doctors aren't particularly familiar with how to do this. These patients feel that they are in safe, legitimate recovery because of the relief and healing cannabis has given them. They view cannabis not primarily as a damaging drug but more as a wellness and enhancement aid.

This concept of cannabis-facilitated or cannabis-inclusive recovery is sometimes referred to as "Cali sober," as the idea became popularized in California. Recovery should be a large enough tent to fit in people with different definitions of their own recovery, not an all-or-nothing proposition that has no scientific evidence to back it up.

With the spread of the philosophy of "harm reduction" and the decline of stigma, I suspect that these broadened conceptions of recovery will continue to become more widely accepted.

In a related issue, the American Society of Addiction Medicine (ASAM) recommends "great caution"[26] when recommending cannabis for any reason to someone who has a substance use disorder. As a clinician, I certainly do exercise discretion in these circumstances, out of an abundance of caution for all drugs and medicines. We always want to "do no harm," and I have firsthand knowledge of how nuanced and destructive an addiction can be. How dangerous is medical cannabis, truly, in people who suffer from, or who have suffered from, substance use disorders? The original rationale for avoiding cannabis was based on the "gateway" theory, which turned out to be a big nothingburger of U.S. government anti-cannabis propaganda.

First, do people substitute addictions in general? As there's not that much consistent literature on this subject, I don't think this has been scientifically proven, despite it being long-standing AA lore. It was pounded into our heads when I was at rehab, but rehab is, or at least has been, mostly based on AA, with, in my experience, very little actual science filtering in.

According to the National Institute of Drug Abuse, in response to a request for comment from the website Tonic:

"a previous substance use disorder is a risk factor for future development of substance use disorder (SUD)," but "it is also possible that someone who once had an SUD but doesn't currently have one has a balance of risk and protective genetic and environmental factors that could allow for alcohol consumption without developing an AUD [alcohol use disorder]."[27]

Leave it to NIDA to answer, "Yes, people are at increased risk, but not with alcohol, which is the one drug we approve of and use in our own personal lives." By this logic, cannabis should be even safer, as it is less addictive than alcohol.

One study published in *JAMA* in 2014, "Testing the Drug Substitution Switching-Addictions Hypothesis: A Prospective Study in a Nationally Representative Sample," found that,

> as compared with those who do not recover from an SUD, people who recover have less than half the risk of developing a new SUD. *Contrary to clinical lore*, achieving remission does not typically lead to drug substitution, but *rather is associated with a lower risk of new SUD onset*.[28] (emphasis added)

The authors of this study suggest that factors such as "coping strategies, skills, and motivation of individuals who recover from an SUD may protect them from the onset of a new SUD." By making the life-affirming transition from addicted to recovered, we gain a recovery "toolbox" that helps us navigate life's stresses and challenges in a healthier way. We learn to connect with people and to ask for help if we need it—which requires pushing our egos to the side. We learn more effective ways to tolerate distress. Thus, when faced with stressful situations that formerly would trigger us to drug or drink, we might now respond by calling a friend or exercising rather than reaching for a substance. In other words, we supplant addictions with healthier activities that perform the function that the drink or drug used to, in a way that protects us from a substitute addiction.

Back to the "use great caution" issue, one might reasonably ask, if people have transitioned, or wish to transition, from more dangerous drugs to cannabis, why would we withhold medical cannabis? Are these not exactly the people to whom we should be providing access, guidance, and support, as well as legal cover and a safe product? If we don't help treat them, they just treat themselves and end up in the illicit market, consuming unregulated weed, which is more dangerous. This is Harm Reduction 101. They will do better if we engage with them than if we turn them away. We still, of course, would explain to them that there are more convincingly proven medications to treat opioid use disorder such as buprenorphine (Suboxone), and we might discourage them from using solely cannabis instead of using it as an adjunct to buprenorphine, as there is more evidence for the latter (see chapter 15).

Where is the evidence that treating people who suffer from substance use disorders with legal, regulated, tested medical cannabis—working with an experienced cannabis clinician—is making alcoholism or opioid use disorder worse, or is causing relapses or overdoses? There is none. Cannabis users don't have worse retention or outcomes in Suboxone programs (see chapter 15). Cannabis can't physically contribute to overdosages in the way that alcohol or sedatives can, as it doesn't affect the respiratory center of the brain, so it is not additively dangerous in a physical sense.

One concern is that latent addictions could be reignited. Cannabis *is* reinforcing and euphorigenic; it does trigger the reward center of the brain. If this feels good, wouldn't the drug of choice feel better? I have seen that happen, though rarely, and never in a person who is in stable, long-term recovery or who has been under the care of a knowledgeable cannabis clinician. Personally, I've never felt cannabis to be remotely triggering or to in any way threaten my recovery from opioids.

Another concern is that the past tendency toward addiction makes patients more liable to get into trouble with cannabis. In one 2017 study, "A Prospective Observational Study of Problematic Oral Cannabinoid Use," the strongest predictor of problematic prescription cannabis use (such as synthetic THC, which they were using medically) was past year substance misuse.[29]

I think how much caution you believe you need depends on how you view cannabis. If you are a group such as ASAM or the AMA, which are fundamentally opposed to cannabis and which have predominantly promoted negative articles about cannabis to its members for generations, then it makes you think you need "great caution" even if there isn't a huge amount of evidence to support this.

If you think cannabis is wholly benign, then minimal caution is warranted. Hopefully, people in recovery are humble enough to show caution toward everything, with an open mind, and are flexible enough to realize that cannabis isn't entirely benign or wholly evil.

From a moderate, in-the-middle position, such as that of yours truly, *some* caution is indicated. In medical terms, this is a relative contraindication, not an absolute one. We have to take each case on an individual basis and see if the cannabis is helping or harming the patient. For example, someone who has been in recovery for twenty years is obviously less at risk than someone who is just in their third week, is still in a haze, and is grasping for comfort. As a person in long-term recovery from opioid addiction, it is very difficult for me to view cannabis as being in the same league, as it isn't nearly as rewarding. Maybe it is for some people. As with other aspects of medicine, it comes down to a delicate balancing act of harms versus benefits. It's important to remember that, in these cases, there is often as much harm in exercising too much caution as too little, because you will lose your audience and fail to utilize potentially valuable tools. If you are too closed-minded, the patient will go elsewhere for care.

For the gulf between the cannabis community and the addiction community about how addictive versus helpful cannabis is, I have some ideas. My recommended cure for the medical community, to address all this confusion over cannabis addiction and flat-out ignorance about medical cannabis in general, is humility. Question and reevaluate your knowledge base from scratch. Could any of your negative perceptions have been unduly influenced by the War on Drug, by your funding sources and professional societies, or by institutional biases against cannabis? Start learning and thinking about cannabis with an open mind. Talk to your patients who are cannabis users and ask them why they use it and what it does for them, and what harms they experience. Be curious. Read more varied sources of information, not just the anti-cannabis articles that dominate our medical literature. If you have time, look deeply into these studies, as they often don't say or prove what they claim in the conclusions, or they skip over benefits that they have uncovered. Read literature from Europe and Israel, where they are more independent and advanced on this issue. Incorporate lived experience. Inhale (figuratively if not literally).

I'd also stop trying to hammer cannabis into the rubric of the other addictions, as is done in the 2018 paper "Cannabis Addiction and the Brain: A Review," written by several authors including Dr. Nora Volkow, the head of NIDA. Sure, there are many broad similarities. Cannabis can be addictive and can trigger some overlapping parts of the brain. But when you start saying things like, "the effects of cannabis withdrawal seem to parallel withdrawal in other drugs of abuse,"[30] you have lost touch with reality. That statement is downright offensive to anyone in recovery from opioid addiction! They are trying to force a square peg into a round hole. This is where including people's lived experience would be quite helpful. Or, when Dr. Volkow says things like, "People take marijuana for the same reason they take other drugs: They make you feel good."[31] That's like saying, "People eat filet mignon and lobster for the same reason that they eat dirt when they are starving and are iron deficient: They are hungry." It misses the all-important *why* of cannabis use and flat-out ignores the multifaceted benefits people receive. Yes, some humility is needed here. In fact, a lot of humility is needed. Through humility comes knowledge.

My recommended fix for the members of the cannabis community is to try to let go of the past. Much more of the newer science that is being done with cannabis is more neutral. You have to educate yourself about the harms as well as the benefits of cannabis—including addiction potential—to keep yourself healthy and safe. Just because the government exaggerated (and lied) about harms doesn't mean there aren't serious harms that can occur with cannabis use. Give doctors a chance to catch up on this issue. Help them with gentle nudges. Provide them with credible information. Always trust science itself; just make sure each particular sample of cannabis science seems to be legitimate science, not unduly biased. Educate yourself about how to read scientific articles. Every time you see a study or an article about the harms of cannabis, look at it with an open mind. Don't just dismiss—this is dangerous. Read through it and figure out where the flaws are, if any. If there are valid safety concerns, pay attention to them. Ask for help if you need to. If you can't find any flaws in it, it's probably valid. Don't idealize cannabis, because it has its drawbacks, just like everything else does, including the potential for addiction and withdrawal.

## Addendum: Java Madness

As a coda to this chapter, I'd like to discuss "caffeine use disorder." The psychiatrists who wrote the DSM-5 would never put in a diagnosis that needlessly pathologized most Americans for using a relatively safe plant-based medicine that enhances many of our lives with modest harm. Um, wait.

They put caffeine use disorder in the category of "a condition for further study." So grab a cup, and let's see who's addicted. I'll go first:

According to the DSM-5 (*Diagnostic and Statistical Manual of Mental Disorders*, 5th edition), if you substituted caffeine for cannabis, it might look like this:

1. Use of caffeine for at least a one-year period, with the presence of at least two of the following symptoms, accompanied by significant impairment of functioning and distress.

Yes! More like forty years, and my functioning is impaired without it—no mental activity whatsoever; I can't even speak. With it I do have some symptoms of distress: anxiety, nervousness, insomnia, heartburn, and palpitations.

2. Difficulty containing use of caffeine—the drug is used in larger amounts and over a longer period than intended.

Yes—my sleep doctor has been working on this for a decade. I have failed to abide by his recommendations to stop by noon and to keep it to one to two cups a day. (Dear sleep doctor: if you are reading this, this book has been mislabeled and is actually a work of fiction.)

3. Repeated failed efforts to discontinue or reduce the amount of caffeine that is used.

Yes, unfortunately. I've tried to quit and cut down many times. I did manage to hold out for up to an hour or two on several occasions.

4. An inordinate amount of time is occupied acquiring, using, or recovering from the effects of caffeine.

Yes, I can't do anything in the morning until I've had caffeine, so that is always my first task, no matter if it takes me a minute or if it involves driving to another state or walking through a blizzard. I spend the rest of the day dealing with heartburn, palpitations, nervousness, and insomnia (and frostbite, if there is a blizzard). Typically, I stand by my coffeemaker and watch it brew in the morning, unable to do anything until I have at least half a cup in hand.

5. Cravings or desires to use caffeine. This can include intrusive thoughts and images, and dreams about caffeine, or olfactory perceptions of the smell of caffeine, due to preoccupation with caffeine.

Cravings for caffeine can be as intense as they are for opioids, especially right when you wake up and remember, just as your head starts pounding, that you are out of coffee.

6. Continued use of caffeine despite adverse consequences from its use, such as criminal charges, ultimatums of abandonment from spouse/partner/friends, and poor productivity.

How about an ultimatum from my spouse to stop whining about the heartburn, anxiety, palpitations, and insomnia that caffeine is giving me. It's difficult to be productive after a full night's insomnia due to caffeine.

7. Other important activities in life, such as work, school, hygiene, and responsibility to family and friends, are superseded by the desire to use caffeine.

Is this a trick question? Getting coffee *is* an important life activity. If I haven't had that first cup in the morning, that will supersede all else. For example, if I'm late for patients but the line at Starbucks is moving at a glacial pace, I will wait rather than try to go through clinic muzzy headed without caffeine.

8. Caffeine is used in contexts that are potentially dangerous, such as operating a motor vehicle.

After a huge tree flattened our home in 2017 and the police condemned it on-site, I snuck back into the potentially unstable structure to rescue my cup of coffee. I routinely spill my scalding coffee onto my lap when driving and swerve out of my lane.

9. Use of caffeine continues despite awareness of physical or psychological problems attributed to use.

I just chomp on acid blockers, beta blockers, anxiety medications, and sleep aids and continue to chug away. I am powerless.

10. Tolerance to caffeine, as defined by progressively larger amounts of caffeine needed to obtain the psychoactive effect experienced when use first commenced, or noticeably reduced effect of use of the same amount of caffeine.

I epitomize tolerance. It takes a good stiff cup in the morning just to wake my digestive system up enough to absorb the second cup. I was up to fourteen shots a day, quivering in blissful mania, until my sleep doctor read me the riot act.

11. Withdrawal, defined as the typical withdrawal syndrome associated with caffeine, or caffeine or a similar substance is used to prevent withdrawal symptoms.

By ten in the morning, if I don't get my fix, my head feels like Bigfoot is jumping up and down on it, and I'm so sleepy I feel like I've been dosed with barbiturates.

So, I appear to qualify for all eleven criteria, as I'm sure many of you do. Is there even a category for eleven out of eleven? I feel like I'm channeling Spinal Tap: "It goes to eleven." Mild, moderate, severe, and *hopeless*? My soul mate is clearly Honoré de Balzac, who had an epic caffeine addiction, as described in his humorous essay "The Pleasures and Pains of Coffee."

Imagine how much more dangerous caffeine would be if it were illegal and if the government were trying to stigmatize it like cannabis. There would be no quality control, and each cup could be contaminated with fentanyl or pesticides. People would have to risk criminal records just to have their morning cup of joe, which they would use anyways, just with more health and legal jeopardy. Teenagers wouldn't believe us about the dangers. Any studies done on its harms and benefits would have results that skewed toward harm due to the consequences of prohibition. As such, it would *seem* much more harmful than it is. Does this remind you of anything?

One might ask if it is just a coincidence that the "Arbiters of What Is and Isn't Addictive" left out coffee. Was it an oversight? Or did just an iota of hypocrisy and self-serving thinking creep in so that *they just happened to skip the one substance that most of them are addicted to, that doesn't contribute to moral panic, and that they can't bill people $450/hour for treating?*

On what grounds is caffeine less addictive than cannabis? Surely not on percentages of people addicted—not even close, as many more people are addicted to caffeine. Not on deadliness: people die from caffeine, such as athletes trying to get a competitive edge, or teens screwing around with energy drinks. We're still waiting for a direct death from cannabis, as it is impossible to die from overconsumption. If anyone thinks it's on grounds of cravings or withdrawal, just try getting between me and my coffeemaker first thing in the morning.

Enough of the hypocrisy about caffeine and cannabis!

## CHAPTER TEN

# WHAT ABOUT DURING PREGNANCY AND BREASTFEEDING?

Is cannabis safe during pregnancy? While many are naturally cautious about ingesting anything that can interfere with a developing fetus, this is another area where the disconnect between the Cannatopians and the Pessimists has had a corrosive impact, with some assuming that any cautionary warnings from our government are just part of the same anti-pot noise. Thus, many are acting as if cannabis use is known to be safe during pregnancy and while breastfeeding. The use of cannabis during pregnancy has recently been climbing and is currently used by between 3 and 16 percent of pregnant women in the United States. One study shows a 64 percent increase in maternal cannabis use from 2001 to 2016.[1]

As a primary care doctor for twenty-five years and counting, one of the things I am most consistently conservative about is considering the risks of different medications during pregnancy and breastfeeding. We are supercautious about prescribing *anything*, even in cases where a female patient *might become pregnant* at some point. For example, we automatically prescribe medications to lower cholesterol and protect kidneys in all diabetics *except* in women of childbearing age, who might become pregnant, as these medications can cause birth defects. We are extremely cautious with drugs of known and unknown toxicity alike.

It has not been conclusively demonstrated that cannabis is (or isn't) safe during pregnancy or breastfeeding. As such, *the prudent thing to do is to presume that cannabis use, especially regular, heavy cannabis use, is unsafe during pregnancy and breastfeeding until we uncover reasonable evidence that it is safe.* Given what's at stake, the burden of proof is on cannabis in this case. That means cannabis ought to be avoided or minimized by anyone who is pregnant or breastfeeding. Women who might become pregnant

SEEING THROUGH THE SMOKE

need to be carefully educated about the risks. (Though let's avoid Drug War nonsense like, "Alabama Senate Committee Approves Bill to Force Women Who Want Medical Marijuana to Show Negative Pregnancy Tests."[2] What would this accomplish? The woman could be pregnant two weeks later. Also, we don't give pregnant women breathalyzer tests . . .).

We particularly don't know the safety of heavy, daily use, as opposed to occasional use. Most obstetricians would vigorously discourage chugging daily vodka during pregnancy but would give a less dire warning against a monthly glass of wine with dinner. Ideally, one avoids as many, if not all, potential toxins when pregnant, but women are not robots. Certainly no one should be penalized for the choices they make.

The data on safety is contradictory, and, to further complicate matters, virtually all of the studies have been done on illegal cannabis. Legal cannabis is clearly safer, as it is regulated and tested for mold, metals, and other contaminants. It's unclear to what extent some of the old studies, which purport to show that cannabis is dangerous in pregnancy or breastfeeding, even apply to the new world of safer, legal cannabis, which can be applied with topicals or by skin patches, or with tinctures, under the supervision of a medical cannabis expert, in the open, working closely with the primary care doctor (ideally, at least). We are moving very far away from the days of taking "whatever the drug dealer had to offer," be it paraquat-soaked cannabis from Mexico or fungus-laced goop that has been sitting around in someone's basement for three years.

When a drug like cannabis is used by a pregnant or breastfeeding woman, the delicate, newly developing fetal systems, including the endocannabinoid system, are exposed to relatively large doses of external chemicals, in this case cannabinoids. Even if you're a believer in the general benefits of cannabinoids, we truly don't know what effect this massive bombardment on these developing receptors and systems would have on a developing fetus or newborn. It is not unreasonable to ask, would we experiment with this?

There are some conditions and circumstances where the choice to use cannabis during pregnancy is understandable, such as when none of the conventional treatments are effective, or when the conventional treatments are more toxic than the cannabis would be. An example of this might be a particularly severe case of hyperemesis gravidarum (uncontrollable vomiting during pregnancy), for which cannabis is effective and which requires some fairly heavy-duty medications to control, which themselves aren't ideal in pregnancy.

Despite the unknowns, or due to "the medical establishment that cried wolf" about the risks of cannabis in general, many people will continue to choose to use cannabis during pregnancy. That is their decision. Nothing terrible is going to happen to their children from cannabis, especially with modest usage of legal, regulated cannabis. There isn't a "fetal cannabis syndrome" like there is with alcohol. According to a 2017 study by the National Academies of Sciences, Engineering, and Medicine (see below), cannabis isn't known to cause birth defects, DNA damage, or most of the other concerning outcomes that were feverish creations of U.S. drug policy.

Most importantly, let us not judge, report, drug test (unless with consent), criminalize, or exaggerate any of this, as historically this stigmatization and punishment quite plausibly have been more damaging than the cannabis has been, to all parties involved. The use of cannabis during pregnancy must not be criminalized, used as legal evidence of poor parenting, or used to disrupt a family unit. Reporting requirements, such as to family services, must be changed so that they do not discourage patients from discussing their cannabis use with their doctors and so that they don't put their physicians in the role of policeperson.

Establishing the safety of drugs during pregnancy is somewhat inferential for several reasons. First, it is unethical to directly experiment on humans. You can't just give a thousand pregnant or breastfeeding women cannabis and a thousand women placebos and see if their children are harmed—that would be against our code of "do no harm"! We are allowed to study on animals (to some, this is of debatable ethics as well), though the results of animal studies don't always directly translate accurately to humans.

For human studies, we mostly have "observational" studies—studies in which a sample of the population is observed with differing variables (e.g., cannabis use during pregnancy versus no use), and from which inferences are drawn that, hypothetically, apply to the population at large. The conclusions of these studies can be clouded by other variables that can be difficult to control for, such as whether people who use cannabis also use more tobacco, alcohol, and other drugs, which obviously would impact the results. There are many other "confounding" issues such as poverty, education, trauma history, mental illness, and racism. It is difficult to anticipate and account for all of these factors or to know if there are other ones you haven't even thought of. As mentioned, most of these studies were on illegal cannabis, without the patients receiving any medical guidance, which further diminishes their applicability.

One researcher whose intriguing studies singlehandedly challenged the "cannabis isn't safe during pregnancy" narrative pushed by the medical institutions at the dawn of the War on Drugs is Dr. Melanie Dreher. When Dr. Dreher was a doctoral nursing student at Columbia, she ended up in Jamaica on a NIDA grant studying "amotivational syndrome" in Jamaican workers (unsurprisingly, she didn't find any "amotivational syndrome," as this is merely a fever dream of the U.S. government). At the time, in the late 1960s, she noted that women would give children cannabis tea to keep them healthy and productive, and to help them concentrate in school. She observed that the children who were given the cannabis tea did in fact do better in school, but she was unable to say if this was just a correlation (i.e., that they had very attentive mothers who gave them whatever they needed to succeed at school, including, in this case, cannabis tea) or if the tea was causing the better grades.

To answer this question, Dr. Dreher took thirty pregnant cannabis users and matched them to controls who were as similar as possible, except without the cannabis. Her team followed these mothers through their pregnancy and then followed their babies after birth using standardized tests of neonatal behavior. At three days, there was very little difference between the cannabis-exposed and the nonexposed babies. Then things got more interesting.

At one month, we got very different results. We found that *the babies of the mothers who were [cannabis] smokers did significantly better on every item on the Brazelton Neonatal scale.* This was completely nonintuitive. We just assumed there would be differences, and the differences would be in favor of the non-exposed babies. That was not the case. All of these mothers were breastfeeding. We knew that cannabis passes through the mammary gland barriers and that these babies were getting continued exposure to cannabis, and yet they were really very sociably alert, had high neurological scores, and were doing very well.[3] (emphasis added)

Dr. Dreher studied these children postbirth until age five.

We found that there was no impact of the cannabis at all. *The real issues had to do with children who had better environment for neonatal development than other children.* The environmental factors, familial factors, economic factors were much more powerful than whether they had been exposed prenatally.[4]

Dreher then applied for funds to follow them from ages five to ten—critical ages to study. She was shot down, and this rejection was explained to her with an uncharacteristic honesty. According to Dreher, "That's when I got the call from NIH (National Institute of Health), saying, 'We're not going to fund you anymore.' They didn't like the results of the study, and said, 'Unless you can find something negative or something wrong with cannabis, we can't fund you, because Congress will not like your findings, and we get our money from Congress. And if you could just find one bad thing about cannabis and follow that trajectory . . .'"

What a wasted opportunity! And, in a nutshell, a perfect example of what the War on Drugs has done to cannabis science. It has selectively funded studies that were intended to discover harm. This bias is so broad based, it is unclear how one is supposed to factor it in when interpreting studies. A heavy finger has been on the scale for the last half century.

There's a popular saying: "Just because you are paranoid, it doesn't mean they aren't out to get you." Something similar applies to cannabis research. Just because the U.S. government spiked the research, this doesn't mean that cannabis *isn't* harmful in pregnancy. The criticisms of Dreher's study are that it was just one study (which hasn't been replicated) and that it is very small. Some suggested that the cannabis was much weaker back then and thus doesn't compare to today's weed, though I wonder if the Jamaicans hadn't figured out how to cultivate strong ganja back then.

Dreher's study has been contradicted by more recent studies, though none were able to be controlled studies like hers—directly comparing some with cannabis exposure to others without cannabis exposure. For example, a 2019 study in *JAMA*, "Association between Self-Reported Prenatal Cannabis Use and Maternal, Perinatal and Neonatal Outcomes," examined the association of self-reported cannabis use and birth outcomes of more than six hundred thousand women. They found that the cannabis using moms had a significantly increased risk of preterm birth (birth at less than thirty-seven weeks—this is associated with complications). They also found that those who reported using cannabis were more likely to have other problems, such as placental abruption and babies that were small for their gestational age, with lower Apgar scores (i.e., worse neurological testing at birth), and a higher risk of admission to the intensive care unit.[5]

Buried in the study, it also says,

> Cannabis use was associated with a 0.5% reduction in the incidence of preeclampsia and gestational diabetes, and similar findings have been observed in a recent study from the United States.[6]

They rapidly dispatch this finding as unimportant by saying, "The modest reduction in risk differences *may not be clinically important*" (emphasis added). One of my long-standing complaints, going back to my dad's 1971 book *Marihuana Reconsidered*, where he demonstrated that the magazine *Playboy* was reporting more accurately about cannabis than *JAMA*, is that *JAMA* overzealously reports harms and ignores the benefits of cannabis, commensurate with the AMA's anti-cannabis position. This is more of the same. To confirm a reduction in preeclampsia (severe hypertension of pregnancy) and gestational diabetes! Multiply this 0.5 percent number times a million pregnancies. Wouldn't this kindle curiosity? Can we use it in diabetics? By what mechanism does it work? Why did the editors let this slide? All doctors and scientists should be deeply troubled by this obvious bias in a supposedly objective journal.

The only problem with this pregnancy study (ignoring the diabetes part) is that it is full of holes. It is based on memory of cannabis use, not actual cannabis use. What does cannabis do to short-term memory? It interferes with it! So why base a study on when people remember getting high? There was no confirmatory drug testing, so we don't actually know about any particular individual's cannabis (or other drug) use. The data sets are prone to "misclassification of cannabis exposure in pregnancy." There was no information about the dosage or timing of the cannabis use—two things that are critical when one is attempting to demonstrate causality. It's more plausible that fifteen joints a day throughout pregnancy would cause a problem than taking one puff once, five minutes before delivery, would.

Worst, in their words,

Although the matched cohort was balanced across covariates, including maternal age, socioeconomic status, tobacco smoking, and other correlates of cannabis exposure, it is likely that residual confounding from unmeasured and unknown confounders remain and this limitation cannot be addressed through matching.[7]

In other words, what other things likely affected the cannabis group but didn't affect the other group? Many things, such as other drugs used, contaminants in the then illegal cannabis, or nutritional status. Poverty is shown to affect pregnancy outcomes. Finally, this was primarily done, again, on unregulated illegal cannabis without the guidance of a cannabis specialist, so how can one generalize?

An intelligent and evenhanded commentary in *JAMA* about this study—anthropologists have reported that occasionally such a thing has been sighted—called "Cannabis Use in Pregnancy: A Tale of Two Concerns," puts an interesting spin on the perinatal outcomes study mentioned above. If we look past the glaring problems with the accuracy of the data for a minute,

The issue is not the data but the values that individuals bring to the data and to whom the data are thought to be most relevant. . . . Some might choose to focus on the reported 41% increased relative risk of preterm birth as unacceptably high; others might choose to focus on the 2.98% absolute risk difference to be such that cannabis-related relaxation or improvement in morning sickness may not be worth abstaining from this drug.[8]

Of course the accuracy of the data is also vitally important, as it helps one perform a decision analysis. If you are considering cannabis during pregnancy, it makes a difference if there is a one in fifty million chance of preterm birth or a one in two chance. Many people would risk the former and not the latter.

When the National Academies of Sciences, Engineering, and Medicine (NASEM) summarized the health effects of cannabis in their 2017 megareport, which synthesized data from thousands of other reports, their conclusions were similar to those of this study. The NASEM report is respected by both "sides" of the issue, though of course the report is only as good as the studies it can evaluate, which, as mentioned, have been primarily focused on finding harm. Moreover, the NASEM study only includes research up until 2016. The NASEM report concludes,

- Smoking cannabis during pregnancy *was substantially linked to lower birth weight in the offspring* (though an important caveat: the lower birth weight might be related to the act of smoking, not to the cannabinoids themselves).

- There was (limited) evidence of a statistical association between maternal cannabis smoking and the infant being admitted to the Neonatal Intensive Care Unit, the NICU (though, another caveat: many hospitals have policies that babies exposed to any drug are automatically placed in the NICU, and none of the studies show the kids remaining in the hospital after the moms are discharged).

- The relationship between smoking or using cannabis during pregnancy and other pregnancy and childhood outcomes is unclear.[9]

It's important to note that there are other studies, such as a 2016 meta-analysis published in the journal *Obstetrics and Gynecology* called "Maternal Marijuana Use and Adverse Neonatal Outcomes: A Systematic Review and Meta-analysis," which find that the witnessed drop in birth weight of the infants born to cannabis-exposed mothers entirely disappears when you factor in tobacco and other confounds. Many of the earlier studies didn't sufficiently weight these factors, causing decades of confusion and exaggerated reports of harm. This paper concludes,

Maternal marijuana use during pregnancy is not an independent risk factor for adverse neonatal outcomes after adjusting for confounding factors. Thus, the association between maternal marijuana use and adverse outcomes appears attributable to concomitant tobacco use and other confounding factors.[10]

In the back of my mind, I do wonder if, after a fifty-year hunt, millions of dollars spent specifically looking for harms, with all of this based on the less safe, illegal cannabis of the past, and given how many pregnant women have smoked weed (or have inhaled the smoke around ancestral fires) during pregnancy over the last five millennia, wouldn't more harms have shown up if there were any?

Still, better safe than sorry, and given the amount that we don't know, it's better to abstain or minimize if you can.

As for the plethora of attempts to link maternal cannabis use to later delinquency, the 2017 NASEM report concluded,

> There is insufficient evidence to support or refute a statistical association between maternal cannabis smoking and later outcomes in the offspring [such as] cognition/academic achievement, and later substance use.[11]

That was years ago, and we obviously need to continue monitoring this. To the extent we can, we want to be sure this is the case.

A 2019 Dutch study, "Preconception and Prenatal Cannabis Use and the Risk of Behavioural and Emotional Problems in the Offspring; a Multi-informant Prospective Longitudinal Study," represents the largest longitudinal study of cannabis in pregnancy. These researchers studied ten thousand pregnant women and their children at ages seven through ten. They were clever.

> Assuring that associations between maternal substance use and child psychopathology are not confounded by other factors is difficult. A method that supports causal inference includes comparing the associations for maternal *and paternal* substance use during pregnancy.[12] (emphasis added)

That is, they didn't just test the relationship between the mom's cannabis use and the functioning of the offspring. They also tested the dad's cannabis use as well to rule out environmental factors—which the mom and dad would both be exposed to—as opposed to solely the effect of the drug itself in explaining the findings. They found that cannabis use during pregnancy was associated with behavior problems in children aged seven to ten years old, but that *both maternal and paternal cannabis exposure during pregnancy were related to these findings.* The same was found for paternal cannabis use without any maternal use. Thus, the association is most certainly partly due to shared familial or genetic confounding factors. Shared familial confounding factors, such as socio-economic position and parental behaviors (e.g. poor diet) associated with both parental smoking and offspring behavioral problems, could confound the association of prenatal cannabis use and offspring behavior.[13]

They flat-out conclude,

In our analyses we adjusted for several socioeconomic indicators, and thus it is more likely that the association is due to common genetic factors. Smoking cannabis may be a *marker* for underlying psychiatric problems in parents (e.g. conduct disorder), and *risk factors that predispose to smoking cannabis could be the same that predispose offspring to behavioral problems*.[14] (emphasis added)

One can but wonder why they didn't do something like this in the American version, the 2020 study, "Associations between Prenatal Cannabis Exposure and Childhood Outcomes: Results from the ABCD Study," where they found similar behavioral problems later in kids whose moms used weed. They called it "psychopathology" to make it sound like a super-scary consequence of the cannabis, and they didn't include clever devices like the Dutch researchers did in order to ferret out the social, genetic, and behavioral biases that are possibly/likely contributing to the results.[15] It feels, reading one right after the other, as if one group (coincidentally the American group) is trying to find harm, whereas the other group is trying to find out *if there is harm*; but hey, I'm just a primary care doctor, not an epidemiologist.

One of the authors of the Dutch study, Henning Tiemeier, who is a faculty member at the Harvard School of Public Health, has summarized the situation nicely: "We are saying this again and again: Those that say cannabis is safe during pregnancy do not really know. Those that say it is not [safe] do not know either."[16] He points out that this complex and evolving scientific debate won't be resolved with the results of any particular study, regardless of whether it's a small study from rural Jamaica or a larger one from a cosmopolitan Dutch city.

This humility is refreshing!

One of the more sensible studies I have read about prenatal cannabis exposure and later cognitive effects was a 2020 study published in *Frontiers in Psychology* called "Totality of the Evidence Suggests Prenatal Cannabis Exposure Does Not Lead to Cognitive Impairments: A Systematic and Critical Review." It is not surprising that this was a spectacular paper given that Dr. Carl Hart, a top-tier drug researcher and a courageous social justice advocate, was one of the authors. In this study, the researchers comprehensively evaluate all of the other studies done in this area. They point out that any results that were found in these other studies

> are nearly impossible to determine without knowledge of the expected range of performance for a particular group. Through the use of normative data, whereby individual or mean group scores are compared against a normative database that accounts for age, and educational level, the clinical significance of the differences can be determined. This is a core assessment principle in clinical neuropsychology but appears to be largely ignored in the literature on prenatal cannabis exposure.[17]

This is critical. With studies that supposedly showed a drop in IQ with cannabis use (see chapter 13), this effect vanished when socioeconomic factors are accounted for. This might be all the more relevant to maternal cannabis use, with struggling moms trying to hold things together in chaotic environments. I just look at where I work as a primary care doctor, in an inner-city clinic where many patients have to decide whether to spend money on food or medicine. If I compare it to the affluent suburb where I live, where there are coaches and tutors for everything from potty training and learning to crawl to college admissions, then of course the kids "do better" on, for example, standardized tests. You can't just ignore this stuff or blame it on cannabis use.

When Hart's team went back and evaluated the differences that were found in hundreds of studies, in kids of cannabis-exposed moms of all ages they found that, of over a thousand measures, cognitive performance was only different from nonexposed kids at a rate of 4.3 percent. Sometimes it was worse (3.4 percent of the time), and sometimes it was better (0.9 percent of the time). This was not statistically significant. They conclude,

Despite analyzing studies spanning approximately three decades, we conclude the evidence does not support an association between prenatal cannabis exposure and clinically relevant cognitive deficits.[18]

They add some insightful social commentary. To start, they point out what is implicit in their very study,

A greater understanding is necessary of the fact that many children with prenatal cannabis exposure are also exposed to factors often seen in people with low socio-economic status, such as poor nutrition, parents with lower levels of education and parents who may also use other substances, including nicotine and alcohol, among a host of other confounding variables. While a select few of the studies included in this review assessed and controlled for some of these variables, the majority did not.[19]

Whether the research is valid or not, it appears that if you find harm, you get into the news. This makes for an extremely sexy headline. You would also receive more funding from the U.S. government to continue your research. Hart and colleagues discuss the implications of the type of research they are taking to task. I will add the entire quote:

We are concerned that a misunderstanding of the relationship between prenatal cannabis exposure and subsequent cognitive functioning leads to an oversimplification of the complex relationships between socioeconomic factors and functioning of the individual whether drug use is involved or not. Misinterpretation of the complex interactions of relevant factors in itself can cause harm to pregnant women and their children by leading to punitive policies and enhancing unwarranted stigma. In some cases, intense stigma has resulted in removal of children from their families, and even in maternal incarceration. The rationale for such policies is, in part, that prenatal cannabis exposure causes persistent deleterious effects, especially on cognitive functioning. Findings from this review suggest that this assumption should be reevaluated to ensure that our assumptions do not do more harm than the drug itself.[20]

Amen! Imagine what removing the kid from the mom does to cognitive (and emotional) functioning. A response to this study, "Commentary: Totality of the Evidence Suggests Prenatal Cannabis Exposure Does Not Lead to Cognitive Impairments: A Systematic and Critical Review," makes three points:

We have three primary concerns with the conclusions of the systematic review: (1) the statement "totality of the evidence" is misleading and cannot be interpreted without a meta-analysis; (2) the definition of "clinically significant" findings used to draw conclusions is limited; and (3) the lack of evidence for a harmful association between *in-utero* cannabis exposure and cognitive functioning should not be concluded as evidence for safety.[21]

I'm becoming convinced that people can demonstrate whatever they want, within limits, with meta-analyses, depending on how they pick the studies to focus on. I do agree with the latter point, along the lines of "absence of evidence of harm is not evidence of safety," especially during pregnancy, when we have had so many nasty surprises, from thalidomide in the past to currently Tylenol (see next section).

All of this, of course, begs the question of what is safe in pregnancy? What are women supposed to use if in mental or physical discomfort during pregnancy? Certainly not nonsteroidals like ibuprofen or naproxen. Not regular intake of alcohol—we don't even know if an occasional glass of wine with dinner is safe. For decades we were told to counsel patients that acetaminophen (Tylenol, or paracetamol in Europe) was perfectly safe. Recently, a consensus statement—"Paracetamol Use during Pregnancy: A Call for Precautionary Action"—tells us quite the opposite. According to this, Tylenol, which doctors have recommended with abandon for decades, "might alter fetal development, which could increase the risks of some neurodevelopmental, reproductive and urogenital disorders."[22] Yikes! Why doesn't this get as much attention as all of these dubious cannabis studies did?

As my wife points out, it's easy for men to say to women, "Just don't take anything during pregnancy. Don't drink. Don't smoke pot. No pain relievers. No unhealthy food. Just . . . suffer and breed." This is why it's important not to exaggerate the risks or publicize risks based on biased or flawed studies. The harms of a potential effect on the fetus must be weighed, I suppose, against the relief any substance provides for the mother. A value judgment. Who's value judgment? It depends on who you ask, but I'd say the mom's. It is simply not ethical to take agency away from the mothers, such as in the recent bill in Alabama, mentioned above, that would force women who want medical marijuana to show a negative pregnancy test.[23] Why not use breathalyzers as well every few hours? Or install cameras at home to make sure the moms are eating healthy and exercising?

Values enter in not just on the patient level but on the level of how doctors decide to interpret contradictory or incomplete data—and keep in mind that most doctors have been conditioned for the last fifty years to go along with the War on Drugs. In the 2018 report from the American Academy of Pediatrics, "Marijuana Use during Pregnancy and Breastfeeding: Implications for Neonatal and Childhood Outcomes," the authors go through the flaws of most of the studies on this topic and reasonably summarize,

> The evidence for independent, adverse effects of marijuana on human neonatal outcomes and prenatal development is limited, and inconsistency in findings may be the result of the potential confounding caused by the high correlation between marijuana use and use of other substances such as cigarettes and alcohol, as well as sociodemographic risk factors.[24]

They conclude, "The evidence from the available research studies indicate reason for concern, particularly in fetal growth and early neonatal behaviors."[25]

What is the main reason that women use cannabis during pregnancy? Cannabis is remarkably effective in treating the nausea and vomiting associated with pregnancy, as well as many of the other attendant discomforts, such as backache, anxiety, and insomnia.

A big problem is that there aren't that many safe alternatives for nausea during pregnancy. Prochlorperazine (Compazine) is class C in pregnancy, meaning that "animal reproduction studies have shown an adverse effect on the fetus and there are no adequate and well-controlled studies in humans." Great. The other commonly used medication, ondansetron (Zofran), is class B in pregnancy, meaning that it hasn't been the subject of any well-controlled studies, but we don't know of any major birth defects it has yet to cause. Slightly better, but who knows what we'll eventually find out about ondansetron if even Tylenol, which was class A, "presumed safe in pregnancy," for decades, isn't actually safe. Also, ondansetron isn't consistently effective, leaving many women without useful options if they forgo cannabis.

Morning sickness can significantly impair function in up to one-third of pregnant women. It's severe form, hyperemesis gravidarum, is medically dangerous and sometimes requires hospitalization to treat. It can pose severe fetal risk. Cannabis can be extremely efficacious for this, and it is hard to imagine that cannabis could be all that much more dangerous than the cocktail of heavy-duty pharmaceuticals that patients typically receive intravenously during a hospitalization for hyperemesis.

In addition to the usual caveats about how this needs to be studied further, I'd add that it would be game changing if we could discover those particular components of cannabis that treat the nausea—so we don't have to throw all five hundred chemicals at the problem with whole-plant cannabis. Then perhaps the harms to the fetus could be minimized while we can exploit the medicinal benefits. Or, wouldn't it be great if we developed a cannabinoid-type medicine that we could somehow establish is safe in pregnancy, or which doesn't enter into the breast milk?

Finally, many argue, in favor of its safety, that cannabis has been used during pregnancy and to address the pain of childbirth for thousands of years. Of course, we have many safer and more effective medications now for childbirth than we did in previous millennia. Just because something has been used for thousands of years doesn't mean it is safe. They used to bleed people to cure diseases.

What about the mixed messages that pregnant women are getting? A patient can get a profoundly contradictory message depending on whom they speak to. Many dispensaries tend to give the message that cannabis is OK, even therapeutic, during pregnancy, whereas doctors can paint an apocalyptic picture of harm. There are few evenhanded, middle-of-the-road resources.

In a 2018 study, "Recommendations from Cannabis Dispensaries about First-Trimester Cannabis Use," researchers fabricated a story of being a patient who is eight weeks pregnant and is suffering from morning sickness. They then called cannabis dispensaries in Colorado, pretending to be this patient (how is this remotely ethical?), and flat-out lied to them, playing on their heartstrings (sort of like the DEA did during Operation

Green Merchant, described in chapter 6, pretending to be sick veterans who needed medical care in order to arrest the people who offered to help these "veterans"). Over the phone, they asked if medical cannabis was a recommended treatment for this condition. The dispensaries failed the test: 69 percent recommended the use of cannabis products for morning sickness.

This finding is extraordinarily problematic for a number of reasons. Dispensary workers, or budtenders, aren't health professionals. Why on earth are they making medical recommendations? There isn't even any basic training, course, or licensing required to be a budtender. And why are they opining about safety in pregnancy, when even the top health care professionals don't know whether or not it's safe? At best, they should say, "We aren't authorized to comment on this, but I suggest that you talk to a medical professional." Not to pull rank, but if I can't figure out the answer to the question of the safety of cannabis in pregnancy after studying it for decades, I'm not convinced that a random budtender in Colorado would know the correct answer. Also, it sounds like bad business—a lawsuit waiting to happen.

On the other hand, the authors of this article didn't truly analyze or drill down as to *why* this type of situation has come about, or what role the *medical profession* might have played. It was sort of like, "Tsk, tsk, isn't this awful. They shouldn't be doing that." They didn't deeply question why dispensaries are so comfortable answering this type of question, which is because so many people are asking them instead of their doctors. Why were the doctors not considered valid sources of information? Some of the comments were pretty illuminating, such as, "Maybe you have a progressive doctor that will not lie to you. All the studies done back in the day were just propaganda." This comment is basically true—even though it was put into the article by the authors to illustrate what silly Luddites the cannabis people are. By "lie" I think is meant, "state routine, doctrinaire anti-cannabis advice, without thinking for themselves or reading widely." It pretty much sums up the level of trust and credibility that the medical profession has earned itself from cannabis users, which is what's driving them to the budtenders.

These thoughts are borne out by a 2021 study, "Pregnant People's Experiences Discussing Their Cannabis Use with Prenatal Care Providers in a State with Legalized Cannabis," in which researchers conducted in-depth interviews with pregnant or postpartum women in California—twenty years after medical cannabis was legalized—who had used cannabis during pregnancy. Sadly,

> most participants did not disclose their cannabis use to their prenatal care providers, due to fears of being reported to child protective services (CPS), or fears of provider judgment. Participants reported that few providers initiated any discussions about cannabis use in pregnancy with them; some participants interpreted this omission as tacit endorsement of cannabis use in pregnancy.[26]

The report notes, among other things, that "providers' role as potential reporters to CPS appears to pose a significant barrier to comprehensive, compassionate counseling and education on cannabis use in pregnancy." The study concludes in a rather understated manner, noting that it "documents notable deficits in patient-provider interactions about cannabis."[27]

Are the patients' fears based on reality? What happens when pregnant women do disclose their cannabis use to their doctors? To a certain extent, it depends on the laws of the particular state. According to a 2016 study, "Obstetric Health Care Providers' Counseling Responses to Pregnant Patient Disclosures of Marijuana Use," in recorded visits, ninety patients disclosed their cannabis use to forty-seven obstetricians (which, I might say, given the stigma and perceived risk, was pretty damn brave of the patients!). In half of these cases (48 percent), the doctors just ignored this disclosed information and offered no advice or counseling. In the other half of cases,

> when counseling was offered, it consisted of general statements without specific information on the risks or outcomes related to marijuana use in pregnancy, discussions regarding the need for urine toxicology testing, and warnings that use detected at the time of delivery would initiate child protective services involvement.[28]

My God! These were obstetricians. No wonder patients don't mention it and go to budtenders. Given this, I'm not confident in how secure I'd feel mentioning cannabis use to my doctor if I were pregnant. They might actually call the fuzz instead of offering care, support, and advice.

All participants in this issue, from all vantage points, have room for improvement.

## CHAPTER ELEVEN
# TOKING AND DRIVING
## Don't Stop at the Green Light

It is not safe to drive when under the influence of cannabis. One of the first things I advise people before certifying them for medical cannabis is not to drive under the influence, just as they shouldn't drive after drinking alcohol or after taking other impairing medications such as oxycodone or Ambien, or taking any combination of the above.

Having been a primary care doctor for twenty-five years, to people from many different sectors of society, I feel that I am able to reasonably conclude that not all people are responsible or have common sense—especially after they have consumed intoxicants. Some may disregard proscriptions against driving or the operation of heavy machinery. As states legalize cannabis, the debates over how dangerous it is to drive under the influence of cannabis (relative to other intoxicants) rages on, as do questions surrounding how to detect and enforce safe driving.

Law enforcement and prohibitionists can wildly exaggerate these dangers by touting statistics of people who tested positive for cannabis after fatal car crashes, *knowing full well* that (a) you can test positive for weeks after last use and, (b) as such, a positive test is no indication that the driver was intoxicated on cannabis while he or she was driving. A positive test merely shows that they used cannabis *within the last three weeks* or so and then later got into a car and crashed. It would be dangerous to drive within the next several hours but not weeks later. This is a red flag: anyone who cites statistics such as these is spreading propaganda, not science.

As such, "zero tolerance" laws, where you get into criminal difficulty if you have *any* cannabis in your system, are more about persecuting cannabis users than promoting public safety. As mentioned, you might have used several weeks earlier. Or you might have even just used some nonintoxicating CBD with a trace amount of THC in it, and you can still test positive.

Companies can greatly misrepresent the effectiveness of their "breathalyzers" for pot. None of these have been shown to work well, or to get around the fundamental problem that, unlike alcohol, the levels of cannabis in a person's body fluids (blood, urine, saliva) don't correlate well with levels of intoxication. A medical patient can have a very high level from everyday usage even though, at the time of testing, they haven't used before driving and aren't intoxicated. Conversely, someone who hasn't used much recently might be quite impaired without necessarily having high levels. Therefore, "per se" laws that make it illegal to drive with more than a certain defined limit don't work on either end of the spectrum.

Some cannabis aficionados can trivialize the risks of driving while stoned and are occasionally heard discussing how they are better drivers when high because they drive more slowly and pay more attention. You may think or feel that you are driving better, but this has never been demonstrated in a driving lab. The best you can say is that if you use cannabis frequently and use a modest amount, you aren't nearly as impaired as if you use cannabis infrequently and are stoned out of your skull. That doesn't equate with "safe."

Stoned drivers are likely more aware that they are impaired than drunk drivers are and, to a certain extent, are able to compensate (provided that they aren't stoned out of their skulls . . .). However, a 2022 study, "Driving Performance and Cannabis Users' Perception of Safety: A Randomized Clinical Trial," showed that the *perception* of the cannabis having worn off to the extent that it was safe to drive somewhat preceded the actual normalization of driving function—by a few hours.[1] This disconnect obviously presents a dangerous window of time.

General guidelines are that one should wait four hours before driving after using inhaled cannabis, six or so hours after using a sublingual preparation, and eight hours after using an edible, though these recommendations are highly person and dose dependent, and they also depend on what other medications a person is using. There is a small amount of evidence that CBD helps mitigate the effect of THC on driving, but not enough to allow you safely or ethically to drive.[2]

They say that drunk drivers barrel through red lights and that stoned drivers cautiously stop at green ones. And no, if you are stoned and drunk at the same time, you don't get it just right and wisely assess what to do at a yellow light. They don't balance each other out; rather, you are significantly worse off than with either substance alone. While the intent or instinct to be cautious when driving stoned is appreciated, this falls into the category of "the path to hell is paved with good intentions."

A commonly cited 2016 study, a meta-analysis, "The Effects of Cannabis Intoxication on Motor Vehicle Collision Revisited and Revised," assesses the risk of accidents under the use of cannabis and concludes that cannabis increases your chances of "being responsible for or being involved in" a motor vehicle accident by 1.36 times.[3]

They conclude that the increase is "of low to medium magnitude" and estimate that alcohol, at a BAC rate of 0.10, just over the legal limit of 0.08, increases your risk of an accident by twenty times. Doing the math, alcohol, at a modestly illegal level, is *fifteen* times more likely than cannabis to cause a crash. A 2017 study from Canada, "Cannabis, Alcohol and Fatal Road Accidents," concluded that

> drivers under the influence of alcohol are 17.8 times (12.1–26.1) more likely to be responsible for a fatal accident. . . . Drivers under the influence of cannabis multiply their risk of being responsible for causing a fatal accident by 1.65 (1.16–2.34).[4]

Doing this math, the increased risk from alcohol over cannabis is eleven times higher, which is in the same range of magnitude as the fifteen times number above.

There are several variables that would affect these numbers. The most important variable, I believe, beyond dosage consumed is experience with using cannabis. There is a tremendous difference between a person who gets really stoned once a year and a medical cannabis patient who takes two small puffs of medicinal cannabis (high CBD, lower THC) twice a day. Technically, neither of them should be driving, but the former would be much more dangerous. This is borne out by studies, such as, "Determining the Magnitude and Duration of Acute $\Delta^9$-Tetrahydrocannabinol ($\Delta^9$-THC)-Induced Driving and Cognitive Impairment: A Systematic and Meta-analytic Review," which concluded, "Multiple meta-regression analyses further found that regular cannabis users experienced less impairment than 'other' (mostly occasional) cannabis users."[5]

Multiples of 1.36 and 1.65 don't sound like big numbers, but if you multiply them times a million drivers, that is an incredibly high number of extra accidents, injuries, disabilities, and deaths due to cannabis-impaired driving. One impaired accident is too many. The whole point of cannabis (from a medical perspective) is to lessen suffering, not to increase it in others. It is especially unfair to innocent bystanders (or, in this case, unimpaired drivers).

Which effects of cannabis impair driving? Are there any aspects of cannabis use that might improve driving? (Are we even allowed to ask this? One could imagine that being calm, mindful, gentle, and patient—on a small dose of regular cannabis—might be protective. Or that you might drive better if you had a good night's sleep the night before, aided by cannabis, rather than writhing in pain all night.) There are numerous motor and cognitive skills that need to be simultaneously functioning and coordinated in order to drive safely. Some of these are attention, motor coordination, and memory—all of which cannabis can affect. Driving-related behaviors have been studied in driving simulators, and some of the driving behaviors that were impaired by cannabis were as follows:

- Increased start time in response to light signal (i.e., the driver might be sitting there lost in thought and not notice that the light has changed).

- Increased lateral position errors and lane deviation.

- Increased braking distance/stop time.

Given that it is cannabis research, with many studies focused on harm, one does have to look critically at the dosages used, as well as every other parameter of the study. If you compare the equivalent of twenty puffs of nuclear-grade Sinsemilla to the effect of one beer, the cannabis isn't going to look very good.

In fact, a 2022 study published in *Drug Science, Policy and Law* called "The Risk of Being Culpable for or Involved in a Road Crash after Using Cannabis: A Systematic Review and Meta-analyses" claims to show that the risks of cannabis-impaired driving have been vastly exaggerated because of the way in which they defined the criteria for including studies in the various meta-analyses they have done. In their words:

> We undertook a systematic search of electronic databases and identified 13 culpability studies . . . studies from which cannabis-crash odds ratios could be extracted. Random-effects meta-analyses gave summary odds ratios of 1.37 (1.10–1.69) for the culpability. . . . A tool was designed to identify and score biases arising from: confounding by uncontrolled covariates; inappropriate selection of cases and controls; and the inappropriate measurement of the exposure and outcome variables. Each study was scrutinized for the presence of those biases and given a total "directional bias score." *Most of the biases were inflationary.* A meta-regression against the total directional bias scores was performed for the culpability studies, giving a bias-adjusted summary odds ratio of 0.68 (0.45–1.05) . . . indicating that the summary odds ratio of 1.45 is an overestimate. *It is evident that the risks from driving after using cannabis are much lower than from other behaviors such as drunk-driving, speeding or using mobile phones while driving.*[6] (emphasis added)

Color me shocked that the bias was "inflationary" toward magnifying the risk of cannabis. This still doesn't mean that it is safe to drive high, but that one must use as much skepticism toward the literature on this subject as with any other cannabis-related subject. (Also, if the number 0.68—which is less than 1.00—holds and is replicated, that would suggest that driving after using cannabis usage is protective.)

Studies of the actual risks of accidents can be contradictory. One would expect an increased risk of accidents, and that is what many studies show. However, these studies are far from flawless. One study that is commonly cited is a 2012 meta-analysis from the *British Medical Journal*, "Acute Cannabis Consumption and Motor Vehicle Collision Risk: Systematic Review of Observational Studies and Meta-analysis," which begins by stating,

> Results [of previous studies] have been inconsistent. More than half of these studies have suggested that cannabis consumption is associated with an increased risk of traffic collision, and the remaining studies have found no association or a decreased risk of collision.[7]

By cherry-picking and choosing the right studies, the authors seem determined to rectify this, and in fact they end up concluding that "driving under the influence of cannabis was associated with a significantly increased risk of motor vehicle collisions compared with unimpaired driving, with an odds ratio 1.92."[8]

However, as discussed, having cannabis in one's blood or other bodily fluids does *not* correlate with actual impairment, so they can't truly conclude what they concluded. They just can't say that the drivers were "under the influence of cannabis." They solely know that the drivers used cannabis at some point within the last several weeks. Also, there are many other confounding variables among the many differently designed studies that they picked and squished together to obtain these findings. So it's difficult to say how helpful this study is. My criticisms aren't a "get out of jail free" card for driving stoned. I just wouldn't bet the farm on the number 1.92—this study mostly seems useful as a good case study of the recent commentary on inflationary bias.

One telling study was published in 2016 by the U.S. National Highway Traffic and Safety Administration (NHTSA)—not exactly a bunch of cannabis-loving Rastafarians. Their study, "Drug and Alcohol Crash Risk: A Case-Control Study," collected data over twenty months on three thousand drivers who crashed and compared this with six thousand controls to see what the increased (or decreased) risk of crashing was with various drugs, pharmaceuticals, and alcohol. Unsurprisingly, alcohol posed the greatest risk. For example, at the legal limit of 0.08, people are 3.93 times more likely to crash than someone who is sober. For THC, the active ingredient in cannabis, the initial finding was that the crash risk was elevated—not as much as alcohol, but the chances of crashing were 1.25 times the baseline risk. However, "after adjusting for gender, age, race/ ethnicity, and alcohol, there was no indication that any drug significantly contributed to crash risk. The adjusted odds ratios for THC were 1.00."[9]

When I first read this study, I thought that it just didn't seem plausible that accidents wouldn't rise at least to a certain degree with cannabis. I thought to myself, "Could this whole issue be a creation of prohibitionists to scare people away from legalization?" I didn't know a single person who had crashed or who had been in an accident while having driven stoned, with just cannabis in their system, though my personal experience (having witnessed the legalization movement for half a century) only goes so far. Alcohol always seemed to be the culprit, or perhaps the two combined together.

The day after I read this, another study came out, from the journal *Drug and Alcohol Dependence*, called, "Canada's Cannabis Legalization and Drivers' Traffic-Injury Presentations to Emergency Departments in Ontario and Alberta, 2015–2019," which studied traffic accidents from emergency departments in Canada before and after it legalized cannabis on October 17, 2018, and concluded that "legalization was not associated with changes in traffic injuries in all drivers or youth drivers."[10] They speculate that increased deterrence, enforcement, and education might all be contributing to this outcome.

Another study that came out around the same time, in late 2021, in the *International Journal of Drug Policy*, titled "Medicinal Cannabis and Driving: The Intersection of Health and Road Safety Policy," reviewed the increased crash risk ratio of several categories of commonly prescribed and used medications, such as antihistamines (1.2 times increased risk); antidepressants (1.4); benzodiazepines (1.6–2.3); Z-class hypnotics, your Ambiens, etc. (1.4—give me a break, this has to be higher); and opioids (1.9–2.2). This study references the risks of cannabis-impaired driving ranging from 1.1 to 1.4, noting that "some older meta-analyses have identified higher and lower odds ratios, but these typically failed to control for confounders such as age, gender, alcohol intoxication, and polydrug use."[11]

Of note, the 1.1–1.4 range is well within if not significantly *below* what many patients are driving around with daily on their antidepressants, sleeping meds, antianxiety medications, and even antihistamines. So why are the prohibitionists making such a fuss about cannabis? Is this a largely contrived issue, part of the "moral panic" we need to restrict freedoms? If they are so concerned about crash risk, why aren't they out in the streets educating people not to drive while under the influence of all these other drugs, especially alcohol?

The authors further note,

> The studies discussed above are only of partial relevance to medicinal cannabis as none have differentiated between medical and recreational use. There are several characteristics of medicinal use that may lead to a lower road safety risk among patients than among recreational users.[12]

This is where issues such as lower doses, stable dosage, uniform products, lower THC and higher CBD ratios, daily tolerance, and communication with and guidance from a medical cannabis professional come in. It is also where Dr. Staci Gruber's work from Harvard Medical (discussed in more detail in chapter 12), which demonstrated improved cognitive function in medical cannabis patients, would come in as well. Maybe if chronic pain patients are actually getting a good night's sleep, their driving is better. It is extremely well documented, across dozens of studies, that medical cannabis patients lessen their usage of opioids and benzos, which have a comparable or greater crash liability. This paper concludes that "in medical-only access models there is little evidence to justify the differential treatment of medicinal cannabis patients, compared with those taking other prescription medications with potentially impairing effects."[13]

Finally, a recent study came out in 2022 in the journal *Health Economics* called "Medical Cannabis and Automobile Accidents: Evidence from Auto Insurance," which concluded the following:

> We find that premiums declined, on average, by $22 per year following medical cannabis legalization. The effect is more substantial in areas near a dispensary and in areas with a higher prevalence of drunk driving before legalization. We estimate that existing legalization has *reduced* health expenditures related to auto accidents by almost $820 million per year with the potential for a further $350 million reduction if legalized nationally.[14] (emphasis added)

In other words, the authors of the study think that these decreases may be related to reduced drunk driving in those states that have legalized cannabis, suggesting a possible "substitution effect" whereby people are switching from more dangerous alcohol to less dangerous weed.

Not to sound like a broken record, but despite the above studies, it is *not* safe to drive while under the influence of cannabis. The effects are unpredictable. It's such a complicated drug, there isn't a linear or consistent dose-effect relationship. But if you look at the actual data, not the headlines or the cherry-picked and manipulated statistics from law enforcement (or the prohibitionist advocacy groups they help fund), the data is not nearly as dramatic or clear cut as one might imagine.

As for detection and enforcement, in light of the above studies, one could make an argument that perhaps there is more societal benefit to focusing enforcement resources on drunk driving. Driving while impaired on alcohol is an order of magnitude more dangerous and results in more than ten thousand deaths in the United States annually—about one-third of all traffic fatalities are alcohol related. Or, we would perhaps be just as well served by educating people about the dangers of their other prescription drugs, which, as described above, contribute to the risk of accidents at at least the same rate that cannabis does. Many people don't even think about these substances. Antihistamines, antidepressants, etc.—it is assumed that because the meds are prescribed by the doctor, or over the counter, they must be safe to use before driving.

It is difficult to know how much of a danger cannabis-influenced driving will actually be once it is fully legal and regulated. Legalization tends to make all aspects of cannabis use safer. If the number of 1.36 times increased risk of accident is valid (versus twenty or so for alcohol) with the surreptitious use of illegal cannabis during a Drug War, it should be possible to lower this number with education, transparency, deterrence, standardized products (so people don't accidentally take too much), and changes in patterns of usage. For example, during the decades of prohibition, the THC levels rose, but with legalization, perhaps we can lower the THC doses and increase the CBD so that the impairment is less. Perhaps as cannabis use goes from being an illicit activity to an accepted, open behavior, we can stigmatize not the use of cannabis itself but, specifically, using cannabis before driving. If we could move beyond our current polemical, distorted debate over cannabis legalization, with exaggerated claims flying all around, might not cannabis education be that much more effective? We could focus criminal penalties on the most egregious cases as a deterrent, based on intoxication not on use (as we do with alcohol).

Some worry that the problem of stoned driving will worsen as more states legalize. Their argument is that more people will be using cannabis in general, so, by simple math, more people will be driving stoned. This assumes that the same percentage of people using cannabis will be driving stoned (which can be impacted by education) and that levels of drunk (or medicated) driving won't decline with cannabis legalization (as the above *Health Economics* article implies is already happening).

Certainly, some people, possibly a substantial number, will substitute cannabis for alcohol as people increasingly have a legal choice between the two. We might have the same ratio of irresponsible, impaired drivers overall (suppose a certain stable percentage of people just don't care), but they might be impaired by a less dangerous drug (cannabis rather than alcohol). In an indirect way, this might provide us with some harm reduction. (This line of thought somehow feels less than reassuring . . . please just don't drive while on *anything*!)

The quest for a weed breathalyzer that works is ferociously being fought over by several different companies and academic groups. To market and convince everyone that your particular device is effective has become a cottage industry, replete with snazzy websites and futuristic-looking devices that could fashionably adorn the set of *Star Trek*. There is only one problem: they aren't very accurate, both in that they miss people who are impaired and they falsely implicate people who aren't.

One brand makes a big deal about being able to detect if someone smoked cannabis within the last three hours. A small puff of high-CBD weed by a seasoned medical cannabis patient within this three-hour window would likely result in minimal intoxication. Who wants to arrest this person? It would be better if they didn't drive, but it's probably better than driving after taking a Benadryl or drinking a few beers. Further, someone who has consumed a huge dosage of an edible and is utterly unfit to drive would go completely undetected by this device because they didn't smoke anything.

Numerous studies have evaluated this issue, including a recent study in the magazine *Traffic Injury Prevention* titled "The Failings of *Per Se* Limits to Detect Cannabis-Induced Driving Impairment: Results from a Simulated Driving Study," which flat-out concluded, "There appears to be a poor and inconsistent relationship between magnitude of impairment and THC concentrations in biological samples, meaning that *per se* limits cannot reliably discriminate between impaired from unimpaired drivers."[15] Per se limits are a legal cutoff, such as 0.08 for alcohol. There's just no such limit for cannabis because, as discussed above, it affects people so differently in different circumstances.

Who knows what technology might be developed in the future? As we studied in philosophy class in college, you can't predict the future of technological invention. Recently, they likely have come a little closer at my home institution. In the article "Identification of Δ9-Tetrahydrocannabinol (THC) Impairment Using Functional Brain Imaging," they developed a device that scans brain waves and purportedly detects impairment more accurately than other devices. They gave people huge doses of THC, which may have significantly augmented their findings (up to eighty milligrams orally—I'd be high for weeks; gummies and seltzers often have five milligrams), and it still only identified impairment with 76.4 percent accuracy and had a 10 percent false positive rate, meaning people get sent to prison despite not being impaired, so it's not ready for showtime yet.[16] The fact that these results represent an improvement over the other devices shows how far we are from coming up with an effective device.

If biological tests aren't particularly helpful in identifying roadside intoxication, how effective are "drug recognition experts" (i.e., police staff who are professionally trained to detect and quantify intoxication)? As mentioned, in the same study, "Identification of Δ9-Tetrahydrocannabinol (THC) Impairment Using Functional Brain Imaging," the accuracy of the drug recognition experts was only 67.8 percent, and the false positive rate was 35.4 percent, which is a social justice disaster![17] If I didn't sleep well the night before, was nervous, hadn't had coffee yet, and was having an allergy attack, I would probably flunk whatever tests they gave me. More people with dark skin magically tend to flunk these tests. Also, how do they manage to miss it when people are super stoned? I bet people with tons of lived experience with cannabis would make the best drug recognition experts.

All of this, of course, begs the question: if a detailed evaluation by a highly trained expert in the field can't tell if you are intoxicated on weed much better than a coin toss, how impaired on cannabis could you possibly be? Is this approach pragmatic or punitive?

I want to reiterate that I am against stoned driving. A component of this issue that people don't always think of is that you don't just risk your own health. Just like someone not getting vaccinated for COVID can infect and gravely injure others, you also risk the health of others if you get into a substance-precipitated accident. I am also against Drug War witch hunts, as these ruin lives too. What really matters is whether the driver is impaired, regardless of whether the impairment is due to cannabis, alcohol, or any combination of legal or prescription drugs. If an experienced driver has taken a puff of moderate-strength cannabis an hour ago to treat their rheumatoid arthritis but is driving perfectly flawlessly, do we need to arrest this person just because they used cannabis? Would we arrest them if they took one of their prescription oxycodones but were driving well? Or do we focus on the person who is weaving down the street and mowing down the bicycle riders, regardless of the cause?

**CHAPTER TWELVE**

# ADULTS

## This Is Your Brain on Pot

There's no question that cannabis affects cognition—that's always been a big part of why people use it. It causes a temporary worsening of some brain functions, such as short-term memory, accompanied by a relaxation or improvement in other functions. What are the actual short-term harms? Do any of them persist beyond the intoxication and become long term? What about benefits? Have any studies on the ways in which cannabis improves creativity or personal insight found their way through the U.S. government's fifty-year embargo on studying anything but harms? The literature for the cognitive effects of cannabis on the teenage brain is different (though often overlapping), and teens will be discussed in the next chapter.

Part of the acute effect on cognitive function comes down to such variables as dosage and frequency of use. A person who takes ten puffs of an extremely high-potency concentrate once a month will have a different experience than someone who routinely takes a modest puff of lower THC/higher CBD medicinal cannabis twice a day. Many of the studies of cognitive impairment have been on "heavy" cannabis users, who aren't necessarily typical of most cannabis users. This is like trying to understand the effects of alcohol on cognition by evaluating people who are frequently and utterly inebriated on moonshine—a biased scenario inflating the perception of the harms of cannabis.

There is also the usual historical zeal to find only the harms of cannabis. If you look closely at the language of some of these studies, it is informative about bias. For example, in a study that will be discussed later, *the authors failed to observe* general Δ9-THC induced *memory deficits* across the whole sample. *This negative finding could be explained* by a lower sample size . . . and/or the use of an intermediate oral dosage of Δ9-THC (10 mg; a dosage typically lower than those used in studies quantifying impairments by Δ9-THC content).[1] (emphasis added)

It's not, "Hey, there weren't memory deficits," but rather, "I wonder why we didn't prove our *a priori* assumption that cannabis hurts memory." Also, ten milligrams *is* a respectable dose that would get most modest users quite stoned; they just didn't spike the study by giving a gargantuan dose of THC and, as such, are lamenting the use of an "intermediate" (normal) dosage.

Of course, if you get people impaired enough, by giving them a sufficiently large dose of anything psychoactive, there are going to be harms. If kids drink enough Robitussin, they start "Robo-tripping" and begin to hallucinate alien beings. Try to think of any drug or medicine for which this isn't true. Confirmation bias is defined (thank you, Wikipedia) as the "tendency to search for, interpret, favor, and recall information in a way that confirms or supports one's prior beliefs or values." The language cited above about "failing to observe" what they were ostensibly trying to find could respectably compete in any confirmation bias contest.

Some of the effect on cognition might also have to do with the intention with which a person uses cannabis in the first place, as there is fascinating evidence coming from Dr. Staci Gruber at Harvard Medical, discussed below, that suggests medical patients have *improved* cognitive function, while "recreational" users demonstrated declines (though in chapter 21 we discuss how fine and sometimes arbitrary a line it is between "recreational" and "medical" use).

Another huge elephant in the room blocking our ability to derive clear conclusions about cannabis and cognition is that most of the studies on cannabis and the brain were done with illegal cannabis of unknown quality, content, and safety due to prohibition. The subjects in these studies were not using regulated post-prohibition cannabis, which is carefully tested for impurities and is of (fairly) consistent quality and strength. Moreover, the cannabis was not prescribed and monitored by a cannabis specialist, who would be involved in minimizing harms. As such, there is no reason to assume that *any* of the harms previously found (to the extent they *were* found . . .) would be transferrable to the new era of safer, healthier, regulated cannabis. Again, it's like trying to generalize about the health effects of alcohol by studying people drinking moonshine that they bought from a stranger.

One counterargument against this is that the newer cannabis is actually much stronger, and, as such, we've been potentially *underestimating* the cognitive effects of cannabis. I don't feel this argument is particularly compelling, as people tend to titrate their dosages to their level of comfort and usually have an unpleasant experience if they consume too much. I think the "this isn't your grandparents' weed" argument is vastly outweighed by the benefits of legalization: the labeling; standardization of dosages; screening for mold, heavy metals, pesticides, lack of adulterants, etc.; and the fact that it is all out of the shadows and closer to being integrated into mainstream care.

Another factor to consider is that these studies were primarily done with a specific spotlight on just those areas of cognition that cannabis impairs, as opposed to those it helps or neutrally doesn't impact. For example, the National Academies of Sciences, Engineering, and Medicine (NASEM) report focuses on memory, learning, and attention as three domains *in particular* that many people perform worse in after they consume weed. If researchers had studied, and NASEM had looked at, creativity, humor, and insight, I suspect there wouldn't have been deficits, and people might have done significantly better than the norm.

What does NASEM have to say about cannabis and cognition in their 2017 comprehensive report? They say there is strong data for immediate impairment, but little to no data for lasting impairment,

> within the domain of learning . . . systematic review and the component study highlighted within that review showed strong data for the acute (immediate) impact of cannabis use on learning. However, results from three systematic reviews . . . reflected limited to no support for the association between the sustained effects of cannabis use after cessation and the cognitive domain of learning.[2]

They found the same thing with memory and attention. One thing they do note is that "cannabis users may be engaging a different neural network to achieve similar outcomes during the task (e.g., compensatory efforts)." It's unclear what the significance of this is. Neuroplasticity?

The conclusion seems to be that cannabis can temporarily affect a discrete number of (important) cognitive measures negatively, like short-term memory, but the user's function returns to normal after a few days or a few weeks. I haven't seen anything that convincingly challenges this conclusion. Recently, the respected cannabis researcher Matthew Hill echoes this sentiment. In a 2020 piece in the *Proceedings of the National Academy of Sciences* titled "Cannabis and the Adolescent Brain," Hill is quoted as saying,

> There have been a couple studies that have gotten a lot of headlines that have not replicated well. . . . I don't think there's any compelling evidence that moderate levels of use are going to produce long-lasting cognitive deficits.[3]

One 2022 study that received a lot of media attention is called "Evidence on the Acute and Residual Neurocognitive Effects of Cannabis Use in Adolescents and Adults: A Systematic Meta-review of Meta-analyses." OK, we're getting extremely meta here. It is a meta-analysis of meta-analyses, so you truly have a lot of leeway to decide which articles to accept as valid and to extract data from. (As discussed in chapter 11, it can be difficult to avoid bias such as inflation of harm.) They went through thousands of studies and picked out the ten that they felt best represented the last fifty years of research on whether cannabis causes lasting cognitive harm, which is what they found: "Cannabis intoxication leads to small to moderate deficits in several cognitive domains. . . . The detrimental effects of cannabis persist beyond acute intake."[4]

This study included both adolescents and adults, which, as they mention in the limitations section, are different groups with different concerns. The evidence was deemed to be low to moderate quality. Specifically,

Our meta-review enabled us to show both acute and residual effects of cannabis on many aspects of cognition provided from meta-analyses being generally graded as low-to-moderate quality evidence.[5]

Maybe this is just research speak, but when they say "enabled us to show," it again suggests that they were trying to show something instead of neutrally evaluating if there was anything to show.

They state at the outset that "evidence was largely based on cross-sectional data which limited the quality of the evidence." This chicken/egg problem is enough to make you become a vegan! Did the differences in cognition precede the cannabis use, or did the cannabis use cause them? It's impossible to say anything definitive without following people over time. According to the authors, this "limits the inference of a causal relationship between cannabis use and cognition as well as the generalizability of results." The authors go on to say, "The review has not been pre-registered and thus results should be considered exploratory."[6] What on earth does that mean?

CNN, not to be deterred from a frenzied click-baiting opportunity, had a prominent headline, "Using Marijuana May Affect Your Ability to Think and Plan, Study Says." (Reading poorly conceived headlines like this may also affect your ability to think and plan.) I didn't understand why it was getting so much attention, as it didn't show anything definitive.

Ironically, one of the authors of the study holds the Eli Lilly Cannabis Chair at their university—Big Pharma strikes again! There is now a Canopy Growth Professor of Cannabis Science—Big Marijuana strikes again! The names of the professorships remind me of a funny motif in my favorite work of fiction, *Infinite Jest*, by David Foster Wallace, where the years were all named by corporations, such as the Year of the Depend Adult Undergarment, or YDAU. The Canopy Professor is extremely credible, as I can only assume the Eli Lilly one is. These days they've become much better at shielding the researchers from the agendas of the funding source.

Just a few months preceding the "cannabis causes lasting damage to your ability to think and plan" report that got so much press attention, this same Eli Lilly Cannabis Chair researcher put out a comprehensive review called "Cannabis and Cognitive Functioning: From Acute to Residual Effects, from Randomized Controlled Trials to Prospective Designs," where it was noted that, when meta-analyses focused on more chronic residual effects relative to effects from short abstinence periods, users (generally adults) no longer showed cognitive deficits, or showed significantly milder deficits. This finding was demonstrated by Scott et al., for abstinence periods that persisted for more than 3 days, by Schoeler et al., following 10 days of abstinence, and by Schreiner et al., after ~1 month of cannabis use abstinence. *This suggests that these residual effects have a short-term duration.*[7] (emphasis added)

It was concluded, "Cross-sectional studies on the residual cognitive effects have generally shown that cannabis is associated with cognitive deficits that are relatively small and *seem to abate after a relatively short period of abstinence*"[8] (emphasis added).

Why the opposite conclusion a few months later? I can understand different types of studies using different methodologies, but it does give one the impression that there is a lot of leeway in the meta-meta-analysis process. In order to assess this, you would have to analyze many meta-meta-analysis studies by doing a meta-meta-meta-analysis. I am not going to go there—it sounds like something out of the book *Catch-22*. Somehow in the weaning down from two thousand studies to ten studies they were able to aggregate data in such a way as to, in their words, "enable" them to publish something the press found very interesting. Much less media attention was given to the other, relatively boring assessment that didn't show much in the way of cannabis-related harm. The headline "Cannabis Doesn't Do Much of Anything" will never win out over "Miracle Cure!" or "Menace to Society!"

To digress from meta-analysis to a meta discussion on bias for a moment . . .

I'm not an epidemiologist, but I feel like, in writing this book, I stumbled on a type of bias I had never heard described before, which I'll call "fishing bias." Say, for example, you are anti-cannabis and you work at a prestigious medical institution. In a particular study, you state that you are looking at X, which you are in fact looking for. But, while you are at it, you muck around, ask about all types of potential adverse effects (depression, psychosis, suicide, etc.), and perform cognitive testing to try to uncover problems with things such as memory or performance. To be statistically significant, there generally has to be a less than one in twenty chance that any particular finding would result from chance. So, if you do study after study after study, with your line in the water, trolling for adverse effects or cognitive problems, you will eventually find something, and it will appear to be statistically significant.

Now, when you happen to find something harmful while mucking around, that's guaranteed to be a huge headline across the globe—regardless of the results of what you were ostensibly looking for—due to your visibility in the field. The newspapers scream, "ADVERSE EFFECT FOUND!" or "COGNITIVE DEFICIT FOUND!" But if you test and *don't* find any such harms, that is hardly noticed—it certainly doesn't generate headlines—because that isn't what you were looking for, and it just looks like part of the study protocol. Playing by the rules, these nonfindings will be mentioned, but in passing, in small print, in the middle of the study. Any incidentally found benefits of cannabis are often buried as well. No journalist reports "adverse effect *not* found" or "cognitive deficits *not* found," as these issues were peripheral to the stated aim of the study, which was to look at X. This type of fishing exploits (a) chance and (b) publication bias as a way to introduce findings of harm into the public discussion, without any risk of the findings of "no harm found" getting noticed or added to the ledger of what we do and don't know.

Does this sound far-fetched? I asked several prestigious researchers, and they said things along the lines of, "It's absolutely true. All researchers know this, but people outside of research don't."

Another avenue pursued to attempt to demonstrate that cannabis causes lasting brain damage is with the use of structural and functional neuroimaging. I want to emphasize that chronic, heavy cannabis use *does* physically and temporarily alter the brain. We all have natural cannabis receptors throughout our brains, and in response to heavy cannabis use, these cannabinoid receptors in the brain downregulate, or thin out. That means that you need to use more cannabis to get the same effect. Any external THC or other cannabinoids have to search around in your brain for fewer available receptors to work their magic, or their harm, depending on your perspective. This explains why a heavy, daily user who abruptly stops using cannabis is likely to undergo withdrawal symptoms such as insomnia and grumpiness. The natural endocannabinoids that we produce—and which regulate sleep and mood, for example—have many fewer cannabinoid receptors to work with and as a consequence don't function as effectively. The cannabinoid receptors come back in a matter of weeks, as anyone who has taken a T-break (tolerance break) knows. (This is when you deliberately stop using cannabis products for a few weeks to "reset" your tolerance—this saves money, is healthier, and improves the cannabis experience.)

Does cannabis actually change the physical *structure* and function of the brain, beyond some downregulated receptors, in a way that's measurable or visible with imaging? The studies in this area have been conflicting. According to a 2019 review article, "Cannabis Use in Youth Is Associated with Limited Alterations in Brain Structure," which summarizes the adult and adolescent literature,

> Several studies report associations between frequent cannabis use in adolescents and young adults and reductions in hippocampal volumes. However, other studies do not replicate these reductions, including one longitudinal study. Similarly, orbitofrontal cortex volumes have been examined with mixed results. While three studies found larger volumes of cerebellar structures in adolescent frequent cannabis users, three report equivocal findings or decreases in cerebellar volumes. Frequent cannabis users may also have thinner prefrontal cortex, although several studies have not replicated these findings. Finally, inconsistent results are apparent in amygdala, striatum, and cingulate cortex, despite their high density of CB1 receptors.[9]

Does that clear everything up?

This study concludes, "The present study found predominantly nonsignificant differences in brain structural measures among cannabis nonusers, occasional users of cannabis, and frequent users of cannabis." They do add the caveats that there could be findings for very heavy cannabis users or that there could be small but important changes that they weren't able to detect. They emphasize that they are not saying that cannabis is safe for adolescents. Finally, "in the absence of randomized controlled trials of cannabis, longitudinal data will provide the best test of whether cannabis causes brain structural alterations."[10]

As we'll see, "longitudinal" data—following people over time—is going to be essential.

Dr. Carl Hart is one of the drug researchers whom I trust and respect the most. While his résumé is dazzling, full of items such as being the chair of the Department of Psychology at Columbia University, what I admire most about him is his honesty and his transparency. He is one of a handful of people who sees the drug issue from all sides. To start, he has done research on drugs of misuse (aka drugs that happen to be the ones we've decided to make illegal) for decades, giving thousands of test subjects all varieties of drugs and studying their effects. He has a long-standing inside view of NIDA and the drug research political bureaucracy. Next, he is gifted in explaining the ways in which the War on Drugs affects the research agendas of his colleagues, as well as the hidden consequences of this research. Finally, as a Black man, to be so open and honest about his own "grown-up" recreational drug use in our racist and antidrug society is courageous. In his masterful book *Drug Use for Grown-Ups*, it is instructive to read about how he was able to break out of the anti-cannabis cognitive echo chamber in which he was firmly ensconced as a government-funded drug researcher.

According to a 2020 piece by Dr. Hart, "Exaggerating Harmful Drug Effects on the Brain Is Killing Black People,"

> There is a disturbing tendency among many neuroimaging drug researchers to interpret any brain differences between drug users and non–drug users as deficits representing substantial loss of function (i.e., brain damage). In reality, such differences reflect the normal range of variability found in the human brain. Stated differently, *brain differences do not necessarily equate to brain damage*. So, as you read the brain-imaging literature, be on guard for the inappropriate use of terms—such as alterations, atrophy, deterioration, and reductions, among others—that imply a change has occurred. *In order to measure a real change, multiple brain scans need to be completed at different time points.*[11] (emphasis added)

In *Drug Use for Grown-Ups*, Dr. Carl Hart bluntly points out, "There are virtually no data on humans indicating *responsible recreational drug use* causes brain abnormalities in otherwise healthy individuals" (emphasis added). He goes on to explain,

> Because brain images are typically collected at only a single time point for both [drug using and non–drug using] participants, it's nearly impossible

to determine whether active drug use caused any observed differences. Any differences could have existed before the initiation of drug use.[12]

Hart mentions several other problems with this type of study, including insufficient factoring in of tobacco and alcohol, which skew the results. He points out that there should be a third comparison group, which uses tobacco and alcohol but not cannabis, to see the extent to which these two are contributing to any changes that are seen in the brains, apart from the cannabis.

Also, as most of these tests don't measure behavior, it is impossible to state the importance or significance of any brain differences you might find—you are just speculating. In my experience, as I've discussed, this speculation often involves referring to other studies with similar methodological flaws, creating an echo chamber. As my brother David, who is an astrobiologist and a brilliant writer (and also a fellow of the American Association for the Advancement of Science), put it, "inconclusive studies lead to a body of opinion which is used to justify other inconclusive studies."

As Dr. Hart says (in a different interview), "I'm disappointed that scientists are still able to publish high-profile papers that only look at neuroimaging without a behavioral endpoint." Dr. Hart also comments on the cultural implications of these scary-sounding but less than helpful brain-imaging studies,

> It took me a long time to see the damage my field was doing to communities like the one from which I came. I was too busy for too long being a soldier in the regime, caught up in the cause of "proving" how damaging drug use is to the brain. And because my intense actions aligned with the dominant perspective held at the National Institute on Drug Abuse (NIDA)—my primary funder—I personally benefited. I was awarded multimillion-dollar grants to conduct my research, and I served on some of the most prestigious committees in the area of neuropsychopharmacology. I also was awarded tenure at my university, which, importantly, allows me to speak so freely here and elsewhere.[13]

When we look at the few longitudinal studies that exist—the kind of studies that seem most helpful—what do we see? One study, "Longitudinal Study of Hippocampal Volumes in Heavy Cannabis Users," followed young adults, ages eighteen to twenty-four, with an MRI and a comprehensive psychological assessment for three years. There were changes in the size of the hippocampi, but they were the same in both groups, the group that started smoking cannabis on average at age sixteen and who smoked, on average, five times a week versus the group that never used cannabis. The authors concluded,

> This is the first longitudinal examination of hippocampal neuroanatomical changes in young adults over a three-year time period. *Contrary to our hypothesis, heavy cannabis users showed no significant differences compared to healthy controls in volume nor shape of the hippocampus, neither cross-sectionally, nor over time.*[14] (emphasis added)

This study did the basic things that Dr. Hart says you need to do for it to be informative and resulted in a "no brain change or damage" conclusion.

Taking another of Dr. Hart's suggestions, what if researchers more meticulously controlled for alcohol and tobacco? A 2015 study, "Daily Marijuana Use Is Not Associated with Brain Morphometric Measures in Adolescents or Adults," did just that:

> Groups were matched on a critical confounding variable, alcohol use, to a far greater degree than in previously published studies. . . . The groups were closely matched on an alcohol problem measure (AUDIT) and were not different on many possible confounding variables (e.g., tobacco use, depression, impulsivity, age, and gender).[15]

They studied "structures suggested to be associated with marijuana use, as follows: the nucleus accumbens, amygdala, hippocampus, and cerebellum." What did they find?

> No statistically significant differences were found between daily users and nonusers on volume or shape in the regions of interest. Effect sizes suggest that the failure to find differences was not due to a lack of statistical power, but rather was due to the lack of even a modest effect. In sum, the results indicate that, when carefully controlling for alcohol use, gender, age, and other variables, *there is no association between marijuana use and standard volumetric or shape measurements of subcortical structures.*[16] (emphasis added)

They make several other observations that are helpful. First, as I've alluded to, "The press may not cite studies that do not find sensational effects, but these studies are still extremely important." Hear, hear!

They make a point about confounding variables in cannabis studies:

> Alcohol is not the only potential confounding variable in studies on marijuana. A key difference between marijuana users and control subjects is often the fact that users are willing to engage in a high-risk, illegal behavior while control subjects are not.[17]

Yes, I remember that in high school, it was sort of axiomatic that those of us who used cannabis weren't your typical obedient students.

They even found that different studies were using different software to analyze the brain images and that this could significantly change the size of the effects being observed.

Finally, they contextualize their findings:

> It is important to note that the current study does not "prove" that marijuana has no effect on brain morphology. In fact, it is virtually impossible to prove that an effect does not exist. The point of hypothesis testing is not to prove the null hypothesis, but to reject the null hypothesis, which cannot be rejected in this study.[18]

Or, as they taught us in philosophy class, it is difficult to prove a negative.

Taking into account another of Dr. Hart's suggestions, what happens when you simultaneously study the brains and do cognitive testing? In a 2019 study, "Preliminary Results from a Pilot Study Examining Brain Structure in Older Adult Cannabis Users and Nonusers," the researchers compared long-standing cannabis users versus nonusers. The subjects were in their late sixties. The users had been partaking of cannabis for decades. The study found that "users and nonusers did not differ in terms of total gray or white matter volumes controlling for age and depression symptoms," though there were slight enlargements in certain parts of the brains of the cannabis users. The two groups performed equally on the cognitive testing, and the report concludes, "Cannabis use likely does not have a widespread impact on overall cortical volume while controlling for age."[19]

For the sake of speculation, even if cannabis did change the brain, which has not been established, is this necessarily for the worse? Say it made you smarter or more creative or cognitively flexible and neuroplastic, or just nicer? Is all change inherently bad? In teenagers, this of course makes us nervous, because we don't know what the long-term consequences of any changes might be. It is difficult to argue against the idea that there's no reason to mess with nature and no reason to conduct an experiment on ourselves at an age when our brains are still rapidly developing.

I do wonder why cannabis-using humans would evolve, or if cannabis would evolve with us for so much of our journey, if it truly harmed our cognition more than it helped us adapt. Wouldn't those who used it at a young age (and for much of our history, everyone was at a young age, as people didn't live as long) be at a selective disadvantage if it harmed us?

Maybe some harmful traits are outweighed by other traits that are beneficial. An example of this phenomenon in nature is the evolution of sickle-cell anemia. This miserable, painful condition was adaptive in parts of Africa because the sickled cells are more difficult to infect with the malaria parasite, so people who carried these traits were more likely to survive and reproduce.

Could the cannabis increase in creativity and cognitive flexibility, or some other traits, more than offset the short-term memory loss that cannabis causes? With the Drug War mentality, it has been fraught to even speculate about any positives of cannabis, as you get accused of "encouraging drug use."

In searching for the most dynamic cannabis researchers, I'd start with Dr. Staci Gruber of Harvard Medical's McLean Hospital in Belmont, Massachusetts, not because there is anything special per se about Harvard, except for good branding, but because there is absolutely something special about Dr. Gruber. As is often the case with cutting-edge people in any field, her background is varied, nonlinear, and diverse. Before getting a PhD in experimental cognitive neuroscience and becoming a world-famous expert in neuroimaging and neuropsychology, she studied jazz studies and vocal performance at the New England Conservatory. Among many other accomplishments, she used her neurocognitive expertise to influence a Supreme Court case which resulted in a ruling that made it illegal to execute minors. Score one for humanity. Bravo, Staci!

With auburn hair, overflowing charisma, humility, and a quick wit, Dr. Gruber's magnetic personality gives her a preternatural ability to impart an astounding amount of fairly complex information in a short period of time. She can do this in digestible and understandable language, without losing people—an uncommon skill for neuroscientists, many of whom communicate with each other in an obscure dialect of Nerdese. Dr. Gruber's ability to explain complex concepts is clearly evident in a five-minute clip where she can be seen testifying before Congress about loosening the politicized and antiquated barriers to cannabis research. Even the elderly Republican congressmen—not particularly up to date on cannabis, or science in general, or—for some—anything reality based for that matter—seemed to follow along.

In 2014, Gruber created the MIND (Marijuana Investigations for Neuroscience Discoveries) center, which was dedicated to understanding the effects of medical marijuana on "cognition, clinical state, quality of life, brain structure and function and related measures." Dr. Gruber had been studying recreational cannabis users for decades and decided to assess if medical cannabis patients and recreational cannabis users were comparable in terms of their cognitive functioning. She was curious if medical cannabis users were subject to the same short-term decrements in memory and other measures that she had seen in heavy recreational users. Almost all of the studies done on cannabis have been done on recreational cannabis users, which has generally meant high THC, low CBD, illegal weed with God knows what in it, unknown interface with medical care (if any), and a variety of other potentially significant deviations from the actual practices of medical marijuana users.

In a 2016 study titled "Splendor in the Grass: A Pilot Study Assessing the Impact of Medical Marijuana on Executive Function," Dr. Gruber followed this hunch of hers—that the cognitive effects of cannabis on medical patients might be different. This work was elaborated upon in a 2018 paper, "The Grass Might Be Greener: Medical Marijuana Patients Exhibit Altered Brain Activity and Improved Executive Function after 3 Months of Treatment." In this work, she evaluated the cognitive functioning of patients who started out as marijuana naive and then again after they had used medical marijuana for three months. When subjected to the exact same testing, these patients demonstrated across-the-board *improvement* in their cognitive function after initiating treatment with medical cannabis.[20] Specifically,

> Following 3 months of treatment, *MMJ patients demonstrated improved task performance* accompanied by changes in brain activation patterns within the cingulate cortex and frontal regions. Interestingly, after MMJ treatment, brain activation patterns appeared more similar to those exhibited by healthy controls from previous studies than at pre-treatment, *suggestive of a potential normalization of brain function relative to baseline.* These findings suggest that MMJ use may result in different effects relative to recreational marijuana (MJ) use, as recreational consumers have been shown to exhibit decrements in task performance accompanied by altered brain activation. Moreover, *patients in the current study also reported improvements in clinical state and health-related measures as well as notable decreases in prescription medication use, particularly opioids and benzodiazepines after 3 months of treatment.*[21] (emphasis added)

Why would this be the case? If recreational marijuana use causes a measurable decline in cognitive functioning, at least temporarily, how could medical cannabis use improve functioning? Weed is weed, stoned is stoned, so why should the results swing in the opposite direction?

Dr. Gruber posits several possible explanations. The most obvious one is symptom alleviation. People who contend with less of a disturbance in their mood and sleep, with better-controlled chronic pain, will be less exhausted and anxious and will be thinking more clearly. That's true for any of us after a good night's sleep or when our goddamn headache finally goes away. But, as discussed elsewhere (see chapter 21), many "recreational" patients have always used cannabis medically, and vice versa, so this explanation isn't complete. Is it a question of product choice? The most obvious point of recreational use is to get high, which arguably involves maximizing THC content, but medical users often/ideally select products with more healthful cannabinoids, such as CBD, that have been shown to offset some of the side effects of THC. Maybe they also just use lower amounts of THC as well, as the point is to feel better, not to get stoned. Other possible explanations are that perhaps there was less chronic exposure to the cannabis in these new medical patients—though this implies that chronic exposure is detrimental to adults, in a toxic, brain-damaging sort of way, which certainly hasn't been demonstrated yet. Age of onset might be an alternative explanation, as most recreational users start in their teens, and many medical users start in adulthood. Finally, medical users, due to the relief they found with cannabis, were using fewer other medications, such as opiates and benzodiazepines (e.g., Valium, Ativan), which themselves can greatly interfere with cognitive functioning.

In a 2021 follow-up study, "An Observational, Longitudinal Study of Cognition in Medical Cannabis Patients over the Course of 12 Months of Treatment: Preliminary Results," according to their analysis, the benefits to cognition did persist at twelve months. Using some more detailed analytics, they concluded that the observed benefit is not a direct result of the cannabis but more an indirect effect of clinical improvement. As they say, "patients may think more clearly if they feel better overall." Further, "greater improvement of clinical state over time was significantly associated with increased CBD exposure," which either means that the CBD is healthful, that CBD protects from the effects of THC, or that the cannabis works a lot better with CBD on board.[22]

Assuming the results hold, they inform several aspects of the "is cannabis a safe and effective medicine?" debate. To start, they provide further reassurance about safety in patients that start medical cannabis as adults—there were no indications of worsened functioning. This also sounds like a good harm reduction recipe for making cannabis use safer—lower the THC, raise the CBD, and use cannabis modestly to address your most troublesome symptoms.

While the experts wrestle with these research questions about relative harms and benefits, one thing that reasonable people can agree on is that, with our current level of knowledge (or lack thereof), cannabis is too risky for young developing brains without an overriding medical indication. For all the adolescents out there, the best advice I can give at present is to "just say wait," which, unfortunately, is *exactly* what adolescents aren't good at doing.

## CHAPTER THIRTEEN

# TEENS

## Just Say Wait

If cannabis appears not to be particularly harmful to the cognition of people who started as adults and who use it modestly or medically, what about for teens? The data has been interpreted as more concerning for teens than for adults, though the issue hasn't been definitively settled because much of the data is contradictory, biased, or inconclusive. However, because there are so many unknowns, and since there does exist some evidence that it may harm the brains of teens, *it is strongly recommended that teens avoid weed*. Ideally, we'd convince them to "just say wait" until twenty-one, but more realistically, and most crucially from the brain's perspective, at least until eighteen. Waiting until twenty-five—when the brain actually stops developing—is a hard sell. This is particularly true because the legal drinking age is twenty-one. As alcohol is more harmful than cannabis on virtually all parameters, and as our society couldn't function without alcohol for five minutes, few would be inclined to take a legal age for alcohol or cannabis use of twenty-five seriously.

Potential harm to the teen brain isn't an effective argument in favor of continued prohibition or criminalization. Teen rates have *not* been rising in states that have legalized. In fact, some evidence has these rates going down, as drug dealers don't bother to check IDs, but dispensary staff are required to. Even the head of NIDA, Nora Volkow, has recently conceded that teen rates haven't been rising in legal states.

I have colleagues who cite the uncertainty of the effect on teen brains as an argument against legalization: "The policy [of newly re-legalizing cannabis] is ahead of the science." This begs the question: is our current policy—of arresting teens, arresting young moms, separating families, giving teens criminal records and exposure to actual criminals and harder-core drug users, impoverishing minorities or their families who use cannabis via asset forfeiture, and exaggerating the harms so that no one truly believes in them—any better for teen brains? Why should this punitive, destructive system be the default? It seems that it should be the opposite, both ethically and pragmatically.

Cannabis has (almost) always been readily accessible, independent of prohibition or legalization. It has long been easy for teens to get weed, even at the height of the Reagan years—believe me; I was a teenager then. It was a buyer's market at Wellesley High School when I was there from 1980 to 1984.

Unfortunately, "just say wait" conflicts with the natural teen tendency to explore, rebel, and take risks. From the point of view of curious, mischievous teens, cannabis is extraordinarily tempting. It's not a big secret that weed enhances your sensations in a pleasant and interesting manner, and its occasional use likely isn't *that* dangerous compared to other ways to rebel, such as binge drinking or risky sexual behavior (as long as you don't drive under the influence of cannabis or participate in risky sexual behavior). I don't believe that by acknowledging the benefits of cannabis—which teens already know about—you are encouraging its use. I feel we come across as more credible when we acknowledge what has been common knowledge for several generations (actually millennia) and then explain why it might not be a good idea to use cannabis *just yet*.

What is more dangerous is if, during the process of simple experimentation, a teen learns to reflexively use cannabis to make their teenage angst, insecurity, loneliness, boredom, and other problems temporarily disappear. This can be awfully alluring as, now, with one discreet vape pen hidden in your pocket, you can so easily switch a bad feeling for a good feeling. This is a hallmark of how many addicted people learn how to not cope with their feelings. It is one reason why weed may be particularly addictive for teens, as they can rapidly learn to self-medicate feelings that need to be tolerated or addressed, not medicated.

So, how to best keep teens off weed? I vote for honest communication and truthful education, sort of like an anti-DARE program where we give reality-based information and offer nonstigmatizing help to kids who get into trouble. Let's bring it all out into the open. That might make it less fun and exciting for the teens too.

Why might cannabis be more harmful for teens than adults?

The teenage brain is rapidly growing and reorganizing during adolescence and beyond. It is felt to be particularly vulnerable to all types of outside insults, regardless of whether it is cannabis, alcohol, environmental toxins, or various other legal and illegal substances that people commonly consume. The endocannabinoid system is particularly important to many aspects of the neurodevelopmental process. Cannabis use in adolescents is hypothesized to interfere with synaptic "pruning," the process by which developing brains eliminate unneeded connections and pathways.

The concern is that heavy cannabis use may affect the structure and connectivity of certain parts of the brain, such as the prefrontal cortices, which are critical for executive function, or the hippocampi, which are where our memory consolidation takes place. The worry is that this might cause lasting damage. The worst scenario, according to some studies, is heavy use before sixteen. The longer you wait, and the less you use, the better off you are.

How harmful is it?

We don't actually know how harmful, or even if, truly, cannabis is harmful, for the teenage brain. The reasons for this are nicely summarized by a 2020 article in the *Proceedings of the National Academy of Sciences*, "Cannabis and the Adolescent Brain." According to this piece,

> Many observational studies have *suggested* that adolescent cannabis use *may be linked* to long-term harms, including cognitive impairment . . . but in almost every area that researchers have examined, *results have been inconclusive* regarding the precise nature and strength of these associations. In particular, there's *little consensus* as to whether cannabis directly causes long-term health harms in people, whether it's one of a number of risk factors, or whether it simply correlates with other root causes.[1] (emphasis added)

Observational studies aren't as effective because it is unclear if the differences between the cannabis users and nonusers existed before the cannabis use, making it difficult to say if the differences are *due* to the cannabis use.

Other obstacles to knowing the full dangers of cannabis to teens include that it is unethical to run tests on actual adolescents (as much as some of them might appreciate the free weed . . .). Doctors and researchers generally aren't allowed to deliberately give people substances that might be harmful in order to see if they are harmful, except under highly specified circumstances.

Another factor to consider when looking at the studies that have been done on teens and cognition is that most were done on illegal street cannabis. They might not reflect the effects of or actual harms of legal, regulated cannabis. It's like studying the effects of moonshine on the teenage brain—who knows what it's contaminated with and how much they are actually using. Obviously that wouldn't be considered very helpful research in terms of illuminating the effects of legal alcohol.

I mostly take care of adult cannabis patients. With the teenage cases that I am involved with (as the second doctor—the first being a pediatrician, per Massachusetts law), it seems like a very different process that would result in much less harm than the de facto process of teens self-medicating and not telling their parents, which happens so frequently. Within the legal rubric, dosages are monitored, weed is procured from a legal dispensary, parents are involved, and use is well thought out, with predetermined goals, contracting, and follow-up. We supplement with CBD and evaluate if the cannabis is helping or harming different aspects of their lives, including schoolwork. It is important to remember that *none* of the studies on harm in teens reflect this paradigm. It is all based on kids procuring God knows what illegally, with no monitoring.

What does the 2017 NASEM study say? Basically that we don't know, because in most of the studies, adolescents were mixed in with adults—which might sufficiently dilute any findings for the adolescents so that they don't show up. Also, again, these studies were observational in nature. NASEM says, "The evidence for an association between cannabis use and effects on cognitive development during adolescence is limited at this time." But they are quite eager to find out, for the following reasons, all of which are also excellent reasons to err heavily on the side of caution with cannabis and teenagers:

> Data in the cited systematic reviews and elsewhere continue to indicate that an early age of initiation [of cannabis] tends to be connected to bigger differences in brain function during adulthood. Second, the brain does not complete development until approximately age 25, and data

from the field of alcohol use reflect that substance use exposure during this period when the brain undergoes rapid transformation could have a more lasting impact on cognitive performance. This interference in cognitive function during the adolescent and emerging adult years, which overlap with the critical period in which many youths' and young adults' primary responsibility is to be receiving their education, *could very well interfere with these individuals' ability to optimally perform in school and other educational settings.*[2] (emphasis added)

"Could very well" sounds speculative. If there is an impact on cognitive performance, I don't think it is likely to be pronounced enough to materially interfere with education during the "emerging adult years." Possibly in mega-stoners, who are stoned throughout the school day, but they obviously have other problems, and who knows to what extent the cannabis is contributing. Cannabis helped me write papers in high school. We smoked acres upon acres at Swarthmore College, and everyone went on to become a leader in one field or another. Some people use cannabis to self-treat their ADHD, and it enables them to function in school (see chapter 19). Others get into trouble with cannabis and use it to smoke away their emotional challenges or boredom. You just can't generalize, stereotype, or put everyone in the same bucket.

Since the NASEM report came out in 2017, there have been a number of studies that have added to the conflicting nature of our data base. A recent longitudinal study—exactly the type of study we need—from Germany, in the journal *Cognitive Development*, called "Residual Effects of Cannabis-Use on Neuropsychological Functioning," studied eight hundred matched adolescent cannabis users versus nonusers at age fourteen and then nineteen. It comes up with some surprising conclusions:

> Cross-sectionally, we detected no significant neurocognitive differences before initiation of drug use. However, after controlling for confounders, light cannabis use as well as late-onset thereof was associated with *increased decision-making skills* both cross-sectionally at follow-up as well as longitudinally compared to non-using controls.
>
> In summary, our data suggests that *decision-making is not impaired when cannabis is used in moderation and onset of use occurs after the age of 15.* In addition, we find no evidence to support the presumption that

cannabis consumption leads to a decline in neurocognitive ability.[3] (emphasis added)

This goes back to my earlier comment, in the previous chapter, that whether cannabis improves or worsens cognitive abilities depends on *which* abilities you test for and how you test for them. Cannabis changes your thinking, but who's to say, really, with what we know so far, if the changes, on the whole, are for better or worse (assuming the brain isn't being harmed)?

In their discussion, they elaborate,

> When looking at the adjusted means, decision-making skills in light cannabis users improved from age 14 to 19 while control group performance remained approximately the same.[4]

They refer to other studies that show stable or improved decision making with cannabis. After controlling for confounders, "we found no evidence of effects of cannabis on the remaining neurocognitive variables such as attention, working memory, short-term memory and risk-taking."[5]

In essence, we are presented with a bunch of American (Drug War era) observational studies that show harm and a well-done, more recent, non–Drug War era longitudinal German study that shows no harm and possible benefit. Where does that leave us? Close to where we started: we don't know, but we're more open-minded about an alternative narrative that maybe too much attention has historically been given to observational studies claiming that cannabis harms teens.

Several studies show that cannabis causes at most a small, short-lived cognitive effect that resolves in a matter of days or, at the most, weeks. A 2018 study, published in *JAMA Psychiatry*, called "Association of Cannabis with Cognitive Functioning in Adolescents and Young Adults: A Systematic Review and Meta-analysis," studied sixty-nine studies of 2,152 cannabis users with an average age of twenty. They found a "small overall effect size" on cognition between the heavy cannabis users and the nonusers. Importantly, this "did not vary by sample age or age at cannabis use onset." And here's the kicker: *in studies requiring an abstinence period of longer than seventy-two hours, the cognitive effects disappeared.* They mention that "reported effect sizes may actually be overestimates, considering results from measures of bias." For example, they cite publication bias, "in which statistically significant findings are more likely to be published." Finally, "reported deficits may reflect residual effects from acute use or withdrawal."[6]

Even the not particularly pro-cannabis addiction department of my home institution came out with a 2018 randomized controlled trial, "One Month of Cannabis Abstinence in Adolescents and Young Adults Is Associated with Improved Memory," where they took young cannabis users (ages sixteen to twenty-five) and had a random group of them stop using cannabis, which they verified with drug testing. They concluded,

> This study suggests that cannabis abstinence is associated with improvements in verbal learning that appear to occur largely in the first week following last use.[7]

Unfortunately, they didn't have a non–cannabis using control group, so it's hard to say what came first and what caused what. According to the study,

> Without comparison to a non-using sample or knowledge of performance prior to the initiation of cannabis use, it is difficult to interpret the role of cannabis in affecting domains that did not improve more among abstainers compared to non-abstainers, such as tasks of attention, visual span capacity, short-term visual recognition memory, and verbal delayed recall. There are several possible explanations . . . [including that] cannabis does not adversely impact attention or these other domains, thus no improvement over practice effects would be evident with abstinence.[8]

It would also have been interesting if they had included a task that some people do better on with cannabis—such as creative writing, art, or some other right-brained creative or intuitive activity—and see if that got *worse* with the people who abstained for a month. If you only look in one direction, you might not see interesting things in the direction you aren't observing.

Many are pinning their hopes on the ongoing NIH-funded ABCD (adolescent brain cognitive development) study, which takes advantage of the fact that, while we can't experiment on teens, they have an unfortunate penchant for experimenting on themselves, with cannabis and other substances. This description explains the ABCD study's methods and goals:

The ABCD study completed enrollment in 2018, recruiting nearly 12,000 children aged 9 or 10, and will follow the children through roughly age 20. Researchers . . . have already collected the baseline brain images, genetic information, and neuropsychological, behavioral, and many other health measures. Over time, the project aims to characterize normal adolescent brain and cognitive development and tease apart multiple factors that can influence those processes, such as screen time, sports injuries, and—importantly—substance use.

By starting at a relatively young age and taking a diverse demographic, geographic, and socioeconomic sample, researchers intend to capture detailed information on circumstances that precede substance use and could influence risks. And by including 2,100 people who are either twins or triplets, they plan to compare many cannabis-using and non-using siblings, to isolate the effects of genetic and family factors. Such comparisons could also help reveal whether some youths are more predisposed than others to use cannabis or are more vulnerable to its effects on the brain.[9]

Hopefully, they won't find a way to put a finger on the scales of this U.S. government funded and administered study to nudge it toward inflating harm. If there were benefits, which could be parlayed into medical treatments, would the tools they are using show them, or are they just organized to find harm? Also, does it distinguish between legal states versus illegal cannabis? Does it include any kids who are working with cannabis clinicians and have their medicine prescribed for them and monitored, with the parents involved?

When I saw that they were using the Marijuana Adolescent Problem Inventory (MAPI) to gauge whether the adolescents are having difficulty with cannabis, it reminded me of the experiment in 2004 where they gave people huge doses of IV THC and then defined "psychosis" as "anxiety, tension, depression, or uncooperativeness" using the Positive and Negative Symptoms Scale (PANSS). According to the PANSS, I'm psychotic every single day I go into my primary care clinic and try to be an effective doctor (even when I've had no cannabis for five years)!

The MAPI asks questions like those in figure 13.1.

| Item # | Item | Loading |
|--------|------|---------|
| 01 | Not able to do your homework or study for a test | 0.61 |
| 02 | Got into fights, acted bad or did mean things | 0.53 |
| 03 | Missed out on other things because you spent too much money on marijuana | 0.66 |
| 04 | Went to work or school high | 0.40 |
| 05 | Caused shame or embarrassment to someone | 0.55 |
| 06 | Neglected your responsibilities | 0.66 |
| 07 | Relatives avoided you | 0.40 |
| 08 | Felt that you needed MORE marijuana than you used to in order to get the same effect | 0.59 |
| 09 | Tried to control your marijuana use by trying to smoke only at certain times of the day or certain places | 0.18 |
| 10 | Had withdrawal symptoms, that is felt sick (irritated or anxious) because you stopped or cut down using marijuana | 0.64 |
| 11 | Noticed an ongoing or unpleasant change in your personality | 0.67 |
| 12 | Felt that you had a problem with marijuana | 0.71 |
| 13 | Missed a day (or part of a day) of school or work | 0.53 |
| 14 | Tried to cut down or quit smoking marijuana | 0.49 |
| 15 | Suddenly found yourself in a place you could not remember getting to | 0.52 |
| 16 | Passed out or fainted suddenly | 0.38 |
| 17 | Had a fight, argument, or bad feelings with a friend | 0.60 |
| 18 | Had a fight, argument, or bad feelings with a family member | 0.53 |
| 19 | Kept smoking marijuana when you promised yourself not to | 0.62 |
| 20 | Felt you were going crazy | 0.60 |
| 21 | Had a bad time | 0.52 |
| 22 | Felt physically or psychologically dependent on marijuana | 0.71 |
| 23 | Was told by a friend or neighbor to cut down on smoking marijuana | 0.59 |

**Figure 13.1. Marijuana Adolescent Problem Inventory (MAPI).** *Source:* Ashley A. Knapp et al., "Psychometric Assessment of the Marijuana Adolescent Problem Inventory," *Addictive Behavior* 79 (April 2018), https://www.ncbi.nlm.nih.gov/labs/pmc/articles/PMC5851012.

I wonder if, anywhere, there exist kids who have never used cannabis but

- had a bad time;

- caused shame or embarrassment to someone;

- had a fight, argument, or bad feelings with a friend or family member;

- was not able to do their homework; or

- neglected their responsibilities.

These questions don't seem particularly specific for cannabis. They seem more specific to "being a teenager." To have overly inclusive criteria to detect cannabis-related harms is one way to put a finger on the scale.

It is important to watch out for bias for a number of reasons. As discussed, bias has been baked (pun probably not intended) into so much of this research in the form of confirmation bias, publication bias, "fishing" bias, and cultural and financial pressure to find negative things about weed. On a practical level, if this study is viewed as not entirely neutral, people aren't going to believe the results, especially the millions of cannabis users and supporters who are suffering from "boy who cried wolf" syndrome (or "boy flat-out lied and fabricated the existence of a wolf" syndrome) about U.S. government–funded studies on cannabis-related purported harms.

Some of the researchers already appear convinced that cannabis causes deficits, and this could plausibly introduce a degree of confirmation bias. As reported in Medscape,

> "My work, as well as the work of a lot of other colleagues, has shown that younger kids do have more negative consequences from more regular cannabis exposure," said Krista Lisdahl, PhD, director of the Brain Imaging and Neuropsychology Laboratory at the University of Wisconsin–Milwaukee and principal investigator in the National Institutes of Health's ongoing Adolescent Brain Cognitive Development Study. "What we tend to see is mild to moderate reductions in verbal memory, complex attention—like cognitive control—problem solving, and psychomotor states."[10]

No slight intended to Dr. Lisdahl, but it would be more scientifically helpful if people went into the ABCD study with a blank slate of expectations. They could ask, from scratch, is cannabis harmful or helpful? That is, let's not merely confirm our beliefs that cannabis is harmful (along with the cultural and socioeconomic biases that these beliefs are often based on, as per the above discussions).

I'm not accusing anyone of anything. I'm just saying let's be careful not to repeat the mistakes of the past. There is very little room for error if this study is going to be widely accepted and believed.

Does cannabis lower IQ? This has been a persistent propaganda point against cannabis since the dawn of the Drug War. This idea was given new life by a 2012 study, "Persistent Cannabis Users Show Neuropsychological Decline from Childhood to Midlife," by lead researcher Madeline Meier. Dr. Meier was able to "show" a drop in IQ from adolescence to adulthood: "Persistent cannabis use was associated with neuropsychological decline broadly across domains of functioning." Even worse, *"Informants also reported noticing more cognitive problems for persistent cannabis users."*[11] (This sounds profoundly unobjective—about as far from the objectivity of an RCT as you can get while remaining on planet Earth! Discussed a little later.) Even worse,

> Impairment was concentrated among adolescent-onset cannabis users, with more persistent use associated with greater decline. Further, cessation of cannabis use did not fully restore neuropsychological functioning among adolescent-onset cannabis users. *Findings are suggestive of a neurotoxic effect of cannabis on the adolescent brain.*[12] (emphasis added)

This study received a phenomenal amount of attention, with news headlines across the world decrying the fact that "Teen Cannabis Use Lowers IQ."

The only problem was that there were terminal problems raised about the methodology. A year later, an article came out called "Correlations between Cannabis Use and IQ Change in the Dunedin Cohort Are Consistent with Confounding from Socioeconomic Status," which showed that "existing research suggests an alternative confounding model based on time-varying effects of socioeconomic status on IQ."[13] In other words, Meier didn't accurately and adequately factor in socioeconomic factors (i.e., disadvantaged kids tend to do worse on standardized tests). When this was factored back in, the IQ drop disappeared. Needless to say, these boring, if vital, corrections of exciting studies don't get a fraction of the press that the original studies do, however erroneous.

By 2017, Dr. Meier was back at it, with another longitudinal twin study, "Associations between Adolescent Cannabis Use and Neuropsychological Decline: A Longitudinal Co-twin Control Study," which concluded:

Short-term cannabis use in adolescence *does not appear to cause IQ decline or impair executive functions*, even when cannabis use reaches the level of dependence. *Family background factors explain why adolescent cannabis users perform worse on IQ and executive function tests.*[14] (emphasis added)

Twin studies are particularly powerful, as twins share genetics and often upbringing as well. According to NIDA director Nora Volkow and others,

This study was particularly insightful because of a large sample size ($n = 1989$) and IQ assessments prior to the onset of cannabis use (IQ obtained at age 5, 12, and 18). It demonstrated that adolescents who used cannabis had a lower childhood IQ and a lower IQ at 18 than non-users, but that *there was no decline in IQ from pre- to post-cannabis use.*[15] (emphasis added)

Volkow goes on to speculate that "lower IQ may be a risk factor for cannabis abuse rather than the use of cannabis resulting in neuropsychological decline."[16]

After fifty years of assuming that cannabis lowered intelligence and then "proving" it with these observational studies, through a path littered with thousands of harmful, stigmatizing newspaper headlines about "brain-damaged youth" along the way, it looks like the relationship might go the other way: lower IQ (often related to poverty and other socioeconomic disadvantages) is a risk for cannabis use.

Does this sound familiar? This is reminiscent of an evolution of thought detailed in chapter 8 where, according to the reality painted about cannabis by the U.S. government, "cannabis caused schizophrenia" for fifty years until it started looking more like the genetic tendency toward schizophrenia might also be causing the propensity toward excess cannabis in these patients (or that cannabis may be one of many factors that can predispose toward psychosis, including stimulants, tobacco, etc.).

One question is: why do people keep citing the now obsolete (discredited) 2012 Meier study? Dozens of articles I've read researching this book cite the flawed 2012 study, not the more credible 2017 study. Is it deliberate that people are using the wrong study, for propaganda points, or is it because the rebuttals and the negative studies get so much less press and attention? At my hospital, after hearing an addictionologist speak about cannabis and listening to him discuss the infamous IQ drop, I sent him the 2013 rebuttal and the 2017 study showing no decline. He replied, "I had no idea." (Brief editorial: this is a consequence of the American Society of Addiction Medicine and other such groups almost exclusively publicizing studies that have anti-cannabis conclusions and perhaps is an indication that their members would be better equipped if exposed to a more balanced menu of information.)

How do teenager cannabis users fare as adults? This is another area of disagreement between the cannabis community and the research community. NASEM states, "Cannabis use during adolescence is related to impairments in subsequent academic achievement and education, employment and income, and social relationships and social roles." Keep in mind Dr. Volkow's statement above that "it looks like the relationship might go the other way: lower IQ is a risk for cannabis use." Hmm . . . I wonder how having a lower IQ (and the social conditions—poverty, racism—that result in low IQ tests) could *possibly* affect subsequent academic achievement. Could it be that cannabis is, again, blamed erroneously?

How can you truly factor out poverty, trauma, and so many of the other issues that may alternatively explain these outcomes that co-occur with cannabis use? What about tobacco? A 2016 study, "Are IQ and Educational Outcomes in Teenagers Related to Their Cannabis Use? A Prospective Cohort Study," showed that,

> after full adjustment, those who had used cannabis ≥50 times did not differ from never-users on either IQ or educational performance. *Adjusting for group differences in cigarette smoking dramatically attenuated the associations between cannabis use and both outcomes, and further analyses demonstrated robust associations between cigarette use and educational outcomes, even with cannabis users excluded.* These findings suggest that adolescent cannabis use is *not* associated with IQ or educational performance once adjustment is made for potential confounds, in particular adolescent cigarette use.[17] (emphasis added)

Even if disadvantaged kids—poverty, tobacco use, worse health care—*are* shown to be more likely to use cannabis and subsequently to have lower educational outcomes, this doesn't show that cannabis *causes* the lower educational outcomes.

A 2021 study, "Associations between Adolescent Cannabis Use and Young-Adult Functioning in Three Longitudinal Twin Studies," combined three longitudinal twin studies, to give it significant statistical power, and concluded:

> We observed few instances in which cannabis use remained associated with difficulties in other domains once familial factors were accounted for. *These findings thus provide evidence against the notion that adolescent cannabis use has substantial, long-term effects on emotional and cognitive functioning*, suggesting instead that most negative effects on young-adult well-being are likely to proceed through educational pathways.[18] (emphasis added)

The theory promulgated here is that cannabis causes kids to "disengage from their education." The theory is that if you are stoned instead of doing homework or fuzzy the next day from being really high, you won't do as well in school or sports. This in a way makes sense, but it seems like it would only apply to daily, heavy stoners who did this to the exclusion of other activities. In these cases, cannabis is perhaps more of a symptom than a cause. Most of the longer-term casualties from my high school days seem to have been from alcohol, not from cannabis.

Madeline Meier—yes, the same Madeline Meier who seems to be trying to prove both sides of this issue—came up with a similar conclusion from a longitudinal study that she performed: that it was the environment not the pot. In a 2020 piece, "Cannabis Use and Psychosocial Functioning: Evidence from Prospective Longitudinal Studies," she noted that cannabis use was associated with poorer psychosocial functioning in some domains but that "associations are likely attributable to a combination of causal and non-causal mechanisms, *with causal mechanisms likely to be social, not neurotoxic in nature*"[19] (emphasis added).

By 2022, Dr. Meier was again attempting to demonstrate that cannabis lowers IQ, in a piece titled "Long-Term Cannabis Use and Cognitive Reserves and Hippocampal Volume in Midlife." She violated most of Dr. Carl Hart's sensible suggestions about how to conduct helpful drug research. Nevertheless, it got robust, loud headlines: "Cannabis Causes IQ Drop." It's not a twin study, so it is prima facie less valid than her previous study. Per its "limitations" section, it was plagued by low numbers and a lack of statistical power. She again relied on "informant-reported memory and attention problems." Why would Dr. Meier need to put this into her study (unless the numbers themselves weren't adequate to prove her point)? It's the least scientific thing I've ever heard of. As an example, every time my ex-wife was mad at me, for anything, she thought I had "memory and attention problems." Does that lend evidence to the idea my IQ is lower from my past cannabis use?

Further, they found "smaller hippocampal volumes," but this was, again, studied only *at one point in time*, at age forty-five, so you can't say anything about cause and effect. Remember Dr. Hart's reminder:

> Because brain images are typically collected at only a single time point for both [drug-using and non–drug using] participants, it's nearly impossible to determine whether active drug use caused any observed differences. Any differences could have existed before the initiation of drug use.[20]

Further, according to the Meier study, "smaller hippocampal volume did not statistically mediate associations between persistence of cannabis use and cognitive deficits." So it wasn't the same people that had both lower IQ (purportedly) and a smaller hippocampus? It is guilt by association?

Finally, most damaging in my opinion, from Meier's study,

> Long-term cannabis users also use tobacco, alcohol, and other illicit drugs. Disentangling cannabis effects from other substances is challenging. We did not limit analyses to cannabis-only users because they are unrepresentative of cannabis users.[21]

What possible reason could there be for not testing the "cannabis-only" people separately if they are trying to find out whether *cannabis* and not *cannabis along with other behaviors* is responsible for any changes in IQ or cognition that you find? Unless they didn't have the numbers to reach statistical validity. If this is the case, just say that—but then, no headlines, no glory, no funding. There are also a lot of problems with IQ testing in general (i.e., it's not very accurate and is sensitive to many variables such as poverty). More specifically, when Meier says that these cannabis users have "below-average IQ as adults"—the range for normal I.Q. is 85–115 (i.e., one standard deviation), and the purported drop she shows is to 93.8 (despite all of her methodological flaws)—this is not an accurate statement.

This study was published in the *American Journal of Psychiatry* and will be piped directly into the brains of today's psychiatrists, who will "have no idea" about the nuanced ways in which this data doesn't support what is proclaimed in the headlines. Meier also tried to link this IQ drop to a propensity toward dementia to make it sound even scarier.

What is the best strategy to keep teens away from cannabis? All this uncertainty tells us is that we still don't know definitively if cannabis is bad for teens, or how bad it is (if it is bad). This doesn't exonerate cannabis or prove that it is safe for most teens—remember our null hypothesis. Until the critical question of harm to teens is finally and fully cleared up, we need to uniformly discourage teen usage. And while some experimentation isn't shocking to any parents who understand teens, it is hard to envision a future circumstance when we would not discourage teens from using cannabis for a whole host of reasons, even as it doesn't prove to be neurotoxic. (The short-circuiting of "learning how to cope with unpleasant emotions" by hitting the vape is what worries me the most, personally.)

Reflex censorship isn't effective.

I tweeted a study, from the Spanish journal *Healthcare*, "The Influence of Cannabis and Alcohol Use on Sexuality: An Observational Study in Young People (18–30 Years)," which was represented by the headline, "Young People Who Use Marijuana Have Better Orgasms and Sex." I added the comment, "Study proves what humans have known about cannabis for 5,000 years. . . . Rumor has it, it's not just young people." In response, a pediatric psychiatrist (whom I like and respect) responded with an angry tweet: "Stop promoting cannabis for youth. You're a freaking doctor for God's sake."

My pediatric psychiatric colleague apparently was worried that I was undermining the long-standing strategy of pretending that cannabis doesn't have benefits and isn't enjoyable so that teenagers won't ever find this out. In effect, he was saying, "Don't share this information because some of the subjects, who are under 25, when the brain stops fully developing, might read it and be encouraged to use cannabis."

Of course, half of teenagers will have tried cannabis, and since they do tend to speak with the other half, most of them will have figured out that it can be fun and has some benefits. This is consistent with "just say wait." It strikes me as somewhat paternalistic, old-fashioned, and, most of all, a needless squandering of adult credibility to try to control what teenagers do by restricting or manipulating the information they have access to—particularly in this day and age. This attitude is reminiscent of when MTV would blur out the cannabis images, which only made them more enticing, or radio stations would blur out the word "joint" in the Tom Petty song "You Don't Know How It Feels."

I can understand the logic that states there's no reason to gratuitously contribute to a teenager's positive view of cannabis. It has been shown that teenagers' perception of cannabis is becoming less characterized by fears of harmfulness as we are generally having more truthful discussions with them about this subject. Teen consumption rates have been holding quite steady in the legalized states, but the concern is that if teens view pot with a decreasing respect for its dangers, they might be more tempted to indulge.

The problem is that this strategy of misleading teens, or curating what they are exposed to, doesn't work, because teens are smart and read about things themselves. The best example of this is the DARE program, an antidrug education program started in the Reagan era that saturated public schools for many years, where the harms from cannabis were vastly exaggerated and its use was stigmatized. Teens knew from their collective lived experience that much of what DARE was presenting to them was distorted, exaggerated, or fabricated. This immediately discredited the entire DARE message, including what it was saying—which wasn't as inaccurate—about harder drugs like heroin, or more dangerous drugs like alcohol. DARE either accomplished nothing or raised drug usage—at the expense of more than a billion dollars and wasted time.

A study assessing the efficacy of the DARE program concluded, "Greater exposure to the campaign was associated with weaker anti-drug norms and increases in the perceptions that others use marijuana."[22] According to a 2006 article in *Slate*, "A White House Drug Deal Gone Bad," "more exposure to the ads led to higher rates of first-time drug use among certain groups, like 14- to 16-year-olds and white kids."[23] DARE is also responsible for some of the stigma our society has against the millions who are struggling with addiction, which is costing lives. A failure from beginning to end.

My belief is that the best strategy for dealing with teens, radical and groundbreaking as this may be in the drug realm, is to *tell them the truth*. Have open, honest conversations with them. Don't pretend that cannabis isn't enjoyable and doesn't have benefits. That would be like running an abstinence program by explaining that sex doesn't really feel good and people don't enjoy it. Abstinence programs have a near zero percent success rate as it is.

Instead, explain to the teens, in detail, why we think it is dangerous to the developing brain, so they need to wait. Answer their questions honestly, even about your own use. Especially about your own use. If they try to paint you as a hypocrite, remind them that we didn't know as much back then about the harms. This approach has the added benefit of establishing open communication so that, if they do get into trouble with cannabis (or anything else), you are viewed as a trusted partner, not a dishonest jailer. This approach has worked for tobacco and alcohol, both of which are declining in teens. We don't lie to kids about alcohol; they would see through that in a second. Same with weed.

I was consulted on the case of a sixteen-year-old who was having emotional problems and trouble at school. The parents were wondering if cannabis would help, as he had used it on his own and said that his mood was much better regulated and his concentration more improved than it had been by all the pharmaceuticals he'd been put on. I started to discuss the pros and cons of treatment with medical cannabis with the parents, and the interesting thing about this consultation was that the sixteen-year-old had read many of the articles and already knew many of the potential harms and benefits of cannabis. *He was citing specific studies.* This is a kid who was struggling in school, and I had a more informed discussion with him about cannabis than one might have with most doctors. This not only shows that teens are motivated in things they are interested in, but it demonstrates how futile and counterproductive it is to dissemble about cannabis. Had I started exaggerating or trying to scare, he would have completely tuned out in a millisecond and not engaged in what turned out to be a productive, balanced, and nuanced discussion of caution versus the potential benefit of medical use.

The best "just say wait" strategy is to openly explain to teens the harms without drama or exaggeration. Explain that we think it might harm their cognitive development if used heavily, and there's some data to suggest teens are more likely to get addicted. What's the rush? Life is long. Just don't use cannabis *now*, when your brain is vulnerable. A good resource on stigma-free, honesty-centered drug education was put out by the fantastic nonprofit Drug Policy Alliance called "Safety First: Real Drug Education for Teens."

Often teens are self-medicating with cannabis. We need to engage them in discussions to see *why* they are using cannabis, what needs they are helping to address, that we are apparently failing to address—such as social anxiety—and how they can meet those needs in a healthier way. If you shut it down without discussion or just lecture, you lose a vital opportunity.

## "Addiction for Profit" Concern

With even Nora Volkow, the head of NIDA, concurring that teen use isn't rising in legalized states, and with a broad and unified consensus that teens shouldn't be using cannabis, why are the Reefer Pessimists still so concerned about teen use rising in the future? It comes down to their distrust of the new cannabis industry. The concern is that the cannabis industry will follow in the footsteps of the alcohol and tobacco companies that targeted youths with their ads with such disastrous efficacy. Teens are already more vulnerable than adults to substance misuse and addiction of all kinds, so it is not difficult to imagine the temptation on the part of some profit-hungry corporatists to try to associate their products with the dopamine receptors of our nation's teens. There are restrictions on advertising, such as not allowing advertising near schools, but these aren't particularly effective, as content is widely shared on social media.

The fear of corporate exploitation of teens is given life by the fact that a portion of the cannabis industry is being peopled by business types who formerly did work for Big Alcohol, Big Tobacco, and Big Pharma. Why would "Big Cannabis" be any different? Are these people expected to be more ethical than they were with alcohol and tobacco, just because they are now working with weed, which is groovier? No way. They need to be monitored and regulated.

219

As a counterbalance to this concern, there is an unusual concentration of highly prosocial people from the cannabis legalization social justice movement who are now working within the cannabis industry. Will these more ethical types be able to rein in the corporate excesses? Does the fact that cannabis isn't nearly as addictive or destructive as tobacco or alcohol make this "addiction for profit" strategy less effective for cannabis? It certainly makes the Reefer Pessimists' anti-legalization rallying cry, "Stop Another Addiction for Profit Industry," less compelling than if they were speaking of meth or heroin (or caffeine, for that matter).

It doesn't help the Reefer Pessimist argument when they attempt to paint Big Marijuana with one brush, given that much of Big Marijuana fought—and are still fighting—for social justice, while the Reefer Pessimists were (and many still are) advocating for punitive drug policies that landed so many Black people in jail for simple possession. Or that some of the funding for the Reefer Pessimism "side" has come from Big Alcohol, Big Pharma, and the private prison and rehab industries. It is difficult to view this side, including many elements of the "prohibition for profit" industry, as having the moral high ground, though neither side has an absolute monopoly on hypocrisy.

In some ways, this comes down to a struggle over the future identity of the cannabis industry. The inclusion of people from alcohol and tobacco leaves a sour taste with anyone who wanted to believe that the idealism of the movement to legalize cannabis would dominate the cannabis sphere, including myself. There definitely seems to be a fault line between the "old-school" activists and the newer corporate hotshots that are stepping in. This became apparent to me when I attended a high-end cannabis industry conference in Boston in 2018.

Many of the cannabis events I had previously attended were "business casual" and professionally organized, because the cannabis industry is working hard to gain respectability and legitimacy. Yet nothing had prepared me as I walked into what could have been a shareholder meeting for Anheuser-Busch or Philip Morris. It cost several thousand dollars to attend (I was "comped" in), which selected out many of the less corporate Cannatopians. The room was full of white men in very expensive suits. There were very few women, and I could count the minority participants on one hand.

The word "wellness" was bandied about by the many transplants from the tobacco and alcohol industries, as if a totem to ward off charges of vulture capitalism. One executive did have the decency to make a reference to the tens of thousands of African Americans who were in prison for, essentially, selling cannabis, as everyone there at the conference was trying to do. This was not a balancing act between social justice and profit; this was about profit. The communities damaged by the War on Cannabis were completely absent from any discussion at this conference.

During the conference, they discussed super PACs, EBITDAs, stock options, and "branding." I do not come from a business background at all, and I was sort of lost. My mind kept wandering to the idea that we've come a long way from the grassroots campaigns, such as in California before medical was legal there, when people would risk their freedom to operate "buyers' clubs" for sick patients in order to donate cannabis to those in need. The corporate interests at this conference were, in essence, many of the same overlapping corporate interests that had formerly opposed cannabis in the different statewide referendums. What irony, not to mention hypocrisy! What adaptive evolution.

Is an identity crisis looming for the Cannatopians who now wish to make a living in the new cannabis economy? Do you have to sell a little bit of your soul? Or can we make the prosocial ethos the dominant culture? Of course, this conference represented just one extreme of a sprawling and diverse industry, but these were clearly many of the future decision makers.

Given that the "cannabis industry" is now an amalgam of old-school social justice warriors and modern, corporate businesspeople, can it, on the whole, be trusted to not aim advertisements at minors? In the face of debt, shareholder demands, competition, and financial stresses, it is, at times, going to be awfully tempting. What is the best way to rein this in? Personally, I would simultaneously ban all advertising for cannabis, alcohol, tobacco, and Big Pharma. Ads are intrinsically misleading, especially the pharma ads. All of these industries seem to be doing just fine. Short of banning ads, we need to call companies out, and potentially penalize them with strong regulation, when they cross over the line. As we did with the Cold War, we need to "trust but verify" that they are behaving.

Are there special pediatric cases where the benefits clearly outweigh the potential harms? Obviously if they are dying, like my brother Danny was, what's to lose? It would have been inhumane not to give him cannabis to help with the chemotherapy he was suffering through. What about intractable childhood epilepsy? The word "intractable" answers the question, especially as CBD has proven to be so effective for this indication and has done well on safety studies so far.

More and more cases are entering a gray zone as to whether cannabis might be indicated. Take autism, for example. There is increasingly promising research (see chapter 18) indicating that not just CBD but THC may be instrumental to treating some of the "core" symptoms. We already give autistic kids many unpalatable and potentially damaging medications that aren't particularly effective, which helps explain why CBD and THC are rapidly coming into favor for autistic kids. Or what about when a teen figures out it helps their ADHD? Is cannabis truly worse than Adderall?

This is all the more reason why we must do whatever we can, via the ABCD study or some other mechanisms if that isn't helpful, to truly solve the ongoing mystery of if and how bad cannabis is for teens.

## Part III

# WHAT'S THE BUZZ?
# BENEFITS AND POTENTIAL

## CHAPTER FOURTEEN

# THE ENDOCANNABINOID SYSTEM
## Our Brain on Drugs

Both the cannabis plant and the endocannabinoid system—our natural system of receptors and transmitters that respond to cannabis—far predate *Homo sapiens*. The endocannabinoid system is around five hundred million years old, which is to say, it has been around for roughly two thousand times longer than humans have. The first documented human use of hemp goes back about ten thousand years—a piece of hemp cloth is one of the most ancient surviving artifacts. Hemp is thought to be one of our oldest cultivated crops, for textiles if not for food or intoxication. The first definitive, documented medical use of cannabis is from around five thousand years ago in China. Cannabis has been our companion ever since, for most of our social evolution. One might theorize that a substance that makes us hungry and horny, that both helps us heal and helps us get along with each other, and, crucially, that facilitates creativity would be beneficial to our evolutionary prospects.

What are people currently using cannabis for, besides general wellness, lifestyle enhancement, relaxation, and joy? According to a 2019 study published in the journal *Health Affairs* called "Qualifying Conditions of Medical Cannabis License Holders in the United States," the top five uses in medical states, in decreasing order of popularity, are for chronic pain, spasticity in multiple sclerosis, chemotherapy-induced nausea and vomiting, PTSD, and cancer-related symptoms. About two-thirds of Americans who use medical cannabis use it for one type of chronic pain or another. Other common usages are for epilepsy, spinal cord injury, fibromyalgia, anxiety, irritable bowel disease, and insomnia.[1]

How can cannabis help with so many differing and seemingly unrelated maladies? To answer this, as well as to understand its limitations and harms, it is necessary to briefly confront some of the basic science of the endocannabinoid system (ECS). For some people, "science" is a four-letter word that conjures up endless lectures in middle school, with the clock ticking backward, flies buzzing around, and the teacher endlessly blathering on about cell walls, atoms, binomials, and puberty. But, before you put this book down and hop back on Twitter, keep in mind that, by reading the next few paragraphs, you will probably know more about how cannabis works than almost all doctors and nurses do.

The ECS is an intricate network of transmitters and receptors, which are densely packed throughout our brains and bodies. The ECS is critically important to much of the day-to-day regulation of many of our most important bodily functions. Cannabis, and other cannabinoids, works by hijacking or borrowing the ancient machinery of our ECS.

It wasn't until 1964 that an unstoppable Israeli organic chemist named Raphael Mechoulam isolated the main biologically active molecule in cannabis, known as THC, or tetrahydrocannabinol. Professor Mechoulam obtained some high-end Lebanese hashish from the police, who had confiscated it from smugglers. He dissolved this hashish and isolated dozens of different compounds in cannabis and tested them out, one by one, on a colony of monkeys. One compound caused the monkeys to act, essentially, like a bunch of Grateful Dead fans during Woodstock—the video of this is iconic—and Mechoulam's group deduced that this molecule, THC, or tetrahydrocannabinol, was the active ingredient of marijuana. He proceeded to continue to study its activity for the next six decades (and counting . . .).

Mechoulam's sustained effort led, more than twenty-five years later, to the next earth-shaking discovery: in 1990 it was shown that we have "cannabinoid receptors" in our brains. Instead of cannabis working its magic through actions on other, previously discovered brain receptors, like the opioid receptors, it was now established that there are specific receptors in the brain that interact with cannabis and cannabis-like molecules, as if the brain itself were designed to process cannabis. There are two primary receptors known so far, the CB1 receptor and the CB2 receptor. This was big news and a shot in the arm for cannabis believers who now had more evidence that cannabis was an integral part of our history and evolution—now we even had special, specific brain receptors for this class of molecule.

But wait a second. This earth-shaking revelation begged an even bigger question: what are the actual molecules that are fitting into these cannabinoid receptors that are naturally situated in our brains? Brain receptors take *millions* of years to evolve, so it can't just be the cannabis that we've been using for the last five *thousand* or so years. There must be natural molecules that trigger these receptors. There must be an internal messenger that, like the rest of the ECS, long predated modern, or even ancient, human beings.

Toward the end of 1992, just as I was starting to walk to the mailbox every five minutes, awaiting hopeful news from my medical school applications, a profoundly revolutionary discovery was announced, namely that one of these internal messengers had been discovered. They named it "anandamide." The "ananda" part comes from Sanskrit and means "bliss," while the "amide" part is just the name of a particular chemical grouping. This chemical molecule, and the others that have since been discovered, are called "endocannabinoids" (eCBs) or "internal cannabinoids."

What did this "bliss molecule" do when it attached to these receptors, and what was the resultant effect? What natural roles did it play in health and disease? What do external cannabinoids do to these receptors? These issues are still being untangled and will be investigated for decades to come. We got a late start on this entire avenue of discovery because of the counterproductive funding priorities of the War on Drugs and the ongoing limitations and needless restrictions that remain on cannabinoid research.

The symbolism of these discoveries at the time is hard to overstate. How could cannabis be the toxic, satanic drug that our government and the Partnership for a Drug-Free America were claiming, literally bombarding us with television advertisements about the evils of marijuana, if we have a customized receptor system that mimics and accommodates it? So much for "your brain on drugs"—our brain to a certain extent is the drugs themselves. Or, another way to look at it—our brains have always been on drugs. They have been "on" cannabinoids since prehistoric times. Society's thinking about cannabis—whether we are on drugs or off of them—was about to change.

When we talk about "cannabis" or marijuana, what exactly do we mean? Many of us remember that small, wrinkled baggie that contained oregano-like material, with a lot of twigs and seeds in it, that we surreptitiously procured in high school and that you had to smoke for about twenty minutes to feel any effect. As it turns out, cannabis is vastly complex.

The simple difference between cannabis and hemp—which are the same plant—is the THC content. Hemp, by definition, is less than 0.3 percent THC (in the United States); if there is more than 0.3 percent THC, it is defined as cannabis. Hemp plants have plenty of CBD and other cannabinoids in them.

There are about five hundred different molecules in cannabis, many of which are biologically active, though we are just beginning to understand the effect and importance of the different components. The effects of these more "minor" molecules help explain why the different "strains" have different effects when they are used—some make you sleepy, horny, and hungry; some can make you anxious; and others make you energized and creative.

I will use the word "strains" and "chemovars" interchangeably throughout this book. "Strains" are what is used in common parlance among cannabis users and in dispensaries, though the word "chemovar" is more accurate, because it denotes which actual cannabinoids and other molecules are in your weed. Knowing what exactly you are getting makes it much easier for doctors and patients to predict what the effects will be and how to select a helpful product for whatever is ailing you. For example, you can pick a chemovar with high CBD and a variety of other molecules that facilitate sleep if you are suffering from insomnia.

Strain names aren't particularly reliable. Notice they all have very similar descriptions of their effects, which are generally variations around this theme: "The strain Nonsense Sour Deadhead OG is uplifting with a rush of creative energy followed by a relaxing full body high that is helpful for chronic pain and anxiety." Further, there is little consistency in strains. Sour Diesel in San Francisco likely has little resemblance to Sour Diesel in Boston. One batch of Sour Diesel in Boston might not be very similar to a different batch of Sour Diesel at a different store in Boston. It's better to read the labels and see what is actually in your cannabis—rely on the chemovar and the science, not the advertising of the purported strain effects.

CBD, or cannabidiol, is covered in detail in chapter 20. Less well known are the "minor" cannabinoids. They are "minor" because they are present in minute quantities in the current, commercial strains of cannabis, which have been bred to have high levels of THC. This is one of the unfortunate consequences of the illegality of cannabis: the economic incentives were to raise the THC, at the expense of the other, potentially more medicinal cannabinoids, such as CBD and these other molecules.

Now, as countries—or states, in our case—legalize cannabis and the restrictions on research are lessened or circumvented, we are starting to learn much more about these other cannabinoids. We can breed them back in. We find ourselves at the dawn of a profoundly exciting time, where the medical potential of these molecules can finally be investigated and harnessed. Some of the increasingly well-known cannabinoids that are graduating out of the "minor" league as they are isolated and marketed are:

CBG—cannabigerol; potentially useful to fight nausea, pain, anxiety, inflammation, colitis, and possibly cancer

CBN—cannabinol; potential to help with appetite, inflammation, as an antimicrobial, and, importantly, as a nonintoxicating sleep aid

CBC—cannabichromene; works with other cannabinoids to dampen pain and inflammation, also acts as an anticancer and an antimicrobial agent in the lab

THCV—tetrahydrocannabivarin; controls appetite, promotes weight loss, and prevents insulin resistance

Now that hemp has been legalized by the 2018 Farm Bill, many new hemp-derived products are sprouting up, such as delta THC-8, which allegedly has all the benefits of regular THC but doesn't get you anxious or paranoid. (I tried it—it was sort of boring; it is true that there wasn't any anxiety, but there also wasn't much energy or creativity. It was like being on mental novocaine. What was the point?) We truly don't know the safety of these newly mass-produced molecules as they haven't been tested and the manufacturing is dangerously unregulated, though it is exciting to think of their eventual medical potential.

Cannabis also contains other classes of molecules, such as terpenes and flavonoids, that many practitioners and patients alike feel are critical to its medial benefit. Terpenes are the aromatic oils that give different cannabis strains their distinctive aromas. They are also believed to have medicinal qualities as well. For example, the terpene "alpha pinene," named because of the piney aroma it gives off, is thought to help with memory and anxiety. The most common terpene is myrcene, which smells like hops or beer, and which has a calming effect that can help with sleep and anxiety. Flavonoids are plant nutrients, which help provide color and which are touted for their antioxidative, anti-inflammatory, and immune system boosting properties, though the evidence for any of these having a discreet or measurable effect on human health is fairly preliminary.

In 1998, Professor Mechoulam—the chemist who discovered THC by leading all of those monkeys through the doors of perception—posited the existence of an "entourage effect," which theorizes that the effectiveness of the main therapeutic (and intoxicating) molecule THC is enhanced by the synergistic effects of the different cannabinoids and, likely, terpenes and flavonoids working together. Basically, the action of all these molecules in concert is greater than the sum of the parts, and they are all suspected to work in delicate and ancient harmony to produce their healthful effects. The entourage effect could explain why whole-plant cannabis is near universally reported to be more effective than monotherapy with THC. For example, the synthetic THC called Marinol, available in pill form, that the FDA begrudgingly approved in 1985 as a concession (many thought this was an attempt by the U.S. government to undermine the momentum for full legalization of cannabis) was universally panned by patients as not nearly as effective as whole-plant cannabis. There is not a lot of hard science behind the entourage effect, and in that sense it is still more of a hypothesis, despite being firmly ensconced in clinical cannabis lore.

Some other cannabis medications you may be hearing of in discussions of medical cannabis are:

- Nabiximols (Sativex)—a spray that goes under your tongue that is a roughly equal combination of THC and CBD (legal in many European countries)

- Nabilone (Cesamet)—a synthetic drug that mimics the effects of THC (but more potent)

- Epidiolex—a pharmaceutical preparation of CBD that the FDA approved in 2018 for refractory childhood epilepsy

How important and pervasive is the ECS in our bodies? Of the two known, major cannabinoid receptors, the first, the CB1 receptor, is found in the brain in enormous numbers. In fact, the CB1 receptor is the most common GPCR (G protein-coupled receptor; very important!) in our brains. CB1 receptors are also found in the peripheral nervous system, as well as in other internal organs. The CB2 receptor is predominantly found in the tissues of the immune system, such as the spleen and tonsils. The cannabinoid receptors are widely dispersed all over our bodies, are densely packed, and are involved in many of the most critical life-support activities, such as

- learning,

- sleep,

- feeding,

- decision making,

- reproduction,

- pain control,

- response to stress,

- emotional reactions,

- forgetting harmful memories,

- regulating our energy balance,

- regulating the function of our immune systems, and

- temperature control

to name a few. The ECS is absolutely essential for supporting our life-maintaining "homeostasis," which is, according to Oxford, "the tendency toward a relatively stable equilibrium between interdependent elements, especially as maintained by physiological processes."

Brief rumination: There are so many inane, pointless things they make us memorize in medical school—the names of each bump on the skull, that literally no one has cared about for thousands of years (if they ever did . . .); each vanishingly rare kidney problem, none of which you'd see over the course of ten consecutive careers—and *the ECS* is what they decide to leave out of the medical school curricula? End of rumination.

The location and function of these receptors help explain some of the side effects of cannabis as well as some of its untapped medical potential. For example, a common short-term side effect of using cannabis, which I suspect a few readers may have experienced, is the munchies, which is what engenders stereotypes of cannabis users as willing to go to tremendous lengths to procure ice cream and chips (if and when they can get off the couch . . .). In fact, chronic cannabis users tend to be thinner than nonusers because of long-term effects on metabolism, so there's an irony to this particular stereotype, even if it's true that people do tend to get the munchies and can overeat.

Logically, then, one should be able to block the cannabinoid receptors, lower one's appetite, and create an effective weight-loss drug. This absolutely makes sense, and in fact they tried exactly this with the drug rimonabant, and it was quite effective for weight loss. However, they had to withdraw the drug from the market after a short period because of a terrible side-effect profile, most notably severe psychiatric disease including depression and suicidality. The other side effects, which came from directly blocking the CB1 cannabis receptor, read like a beginner's manual for all of the symptoms that medical cannabis is so effective at treating: anxiety, insomnia, nausea, itchiness, and cramping. This again shows how important the endocannabinoid system is to our bodies' "homeostasis," or ability to regulate itself, and highlights a vast future medical potential for the ECS as drug development progresses (i.e., targeting the appetite parts of the brain while sparing the mood parts).

There is one area of the brain where cannabinoid receptors are conspicuously absent: the brainstem, which is where our respiratory centers are located. This is a big difference from opioids and explains why cannabis is qualitatively safer. As the name implies, the respiratory center establishes the automatic nature of our breathing. (Notice that you just breathe; you don't have to think about it or remind yourself to do so, unless you are reading this sentence.) During an opioid overdose, this center is suppressed and, simply, the person stops breathing. The absence of cannabinoid receptors in the respiratory center explains why no one has ever died from a cannabis overdose, and why cannabis isn't listed in the long lists of other drugs that contribute to opioid overdoses. This is not for lack of effort. But, to consume enough cannabis to stop breathing, one would have to smoke hundreds of pounds within a quarter of an hour. Not even your most die-hard Snoop Dogg fan, desperate to get stoned, who has been starved of cannabis on a desert island for decades, with unusually large lungs, and a bong the size of the Eiffel Tower, could come close to accomplishing that.

Speaking of stoned, that's not a bad description of how endocannabinoids act as they work in our bodies. Other neurotransmitters, like dopamine and epinephrine, generally transmit chemicals forward, from the end of one neuron to the beginning of the next, in the direction of the flow of the signal, just as you might vaguely remember them doing from high school biology class (if you survived the flies and the boredom). This is usually how signals move forward, from the end of one neuron to the beginning of the next. But no! The endocannabinoid system, in line with the hippie culture that followed it millions of years later, has to be nonconformist, and its neurotransmitters do the exact opposite: they release chemicals from the beginning of the further neuron that migrate back to the end of the previous neuron. This is called "retrograde transmission," and it is unique to the ECS. This is critical to explaining how the ECS can modulate the release of other neurotransmitters, as it provides instant feedback, which can turn up or down the output of the other transmitter systems.

If, for example, there is a perception of too much excitement or activity in any particular pathway or system of the body, the ECS can respond to this immediately by sending a backward or "retrograde" signal via the cannabinoid receptors in the brain to dampen down the release of these particular neurochemicals. Is the body too cold? Do you need to generate a fever to fight an infection? Via the ECS, a backward signal is sent, "Hey, we need more heat up here," to all of the different bodily systems that regulate temperature. As such, the ECS works in effect as a "traffic control" system for most of the other systems in the brain.

One theory, first voiced by neurologist and cannabis scholar Dr. Ethan Russo, is that a relative lack of endocannabinoids, or a "clinical endocannabinoid deficiency" (CED), is a way to explain, in part, the pathophysiology of certain diseases. According to Dr. Russo,

> the greatest evidence for CED is present for migraine, fibromyalgia, and irritable bowel syndrome (IBS). . . . All display as yet unfathomed pathophysiological features and remain treatment resistant. Might their underlying nature have been missed?

The ECS, which is so integral to so many processes, and which was only discovered relatively recently, hasn't been given nearly the attention it deserves. It is plausible that our relative ineptitude in treating certain diseases is due to our history of not adequately examining the role the ECS plays in the development of these diseases. Is there evidence for this theory? For migraines,

> Russo cites a study in which it was found that the endocannabinoid anandamide was lower in the cerebral spinal fluid of people who suffer from chronic migraines than in people who don't. This suggests a chronic role that the ECS plays in inhibiting those pain pathways that cause migraines to originate. These levels shouldn't be lower in migraine sufferers unless the ECS had a central and, likely, causative role in migraines.[2]

I would not be surprised if Dr. Russo is proven to be right, at least as a partial mechanistic explanation for these disease states, though the evidence for an "endocannabinoid deficiency syndrome" is somewhat inferential and speculative at this point.

Whether or not there is a defined, etiologic endocannabinoid deficiency syndrome that underpins certain diseases, there's no question that the study of the ECS is going to fundamentally change modern medicine by enhancing our understanding of a huge number of diseases and disease processes. For example, the CB2 receptors, located primarily throughout the immune system, such as in the spleen, tonsils, and thymus and on white blood cells, will prove to be extremely attractive targets for future medicine development. Inflammation is a vital component of our body's response to injury or infection. But inflammation can also become the problem itself, such as with many autoimmune and inflammatory diseases, including lupus or rheumatoid arthritis, or ARDS (e.g., from COVID), to name a few, out of thousands. Turning up or down different components of the inflammatory response system has almost infinite potential to address and alleviate these conditions as we evolve and deepen our understanding of the ECS. The future potential of cannabinoid medicine is limited only by our imagination.

## CHAPTER FIFTEEN

# CANNABIS INSTEAD OF OPIOIDS
## Bigger Isn't Always Better

An extremely common medical usage of cannabis is chronic pain, which plagues tens of millions of Americans, as we, on a population level, get older, more rotund, and consequently more arthritic and pained, year after year. Tylenol (acetaminophen) is widely agreed upon to do little if anything for this (or any) type of pain, except it might cause your liver some pain by damaging it. Few people would be excited to be on opiates these days, even if they could find a doctor willing to prescribe them in this current climate of opiophobia (and, in truth, there is very little data that opiates are effective for chronic pain). Nonsteroidals like Advil, Naprosyn, Aleve, ibuprofen, diclofenac, etc. will destroy your kidneys with enough use, if they don't first bump you off with an ulcer or a heart attack—I see this a lot in my primary care practice. With all of these liabilities associated with the other main types of pain relievers, many are turning toward cannabis, which is increasingly perceived as a safer and effective alternative.

It is a waste of time to debate whether cannabis works for chronic pain. It has been used for this indication for thousands of years. Millions of patients currently are finding relief from chronic pain with cannabis. There are hundreds of studies attesting to its effectiveness. I've had extensive success with thousands of patients who didn't respond well to other treatments. I can tell you from not just the clinical experience of myself and my colleagues but also personal experience, such as for sciatica, migraines, or postsurgical pain—I've used it for decades for this indication: cannabis helps with pain.

Even NASEM concluded, in their landmark 2017 report, that weed treats pain, despite the fact that this report was largely an amalgamation based on only those studies that made it through the Drug War curation, and before the subsequent advent of safer, legal marijuana or of the dozens of real-world evidence papers coming out in favor of using cannabis for pain. NASEM stated, there is "conclusive or substantial evidence that cannabis or cannabinoids are effective" for the treatment of chronic pain in adults, particularly neuropathic pain.

Chronic pain is one of the most challenging conditions for clinicians to treat, as patients tend to say that nothing works and that their pain is an eleven on a scale of one to ten. If the patient says that a particular treatment is working for their chronic pain, why on earth would the doctor question them, regardless of what the treatment is, assuming that it is relatively nontoxic, such as cannabis? (Especially as doctors are now less frequently placed in the gatekeeper role for cannabis, so there isn't much remaining incentive for the patient to be untruthful with us.) In my experience, it's a plus that they aren't asking for something more addictive and rewarding like opioids. These patients, who know what works for them, often have to face the dreaded, huffy, nasal doctor voice: "No, no, marijuana *can't* be working for your pain, because *I* didn't tell you to take it and *we* don't have enough randomized control trials or FDA approval." It's not like cannabis is the latest supplement on the block. Cannabis has been around for thousands of years, and millions of people are consistently saying the same thing about its efficacy. As they teach us in medical school, if it's waddling around, has webbed feet, and is quacking, it's most likely a duck.

How effective is cannabis for chronic pain? It depends on how strong the pain is and, to a certain extent, what type of pain it is. I haven't found much evidence that cannabis is a strong enough painkiller for severe, acute pain, like the kind of pain suffered immediately after breaking a bone, immediately after major surgery, or after being run over by a large bus. For chronic arthritic or nerve types of pain, the kind that causes people to freely consume NSAIDs for years and destroy their kidneys, by most accounts cannabis works well.

There are many different mechanisms by which cannabis treats pain. Both the CB1 and CB2 receptors contribute to this. CB1 receptors in the brain and the spinal cord both work via complementary mechanisms to dampen pain signals, lessen the perception of pain, and make pain a less unpleasant sensation. The CB2 receptors, densely packed on inflammatory cells, help control inflammation, which is often a large component of pain, especially nerve pain. The main limiting factor in treating pain is often the psychoactive effects—the "high" that, in other circumstances, people so eagerly seek out, can be a nuisance for medical cannabis patients who need to be functional. With the availability of newer, more medicinal strains and by manipulating other components such as the CBD content, adding in other cannabinoids, and keeping the dosage of THC low, the psychoactive effects can be minimized, usually without sacrificing pain control.

There are many reasons why the traditional "data" in the lab may not capture the true efficacy of cannabis in treating chronic pain. One factor is that cannabis often alleviates several interconnected symptoms at once—pain, perception of pain, anxiety, insomnia, muscle spasm, quality of life—whereas RCT studies are often oriented to assess one parameter at a time. Another big reason is that many of these studies were mandatorily performed with the substandard government NIDA-grown weed—the Moldy Mush strain, full of twigs, seeds, and stems—rather than the beautiful buds that can be purchased at any local dispensary.

On a personal note, as someone who is in long-term recovery from opioid addiction and who has recovered from major spinal surgery in 2016, I was pleased and relieved to not need to rely on opioid pain relievers for my postoperative pain. For the first few days of exceptionally intense pain, there was no choice but to use opiates, as cannabis just wouldn't have done the trick. To be without opioids would have constituted torture, and hospitals are fairly miserly in dispensing opioids these days. After a few days, I found that medical cannabis was just as effective as the oxycodone the neurosurgeon gave me, but with many fewer side effects. Neither the opioids nor the cannabis made the pain go away completely, but they both dulled it and made it feel as if it were further away from me so that it wasn't as bothersome or interfering. I was eager to avoid the itching, sleepiness, and constipation of opiates, as well as the oblivion. On the cannabis, I was able to get writing and editing done.

My experience is not uncommon. According to a 2017 study by lead author and therapeutic plant specialist Dr. Amanda Reiman, "Cannabis as a Substitute for Opioid-Based Pain Medication: Patient Self-Report," through interviews of almost three thousand medical cannabis patients, respondents overwhelmingly reported that cannabis provided relief on par with their other medications, but without the unwanted side effects. Ninety-seven percent of the sample "strongly agreed/agreed" that they are able to decrease the amount of opiates they consume when they also use cannabis, and 81% "strongly agreed/agreed" that taking cannabis by itself was more effective at treating their condition than taking cannabis with opioids.[1]

There are dozens if not hundreds of studies that corroborate this "substitution effect," with patients, on their own, ditching opioids for cannabis. One wonders how much harm reduction progress we could make if more doctors were active participants in this process, rather than remaining underinformed naysayers.

To what extent can cannabis help us address the current opioid crisis? As I write this, we have lost more than 108,000 people in the United States to opioid overdoses in the last twelve months. Several states have approved cannabis to help address components of this epidemic. Is this sensible? Generally, yes. There are five ways in which cannabis can help alleviate the opioid crisis, four of which I am on board with.

The first way is to offer cannabinoid therapy instead of opioids for patients with new chronic pain syndromes. All doctors should be equipped to offer this option. This practice would lead to fewer patient exposures to opioids and less opioids in circulation that could be diverted by a family member or acquaintance. This is how many addictions to prescription painkillers start, when someone else gets into the leftover opioids.

I'm not at all in favor of undertreating pain patients or in cutting off opioids in patients who need them or who have been on them with benefit, but it *is* amazing how many people don't actually need opioids and do better on cannabis.

The second way to help with the opioid crisis is to transition people who have been on chronic opioid treatment from opioids to cannabis. This must be *voluntary*, as it is wholly unethical and dangerous to force people off of their opioids. Many people have transitioned from opioids to cannabis on their own or are eager to do this. This is especially true if they have access to a cannabis-knowledgeable physician who is able to help coach them, as well as access to safe, legal cannabis. According to a 2019 study, "Pills to Pot: Observational Analyses of Cannabis Substitution among Medical Cannabis Users with Chronic Pain," which surveyed more than a thousand chronic pain patients,

> This article presents results that confirm previous clinical studies suggesting that cannabis may be an effective analgesic and potential opioid substitute. Participants reported improved pain, health, and fewer side effects as rationale for substituting.[2]

I've had success in my clinic transitioning patients from opioids to cannabis, though certainly not with everyone who has tried. In some cases, the pain is so severe they feel the need to stay on opioids. Other patients successfully make the transition off of opioids but have to go back on them because health insurance doesn't cover the cannabis, which they simply can't afford.

My patient Derek is one success story. When Derek first wheeled up to me, he was the recent victim of a drive-by shooting. The specialists had patched him up, but he suffered from severe chronic nerve pain (and PTSD) and had been started on a massive dose of oxycodone. I offered to transition him to cannabis, which he was open to. We worked together on this and, as his opioids gradually came down, eventually to none, his engagement and interest in the world around him increased. He was also doing physical therapy, and time was elapsing, so one can't attribute all of the improvement solely to the cannabis treatment. Though it is difficult to imagine that his remarkable regain of function would have occurred on that gargantuan dose of opioids. He fought his way out of his wheelchair and then off his cane, started a successful small business, and then went on to study economics. He said to me, "If you didn't encourage me to get off of the Oxys, I never would have achieved any of this."

The third way is to utilize cannabis to lower the dosage of opioids required. Cannabis and opioids work synergistically on overlapping receptors, which enables a provider to use less of each when using them together. Dr. Ziva Cooper, the director of the UCLA Cannabis Research Initiative and a superstar cannabis researcher, is one person I listen to at every opportunity because she is smart, ethical, and always right on point. An example of her work is the 2018 paper "Impact of Co-administration of Oxycodone and Smoked Cannabis on Analgesia and Abuse Liability," which is a double-blind, placebo-controlled test of whether subtherapeutic doses of oxycodone—not enough to have an effect—mixed with very low doses of smoked cannabis improve pain. Dr. Cooper's team demonstrated that "cannabis enhances the analgesic effects of sub-threshold oxycodone, suggesting synergy," and that this occurs without an increase in the misuse liability of cannabis.[3] The way Dr. Cooper explains it is that there a "one plus one equals three" effect, which is music to the ears of a harm reductionist.

This result is consistent with the results of a 2017 meta-analysis, "Opioid-Sparing Effect of Cannabinoids: A Systematic Review and Meta-Analysis," in which researchers were able to quantify how much of an opioid dosage lowering could be achieved with the addition of THC. They concluded that "the median effective dose (ED50) of morphine administered in combination with THC is 3.6 times lower than the ED50 of morphine alone."[4] That means you can lower the opioid dose to almost a quarter of what it was without the use of cannabis. For codeine it was 9.5 times lower. Given that much of the harm people encounter with opioids is dose related, the potential health benefits of these combinations cannot be overstated.

A good review, as well as a "how-to" guide on this issue, can be found in the paper "Practical Strategies Using Medical Cannabis to Reduce Harms Associated with Long Term Opioid Use in Chronic Pain" by noted cannabis researcher Dr. Caroline MacCallum. Dr. MacCallum's group concludes,

> When low dose THC is introduced as an adjunctive therapy, we observe better pain control clinically with lower doses of opioids, improved pain related outcomes and reduced opioid related harm.[5]

The fourth way in which cannabis can help us address the current opioid crisis is by virtue of the fact that cannabis can be an unusually helpful treatment for the symptoms of opioid withdrawal. The dozen or so times I've withdrawn from opioids, in the process of surmounting my long-standing addiction, went far beyond what the word "miserable" denotes. It was somewhere between "excruciating" and "apocalyptic." I'd feel sweaty, freezing, flushed, anxious, jumpy, and depressed, and I'd have the worst imaginable nausea, muscle aches, and stomach cramps. Cannabis alleviates many of these symptoms simultaneously. It transformed opioid withdrawal from "I want to die" to "This is awful, but I can (barely) handle it." Few, if any, who have gone through this would disagree, though occasionally cannabis is reported to have the paradoxical effect of making people hyperaware of certain symptoms, which can make their experience of them worse.

It astounds me that addiction specialists haven't picked up on this valuable treatment decades ago. I suspect that it is only due to stigma, narrow-mindedness, bias, and the airtight addiction medicine echo chamber that prevents them from routinely receiving the most up-to-date (or any) information on the medicinal benefits of cannabis. In fact, patients in recovery are commonly tested for cannabis and have been kicked out of their treatment programs, or denied privileges, if they test positive. We have imported a Drug War mentality into addiction treatment, it has settled in, and it continues to harm patients.

A recent example of this shameful bias was when SAMHSA, the "Substance Abuse and Mental Health Services" department of our government, announced that they were cutting off funding to all programs that support medical cannabis patients. According to a great article in *Spotlight PA* by Ed Mahon, "Turned Away,"

> in late 2019, a wrench got thrown into [the treatment] system. The federal Substance Abuse and Mental Health Services Administration told grant recipients that funds may not be used directly or indirectly to purchase, prescribe, or provide marijuana or treatment using marijuana. The agency also warned that the money could not be provided to any person or organization that "permits marijuana use for the purposes of treating use or mental disorders."[6]

Predictably, a patient named Tyler Cordeiro, who had a valid medical cannabis card, was desperately trying to get into recovery and was defunded by this new rule. He subsequently died by overdose. According to the article,

> Tyler Cordeiro was one of the more than 4,700 people who died from a drug overdose in Pennsylvania last year, according to preliminary estimates. His case shows how people at perilous points in their lives can

be negatively affected by the conflict and confusion that exists as states expand access to marijuana, while the federal government still discourages its use.

Who knows how many other people have suffered and died due to this cruel and poorly conceived policy by SAMHSA. If there were any doubts that our government has still been fighting a War on Cannabis, this story should end them.

Was there clinical evidence for denying life-saving opioid addiction treatment to this cannabis-using patient? According to a 2020 paper, "The Relationship between Cannabis Use and Patient Outcomes in Medication-Based Treatment of Opioid Use Disorder: A Systematic Review," which looked at articles in this area,

> there was a small number of studies that produced findings suggestive of a supportive or detrimental role of concurrent cannabis use, but *the majority of studies [of outcomes of opioid replacement treatments] reported that cannabis use was not statistically significantly associated with the outcome.*[7] (emphasis added)

Further, some studies showed benefit, and I would bet anyone a good cup of coffee that, by the end of the decade, legal, regulated medical cannabis will be established as an approved and accepted treatment for opioid withdrawal (unless we invent something better—likely this would be cannabinoid based . . . just better targeted to the specific symptoms).

One final study to cite, "Frequency of Cannabis and Illicit Opioid Use among People Who Use Drugs and Report Chronic Pain: A Longitudinal Analysis," a study of drug users in Vancouver and the impact of cannabis use on their illicit opioid use, stated,

> We observed an independent *negative* association between frequent cannabis use and frequent *illicit* opioid use among PWUD [people who use drugs] with chronic pain. These findings provide longitudinal observational evidence that cannabis may serve as an adjunct to or substitute for illicit opioid use among PWUD with chronic pain.[8] (emphasis added)

Less frequent illicit opioid use will almost certainly translate into fewer overdoses and deaths, because it is the illicit opioids that are, by and large, contaminated with fentanyl.

The final way that cannabis might help the opioid crisis is the most disputed, namely, the idea of using cannabis itself for opioid substitution therapy, along the lines of buprenorphine (Suboxone) or methadone. I have met and heard from thousands of patients who have used cannabis to overcome their opioid addictions in precisely this way, as an "exit drug." Can cannabis be considered as a stand-alone treatment for opioid use disorder? Should people be allowed to try this? Should cannabis clinicians be encouraging it?

I don't feel comfortable recommending cannabis as a primary treatment for opioid use disorder. My hesitancy has to do with the consequences of treatment failure. If someone wants to try cannabis for a migraine, I have a low threshold for assenting to this treatment. If the cannabis doesn't work, the worst-case scenario is that the patient gets a migraine, or a migraine they already have doesn't resolve promptly, and we try something else. Lots of medications do and don't work for migraines. If, on the other hand, a patient tries to use cannabis alone to treat their opioid addiction, and it doesn't work, the consequences may well be overdose and death. We are fortunate that there do exist two medications—methadone and buprenorphine (Suboxone)—that have been definitively proven to reduce overdoses and deaths by 50 percent. Personally, I don't feel it is responsible to prescribe a treatment, cannabis, that hasn't (yet) been proven to save lives when we have access to treatments that absolutely have been proven to do so.

That said, I haven't seen any data showing that the use of cannabis in and of itself, or instead of methadone or buprenorphine, has caused any overdosages or deaths—as far as I know this is a hypothetical risk that hasn't been demonstrated. That said, coming from someone in recovery from a near-fatal opioid addiction, I would strongly recommend going with the proven treatment.

In some states, cannabis is approved as a direct opioid substitution treatment. For example, in Pennsylvania, opioid use disorder is one of the accepted indications for medical cannabis. The Medical Marijuana Advisory Board, when it added "addiction substitute therapy—opioid reduction" to the list of qualifying conditions for cannabis, stated,

Cannabis can offer pain relief and has been reported by patients to ease the symptoms and process of opioid withdrawal. It has been used by patients as an "exit drug" to get off of heroin and other opiates. Given the current state of the opioid epidemic, the Patient/Caregiver Subcommittee recommends allowing cannabis to be used for opioid addiction therapy and opioid reduction.[9]

The addiction people are vociferously opposed to this inclusion, though at this point in history, they ought to agree with the first two sentences "Cannabis can offer pain relief and has been reported by patients to ease the symptoms and process of opioid withdrawal. It has been used by patients as an 'exit drug' to get off of heroin and other opiates." If they can't agree with these weak and general statements, they likely haven't been exposed to current, diverse, unbiased information on this subject and might not be the best resource. It is reasonable to disagree with the last statement, about "allowing cannabis to be used for opioid addiction therapy."

They feel it is dangerous and irresponsible for the states, or the cannabis industry, to suggest that cannabis is a legitimate treatment for opioid use disorder when it isn't evidence based—at least with the kind of evidence they favor. Also, it cuts them out of the process (which, frankly, is part of the appeal to many in the cannabis community who feel that they have been gaslighted about cannabis by the addiction community nonstop over the last half century).

Would most agree that people should be "allowed" to try cannabis? It *is* their choice, *as long as it is an informed choice.* That is the key—the decision has to be based on accurate information—which we are still fighting about. As such, I agree that *the cannabis industry ought not to be advertising or implying that cannabis is a stand-alone or proven treatment for opioid use disorder.* If they do so, they might harm people by implying that cannabis is on par with Suboxone and methadone, which, unlike cannabis, have impeccable evidence behind them. The most I feel it would be reasonable to state is that you can use cannabis to "help with your chronic pain, and with the anxiety and many of the other symptoms of opioid withdrawal, but cannabis is best used in conjunction with a Suboxone provider and not as a sole treatment for opioid addiction." There are plenty of doctors who prescribe Suboxone (myself included) who are aware of the evolution of our understanding of the benefits of cannabis.

When the anti-cannabis advocates over-egg the pudding, it tends to backfire, and the entire message can get lost. There was a recent study in *JAMA*, "Association of State Policies Allowing Medical Cannabis for Opioid Use Disorder with Dispensary Marketing for This Indication," that highlighted this tendency on the part of dispensaries to advertise for this particular indication.[10] They make the important point, which I echoed above, that cannabis isn't an approved or proven "medication for opioid use withdrawal" and that the industry clearly shouldn't suggest cannabis as a stand-alone treatment. Agree.

Unfortunately, due to an overzealousness to indict cannabis dispensaries and to give the cannabis industry a black eye, or due to a misunderstanding of current clinical practice of cannabis medicine by nonclinicians, this study also dismissed the use of cannabis substitution for opioids for chronic pain as well as opioid use as an *adjunct* to treatments for opioid use disorder, such as for withdrawal symptoms. These (helpful and accepted) practices were also criticized as purported examples of bad behavior on the part of the dispensaries, yet, as discussed, these are both highly effective components of alleviating our opioid crisis. This type of gratuitous dismissal of the successful care that hundreds of thousands of people are manifestly utilizing for benefit is insulting to the cannabis community and widens the gap between the two camps.

I'm not sure why it has to be all or nothing with opioids and cannabis, for either side. We can say cannabis is valuable when used for chronic pain and withdrawal symptoms but shouldn't yet be the primary stand-alone substitution medication for opioid addiction. Easy. Take the absolutism out of both sides on this life-or-death issue.

## CHAPTER SIXTEEN

# INSOMNIA
## To Sleep but Not to Dream

O ne of the most common uses for cannabis is for sleep. I am surprised that this is still a (somewhat and decreasingly) contested issue, as it quite obviously makes many people sleepy and helps many people to fall and stay asleep. This is particularly true if you pick a "sleepy" strain or chemovar that features soporific components. I've successfully treated hundreds of patients with cannabis for insomnia. Some people can't even use cannabis socially or as a medicine because it knocks them out. My girlfriend in high school didn't consume (and still doesn't forty years later) because, with one puff, she's out cold, which makes for a pretty boring time at a party, or when out to dinner.

There's also the issue of why patients would say cannabis helps them sleep if it doesn't. If anything, they might say the opposite to obtain addictive and relaxing hypnotics such as Valium or Ambien. It is true that, in the past, in order to legally access cannabis, some patients might have embellished various medical conditions to procure weed, which they may have felt was justified at the time. However, this resulted in some physicians becoming skeptical and distrustful of the entire enterprise. Fortunately, doctors are decreasingly forced to act as gatekeepers; for example, this is not their role in the nineteen states (and the District of Columbia) that have legalized cannabis recreationally as well as medically. (Doctors don't want to be gatekeepers, and they know hardly anything about cannabis, so whoever had the bright idea of making them gatekeepers didn't do any of us a service).

There are dozens of real-world evidence studies showing that cannabis is quite effective for sleep. There are many studies, some cited in other chapters, showing people substituting cannabis for other hypnotics such as benzodiazepines, often as an incidental finding. This wouldn't occur if cannabis didn't have a relaxing and sleep-inducing effect. Even a recent study from my home institution, which fairly transparently seemed intended not to be a pro-cannabis study, showed that weed helps sleep. Named, "Effect of Medical Marijuana Card Ownership on Pain, Insomnia, and Affective Disorder Symptoms in Adults: A Randomized Clinical Trial," the study showed that the statistically significant "improvement in sleep quality" that they found "warrants further study into the benefits of medical marijuana card ownership for insomnia."[1] There was also one randomized controlled trial in 2021, "Treating Insomnia Symptoms with Medicinal Cannabis: A Randomized, Crossover Trial of the Efficacy of a Cannabinoid Medicine Compared with Placebo," which showed that a sublingual mixture of THC, CBN, and CBD "is well tolerated and improves insomnia symptoms and sleep quality in individuals with chronic insomnia symptoms."[2]

If it is not particularly controversial that cannabis helps people sleep, what hasn't been well studied is what actual *effect* cannabis has on one's sleep structure and quality. What does cannabis do to your sleep architecture? Alcohol can make you feel sleepy too and can make some people fall asleep, but alcohol is highly disruptive to the quality of the sleep. What are the long-term effects of using cannabis for sleep? We haven't studied this in humans in detail, but given that there is evidence that people use cannabis instead of alternative sleep medications, including Benadryl, benzodiazepines, and Ambien, all of which quite possibly predispose one to earlier dementia, it's difficult not to see why cannabis is viewed as safer in comparison.

Also, does cannabis help sleep-related disorders such as obstructive sleep apnea (OSA) and restless legs syndrome (RLS)? The nightmares associated with PTSD are discussed in chapter 19.

There are many activities people can and ought to do to improve their sleep before jumping either to cannabis or to a sleeping pill. This is referred to as "sleep hygiene," and it is a profoundly important component of getting a good night's sleep. As a primary care doctor, I know that many people don't wish to be bothered and just want a quick fix, but I insist on at least a brief lecture on these issues.

These healthy habits include limiting caffeine both in quantity and in terms of when you consume, such as keeping it before noon, as it tends to hang around. Exercise is critical, though not right before bed, as that revs your body up. One should limit the activities performed in the actual bed itself to sex or sleeping so that you come to associate your bed with going to sleep, not with watching television, working, plotting the collapse of foreign governments, or whatever else you might be doing in bed. It is important to try to go to bed and to wake up at the same time every day to adjust your circadian rhythm. Finally, avoid using backlit screens (e.g., computer or TV) for at least an hour before bed so your brain doesn't get tricked by the bright light into thinking that it's the middle of the day. Oftentimes, these activities can, by themselves, cure or improve insomnia, and they will make any pharmacological or botanical remedy far more effective.

After all of this, which may have already put you to sleep, the first-line, recommended treatment for insomnia is not medication but cognitive-behavioral therapy (CBT), which has been shown to be effective and which is obviously safer than either sleeping pills or cannabis. The problem is, this is time consuming, it isn't always readily available or paid for by insurance, and most people are busy, stressed, harried, and they just want a good night's sleep, and they want it yesterday. So they either politely decline a referral for CBT or flat-out tell you to take a hike, and you find yourself discussing medications such as melatonin, trazodone, Belsomra, Ambien, or medical cannabis with them.

According to the 2017 NASEM report,

> there is moderate evidence that cannabinoids, primarily nabiximols [an under-the-tongue mixture of THC and CBD], are an effective treatment to improve short-term sleep outcomes in individuals with sleep disturbance associated with obstructive sleep apnea syndrome, fibromyalgia, chronic pain, and multiple sclerosis.[3]

That covers a lot of people. NASEM notes that it makes sense that cannabinoids might help with sleep as the ECS is involved in the regulation of several different components of the sleep cycle. For example, it is known to shorten the time to sleep onset, as many people who feel sleepy after taking a puff can tell you. (For a minority of people, it can do the opposite and is so mentally stimulating that it does *not* particularly help their sleep. This was the effect it had on my dad.)

If we are to expand the evidence we consider to include more accessible real-world evidence, the evidence base becomes drastically more robust. For example, according to a 2019 study, "Use of Cannabis to Relieve Pain and Promote Sleep by Customers at an Adult Use Dispensary," they looked at one thousand adult-use consumers from retail stores in Colorado in 2016. Three-quarters of respondents reported using cannabis to improve their sleep, with 84 percent saying that cannabis was either very or extremely helpful. Further, "most of those taking over-the-counter (87%) or prescription sleep aids (83%) reported reducing or stopping use of those medications."[4] What is striking is that in this study, they excluded medical patients, showing, again, the fuzzy line between medical and recreational cannabis use (as discussed in chapter 21).

A 2018 study, "Effectiveness of Raw, Natural Medical Cannabis Flower for Treating Insomnia under Naturalistic Conditions," looked at more than four hundred medical cannabis users who recorded via an app their perceptions of insomnia severity before and after cannabis consumption. It showed an average drop of 4.5 points on a scale of 0–10. Strains higher in CBD were associated with more relief.[5]

Another study, "Medical Cannabis and Insomnia in Older Adults with Chronic Pain: A Cross-Sectional Study," looked at 128 older patients with chronic pain symptoms to assess the effect of cannabis on sleep. They found that cannabis did have an overall beneficial effect on sleep in patients with chronic pain—which echoes the NASEM findings—but that there may be some tolerance to this effect over time.[6] This is, unfortunately, true for many different sleep medications—the more you use them, the less they work. Sometimes people try alternating between different medications (or different strains of cannabis, with differing combinations of minor cannabinoids) to preserve their efficacy.

Finally, in a 2021 study, "The Use of Cannabinoids for Insomnia in Daily Life: Naturalistic Study," they examined 991 medicinal cannabis users with insomnia across 24,189 tracked cannabis use sessions:

Medicinal cannabis users perceive a significant improvement in insomnia with cannabinoid use, and this study suggests a possible advantage with the use of predominant indica strains.[7]

It makes sense that "in-da-couch"-type sedating strains would put you to sleep better than the energizing sativas (though, as discussed, this distinction may have outlived its benefit).

Another problem that I see in my clinical practice is that once one goes down the road of *any* sleep medications, including cannabis, it can be difficult to get off of them. Patients lose confidence in their ability to sleep without some type of aid. This is why it is critical to focus on "sleep hygiene" and CBT first and not just jump into pills or botanicals.

In a related point, when a heavy cannabis user abruptly stops using cannabis, insomnia can be one of the worst withdrawal symptoms. This symptom can lead to relapse in people who are trying to quit cannabis. It can also be difficult at times to know how much the cannabis is helping a particular patient sleep after they've been using cannabis for a while, versus how much the withdrawal from cannabis is harming their sleep. This is especially relevant as some studies suggest that cannabis can become less effective for sleep over time.

As a lifelong insomniac, I have found cannabis to be modestly effective for insomnia—but *only in very low doses*, preferably with some CBD included. At higher doses, it is way too stimulating. I find myself up very late reading or writing, thinking that I have just discovered something absolutely crucial to the ongoing quest for human knowledge, a novel concept upon which the fate of everything might depend. I stay up late struggling to get it all down on paper. Other people stay up after using cannabis for similar reasons: it can make many routine activities more fun and interesting, so people end up painting, drawing, jogging, organizing their houses, watching TV, listening to music, doing crossword puzzles, gaming, or strumming the old guitar. Who wants to go to sleep and miss out on all this fun? (This is possibly a variation of "revenge insomnia" or "revenge sleep procrastination," which is defined by the National Sleep Foundation as "the decision to sacrifice sleep for leisure time that is driven by a daily schedule that is lacking in free time." I don't need cannabis to be guilty of this almost every night.)

Unfortunately, getting a sufficient amount of sleep is absolutely critical to brain health. Perhaps if you are staying up having life-altering sex, such as can happen when both parties are stoned on cannabis, that might be worth it, but otherwise it sort of defeats the purpose of using cannabis for sleep if you aren't getting any sleep. Keep the doses low.

Another factor to consider, and I'll get crucified for saying this as well because telling the truth apparently is "promoting the use of cannabis": it is a profoundly pleasant way to fall asleep. You are resting mindfully, you feel warm and fuzzy, with a mild sense of euphoria welling up in your chest, as images of your day gently float through your mind's eye. Your muscles are in a deep relaxed state and feel as if they have just been professionally massaged. As you are drifting off to sleep, creative thoughts meander, and pleasant shapes and colors are gently floating behind your closed eyes. This phenomenon is described by astronomer Carl Sagan in an essay that appeared in my father's book *Marihuana Reconsidered*:

> When I closed my eyes, I was stunned to find that there was a movie going on the inside of my eyelids. Flash . . . a simple country scene with red farmhouse, a blue sky, white clouds, yellow path meandering over green hills to the horizon. . . . Flash . . . same scene, orange house, brown sky, red clouds, yellow path, violet fields. . . . Flash . . . Flash . . . Flash. The flashes came about once a heartbeat. Each flash brought the same simple scene into view, but each time with a different set of colors . . . exquisitely deep hues, and astonishingly harmonious in their juxtaposition.[8]

For me, it's just simple shapes and colors—stunningly beautiful, as my brain is nowhere near as intricate, or as generatively creative, as Carl Sagan's was.

Critically, the fact that the *process* of trying to sleep is so much more pleasant with cannabis lessens the anticipatory insomnia that haunts and tortures so many of us insomniacs, and which so drastically worsens our insomnia. You know that you aren't going to be twisting and turning all night, unable to sleep. The main thing that can go wrong is if you start thinking, "Hmm . . . I wonder what types of ice cream I have in the freezer." Flash . . . Flash . . . diet in trouble.

What sleeping medications have I tried over the last forty years? I am a professional insomniac, and it is not an exaggeration to say that I have tried all of them (mostly as and when prescribed by a doctor). All the benzos, several barbiturates, Z-drugs like Ambien (and all the other Z-drugs like Lunesta and Sonata), Benadryl, trazodone, amitriptyline, melatonin and melatonin-based drugs (e.g., ramelteon), Seroquel, gabapentin, Topamax, muscle relaxants like Flexeril, beta blockers, clonidine, hydroxyzine, the new orexin inhibitor Belsomra . . . you name it. Most of these are awful and give you the feeling of a "drugged sleep." That is, you do sleep, technically, but you wake up feeling like a cross between a nuclear waste site and a pithed frog.

Specifically, trazodone and amitriptyline gave me a dry mouth and made me groggy. Melatonin and its analogues didn't do anything, though the gummies taste good, and it's easy to go through a good part of the bottle. Benzodiazepines like Valium are too addictive and made me forgetful at doses high enough to induce sleep. Ambien (zolpidem) and the other sedative/hypnotic medications are habit forming and dangerous, as they are involved in car crashes, overdoses, and strange dissociative events where people wake up to find a pile of dishes and wrappers in their kitchen. "Who ate all this junk and didn't clean up?" Guess what? It was your brain on Ambien. People drive on Ambien as well and don't recall it. It is implicated in a surprisingly high percentage of car accidents. It also might cause or contribute to dementia. Seroquel should be a weapon of war, not a sleeping aid (unless you have an actual indication for it, such as bipolar disorder). Gabapentin (Neurontin) is the most overhyped drug in human history, for all of its uses, not just sleep, along with its cousin Lyrica (pregabalin). (Making you tired and spaced out does not equate with pain control.) Belsomra, if you can actually get the insurance companies to pay for it and the pharmacies to provide it, doesn't do that much to induce sleep until, possibly, the middle of the next day, when the need for a nap can come crashing down on you like a tidal wave. CBD alone does nothing to help me sleep.

All of this is not ideal, especially if you have to take care of lives the next day as a primary care doc. Ironically, the medical boards are hysterical about doctors using cannabis, but typically cannabis doesn't give you this type of hangover unless possibly used in huge dosages, which are rarely needed for sleep. Doctors are allowed to chomp down whatever legal, prescribed pharmaceuticals or over-the-counter meds they like, or alcohol, for sleep or any other indication, despite how brain dead they are made to feel the next day. By comparison to most of these meds, cannabis seems natural, safe, and effective.

There is no evidence that cannabis degrades your sleep in the same way, or nearly to the extent, that alcohol does. However, the long-term effects of cannabis and cannabinoids on sleep have not been well-studied.

The studies of what cannabis does do to the quality and architecture of your sleep are somewhat conflicting, and a crystal-clear picture hasn't emerged yet. Consistent with my experience, low doses of THC can help one to fall asleep faster. Cannabis also increases slow-wave sleep, which is more important as you get older, as this type of sleep becomes increasingly scarce. Higher doses of THC can affect the sleep architecture by reducing stage 3 sleep, aka "deep sleep," and by reducing REM sleep. This latter fact could help explain why one doesn't typically remember dreams as well after utilizing cannabis to fall asleep (and why vivid dreams tend to be a common cannabis withdrawal symptom).

It is important to note that the effects of the dosing of CBD are different from THC. At low doses, CBD can be stimulating and can interfere with sleep. To the extent that lower dosages of CBD do help people sleep, it is thought to be because they help with pain and anxiety. At higher doses, CBD can promote sleep. Painted with a very broad brush, a low THC and higher CBD combo, such as a nice CBD-predominant tincture under the tongue before bed, is likely to be effective for sleep.

I have a relative, in her mid-fifties, who suffers from restless legs syndrome (RLS). RLS is characterized by a seemingly irresistible urge to move one's legs, worse at night, that can interfere with one's sleep (as well as the sleep of one's partner) and lead to leg pain and grogginess the next day. There are a wide range of pharmaceutical products we use to treat RLS, most of which typically don't work that well and have a wide range of unpleasant side effects. My relative, who is no stoner by any stretch of the imagination, was desperate, so she asked me for help. I happen to be good at making medicinal tinctures—except for the one time I temporarily set myself on fire and almost blew up trying to boil off the alcohol, but we'll just forget about that one minor blemish to an otherwise spotless record. I gave her some tincture to take before bed, starting low and going slow, and asked her to report back to me a few weeks later with her progress.

"Gone."

"What do you mean, gone? Do you mean better?"

"It's completely gone."

"Any side effects?"

"No, I just use a little at night, and the only effect is that my restless legs don't bother me anymore. I don't feel the tincture at night because I'm asleep, and I don't feel it the next day."

This is what practicing cannabis medicine is like at times. It makes your impossible life as a doctor so much easier. I truly can't fathom why other doctors haven't caught on to this yet. In any case, I was wondering if this had happened to other patients with RLS, so I dug into the literature. In 2017, the journal *Sleep Medicine* had printed a case study of six patients who had had a similar miraculous-seeming response of their RLS with cannabis. According to "Cannabis for Restless Legs Syndrome: A Report of Six Patients,"

> All patients spontaneously reported cannabis use and total relief of RLS symptoms as well as complete improvement of sleep quality after occasional and recreational marijuana smoking (patients 1–5) or sublingual administration of cannabidiol (patient 6).[9]

Far out. My cousin wasn't imagining the benefit. In a 2019 paper, "More Evidence of Cannabis Efficacy in Restless Legs Syndrome," they found twelve more patients with treatment-resistant RLS who had a complete or near-complete response to cannabis.[10] I don't think we understand the mechanism of RLS well enough to understand how cannabis would treat it except to speculate that it has to do with dopamine and the complex interactions between the ECS and a wide variety of other neurotransmitter systems relevant to movement and sleep. (Or maybe it comes down to Dr. Ethan Russo's theory of clinical endocannabinoid deficiency.)

Four months later, my cousin reported that the RLS symptoms have started to come back, so we're going to try to see how infrequently she can take the tincture to keep these symptoms at bay.

There is evidence that cannabis might help with obstructive sleep apnea on a variety of parameters. This needs to be further investigated because many patients simply can't tolerate that uncomfortable facemask that makes them feel as if an elephant is sitting on their face and farting on them when they are trying to sleep. According to a 2022 review article, "Clinical Management of Sleep and Sleep Disorders with Cannabis and Cannabinoids: Implications to Practicing Psychiatrists,"

> In individuals with obstructive sleep apnea . . . cannabinoids are one of the treatments being considered. In this regard, preclinical investigations have demonstrated that combining the agent oleamide [an endocannabinoid] and THC aids in the stabilization of respiration in all stages of sleep as well as the maintenance of autonomic stability during sleep. The synthetic THC dronabinol was found to lower the apnea-hypopnea index in a clinical investigation and is regarded safe for the short-term treatment of obstructive sleep apnea.[11]

I have several patients who are doing better with their OSA using cannabis, in the context of not being able to tolerate the CPAP masks (which is the standard of care currently and which we would always try first).

As the science progresses, I suspect we'll be able to more specifically target the endocannabinoid system and that we'll be able to develop even better sleeping medications than cannabis itself. We might not need to use all five hundred molecules in the cannabis plant to help us sleep. As we make progress, the Ambiens will become a thing of the past, which is precisely why Big Pharma has been so opposed to legalization. As we succeed in lifting antiquated restrictions on research, exciting things are going to happen.

# CHAPTER SEVENTEEN
# CANNABIS AND CANCER
## Knocking on Heaven's Door

There is little remaining doubt that cannabis is helpful to patients for many of the torturous symptoms that different cancers can cause. Nor is there doubt, even among the most die-hard Reefer Pessimists, as to whether cannabis can help alleviate chemotherapy-induced nausea and vomiting. I have been aware of these uses ever since I saw it palliate my brother Danny's nausea and bring back his appetite after his treatments for leukemia half a century ago. It is no coincidence that almost every state with a medical cannabis program stipulates cancer as a qualifying condition. Cannabis is also increasingly being recognized as useful in end-of-life care. It can help people gently transition to the next world without the heavy-handed stuporousness and constipation of opioids. Many patients prefer the gentle euphoria, the mindful anchoring to the present moment, and the calming philosophical insight that cannabis can give them. Though, at this point, anecdotal claims aside, it has *not* been scientifically demonstrated that cannabis is an effective treatment in humans for the cancer itself.

Because they work closely with patients who consistently use and benefit from cannabis, oncologists, among the different medical specialties, are most supportive of medical cannabis. A 2018 survey of oncologists, "Medical Oncologists' Beliefs, Practices, and Knowledge Regarding Marijuana Used Therapeutically: A Nationally Representative Survey Study," demonstrated that 80 percent of them discuss medical cannabis with their patients, and 46 percent of them recommended it.[1] A different survey showed that only 15 percent of oncologists "did not support medical

257

marijuana use of any sort."[2] I suspect this number is receding faster than my hairline is.

On what grounds would you not support access to medical cannabis for cancer patients? The 2017 NASEM report concluded, "There is conclusive evidence that oral cannabinoids are effective antiemetics in the treatment of chemotherapy-induced nausea and vomiting." Inhaled ones are even more effective. One would have to be dug pretty deeply into a Drug War fallout shelter to not evolve one's thinking on this issue in the face of this, in addition to the ubiquitous testimonials from patients. One thinks of those stories of Japanese soldiers on isolated islands in the Pacific who had no idea the war was over. Maybe these 15 percent of oncologists missed the same memo: cannabis helps with chemo. However, it's a complex ethical issue whether doctors are obligated to prescribe treatments that they don't believe in. (Answer: you have to do what's best for the patient, but it also depends on what the accepted "standard of care" is.)

A more speculative and evolving discussion is the role cannabinoids will play as a preventative or a treatment for the cancer itself. There is abundant laboratory evidence that cannabis kills different cancer cells in a wide variety of ways, and cannabis quite possibly may become an adjunct to chemotherapy regimens in humans.

Unfortunately, some cannabis advocates—often the ones who tend not to be particularly bought into or trustful of the Western science paradigm, tout certain cannabis preparations as a stand-alone treatment for cancer, even at times going so far as to suggest that patients forgo allopathic chemotherapy in favor of high doses of cannabis extracts. This is still in the realm of what I'd consider wishful thinking, as cannabis by itself has never been shown in a legitimate scientific trial done on humans to cure any type of cancer. I believe this advice endangers patients by discouraging them from using treatments that have been proven to be remarkably effective, such as chemo and radiation (and then you use cannabis to control the symptoms).

There are a number of credible people that I know personally who claim that their cancers have resolved with just cannabis. Interesting—but I'd stick with the evidence at large when we are talking about something as deadly as cancer. This is analogous to the discussion in chapter 15 around not using cannabis primarily, or solely, to treat opioid use disorder: the stakes are too high, and the evidence is too thin.

Let's untangle what cannabis does and doesn't do to help treat the symptoms of cancer and the symptoms of cancer treatment. We'll also discuss some potential harms of using cannabis in this population. Finally, we can look into what cannabis might do to help in the battle against the cancer itself.

The most common symptoms that patients with cancer suffer from include pain, nausea and vomiting, poor appetite, mood disorders, anxiety, insomnia, and a sort of gestalt pervasive misery labeled "poor quality of life." The treatment with cannabis of many of these different ailments in patients without cancer has been discussed, and generally the same principles hold, being careful to "do no harm" in this vulnerable population. One thing to keep in mind is the capacity of cannabis to treat several symptoms at once—anxiety, pain, nausea, insomnia, and appetite—and thus provide broad-based symptom relief, globally improving "quality of life." It can also help address "polypharmacy" (when someone is taking an ever accumulating number of medications) and can help decomplexify the treatment regimens, making it easier for patients and caregivers.

Pain is a dreaded symptom of cancer. Opioids, which are currently the mainstay of treatment for cancer pain, don't work for some people, aren't well tolerated in others, are overregulated because of addiction risk (yes, even in dying patients), and can be difficult to procure due to (misguided) governmental pressure on doctors not to prescribe them. Opioids can result in a less than ideal quality of life due to falls, constipation, sedation, itchiness, and other side effects. Many are opting for cannabis instead, or as well, to lower the dose of opioids by co-using them with cannabis.

A 2018 real-world evidence study from Israel, published in the *European Journal of Internal Medicine*, titled "Epidemiological Characteristics, Safety and Efficacy of Medical Cannabis in the Elderly," enrolled 2,736 patients and followed them for six months for pain intensity, quality of life, and adverse events. The average age was seventy-four years, and patients were suffering in equal part from chronic pain and from cancer. After six months of treatment, 93.7 percent of these patients reported an improvement in their condition, with median pain scores dropping from an 8 to a 4 (out of 10). According to the study, a "clinically meaningful pain reduction is defined as a decrease of 2 points on a 0-to-10 numerical pain rating or a 30% improvement in pain intensity." So, this response to pain was deemed "substantial." Also, after six months, eighteen percent stopped using opioid analgesics or reduced their dose. This fact alone might explain why the number of falls was also found to have significantly reduced in this study. Most patients reported improved quality of life. The main side effects of medical cannabis were dizziness and dry mouth.[3]

This study, the results of which have been confirmed by other studies, not only helps demonstrate that cannabis is an effective treatment for cancer pain but also that cannabis, if used sensibly, is a safe treatment in older populations.

Severe nausea and vomiting, as well as appetite loss, can be an accompaniment of either the cancer itself, such as if one develops biliary or pancreatic cancer, or of the treatment for the cancer, including chemotherapy or radiotherapy. Control of the nausea and vomiting is essential. Standard medications for this have improved over the years but still often fall short of the oldest medication. Patients, like my late brother Danny, can have vicious anticipatory nausea and vomiting as well. It is torture.

Many patients find inhalation the most effective way to address waves of extreme nausea. I don't recommend smoking as a delivery method. I am also dubious of the "vape pens," where oil extracts are vaporized, because these contain God knows what other chemicals in them. Even though the EVALI lung outbreak was predominantly *illegal* vapes, it does highlight that a lot of chemicals, which have not been proven safe, are in the cartridges of the vape pens or can leech into them over time. Whenever I have sampled a vape pen, after using it, my poor, asthmatic lungs felt like someone went over them with sandpaper. I needed my inhaler. That can't be good.

The safest method of inhalation is to vaporize organically grown cannabis flower, purchased from a legal dispensary, using a dry herb vaporizer. This device is typically about the size of a small cell phone. It heats the flower to a suitable temperature. This temperature is high enough to extract the medicinal cannabinoids yet is low enough to avoid most of the combustion products generated from smoking cannabis, which occurs at a much higher temperature. Even though cannabis smoking hasn't been linked to lung cancer or chronic obstructive pulmonary disease (COPD), avoiding combustion products such as tar, benzene, and polycyclic aromatic hydrocarbons *has* to be better for your lungs.

Other preparations of cannabis—oral, sublingual, rectal—are also effective for chemotherapy-induced nausea and vomiting and are clearly safer for the lungs. However, they don't offer the immediate relief or ready titration that an inhalational method does.

What about when the cancer is severe and patients are drifting toward the end of life?

An important study on this issue was published in 2018 in the *European Journal of Internal Medicine*. This study is called "Prospective Analysis of Safety and Efficacy of Medical Cannabis in Large Unselected Population of Patients with Cancer," and it followed 2,970 cancer patients who were treated with medical cannabis in Israel from 2015 to 2017. The average age of the patients was fifty-nine, and the most common cancers were breast, lung, pancreatic, and colorectal. Half of the cancers were stage 4, meaning metastatic. The main symptoms that required treatment were insomnia, pain, weakness, nausea, and lack of appetite. While 18 percent stopped treatment for reasons other than dying, of the remaining patients, 95.9 percent reported an improvement in their condition. Further,

> 20% of patients reported good quality of life prior to treatment initiation. Impressively, approximately 70% reported good quality of life after 6 months of treatment, indicating a significant improvement. . . . Over a third of the patients reported a decreased [*sic*] in the drugs consumed mainly in the following medications families: other analgesics and antipyretics, hypnotics and sedatives, corticosteroids and opioids.[4]

The study concluded, "Cannabis as a palliative treatment for cancer patients seems to be a well-tolerated, effective and safe option to help patients cope with the malignancy related symptoms."[5] Who wouldn't want this for their loved one?

As a side note, a study like this is unlikely to be taught at an American medical school due to the lack of interest in and knowledge of cannabinoids, and due to historical stigma. One might also question why the major American medical journals don't as frequently publish these helpful and informative studies about the efficacy of cannabis as European journals do. Or why most American doctors almost exclusively read American medical journals, when there are so many great English-language medical journals from Europe. This is a type of "American medical exceptionalism" that is keeping us ignorant of cannabis, and possibly many other things. (Their medical systems all seem to spend less money per capita than we do but have better outcomes, almost across the board, so I bet there's a lot we could learn from them.)

There aren't an abundance of traditional studies demonstrating that cannabis improves appetite or promotes weight gain in cancer patients. This is one of those areas where the traditional studies might not capture what is actually happening in a naturalistic setting. Some of the studies used low doses of oral THC (dronabinol) as opposed to inhaled whole-plant cannabis, which is widely reported to be more effective. There are "real world" studies which confirm that cannabis improves the appetite in cancer patients. For example, in the study cited above about safety and efficacy of medical cannabis in cancer patients, it was shown that the symptoms of "lack of appetite" disappeared in 25 percent of patients at six months and improved in 62 percent of patients, while only 12 percent of patients experienced no effect or deterioration.[6]

I have had clinical success in using cannabis to stimulate appetite in patients with and without cancer. One patient lost her sense of taste and smell plausibly due to COVID. She was having an extremely difficult time eating—until we tried cannabis. Her weight promptly stabilized as the cannabis gummies she was eating made her feel hungry, even though the food itself wasn't particularly palatable without taste and smell.

Cannabis was demonstrated to facilitate weight gain in HIV-affected patients by the dedicated and innovative cannabis researcher Dr. Donald Abrams. Dr. Abrams, an oncologist with a specialty in AIDS patients, went through quite a multiyear rigmarole in the 1990s to get his study approved. It was approved by the FDA then rejected by NIDA because, according to Dr. Abrams, "I was reminded many times that the organization was called the National Institute on Drug Abuse, not *for* Drug Abuse."[7]

To get approval, he had to evaluate some harm of cannabis. He couched his interest in whether cannabis can facilitate weight gain in an ostensible search for whether cannabis interfered with protease inhibitors, a type of medicine for HIV (which was also important to determine—

cannabis ended up having no negative effect). All of the patients in this study gained some weight (due to being in the study and being fed regularly), but there was significantly more weight gain in the smoked cannabis group over three weeks: 7.7 pounds versus 2.9. Dr. Abrams's perseverance resulted in our having some critical data as this was the first study of its kind.[8]

Dr. Abrams's effort to show a straightforward medical benefit of cannabis is reminiscent of the uphill battle that Dr. Lyle Craker faced some years later. These two cases demonstrate what broad-based roadblocks the U.S. government has put up to prevent research into any benefits of cannabis. Even Dr. Abrams, a scientist, started to wonder.

> "It was unbelievable, the number of 'Catch-22's' I found myself coming up against," Abrams says calmly. "People would tell me in the beginning about these government conspiracies determined to prevent any positive news about marijuana from reaching the public and I would think they were goofy. But after a while, I confess I found myself shaking my head and wondering what was going on."[9]

There are just a few other studies on weight gain and cannabis. One 2018 study, "The Effect of Nabilone on Appetite, Nutritional Status, and Quality of Life in Lung Cancer Patients: A Randomized, Double-Blind Clinical Trial," used nabilone (a synthetic version of THC) and showed that patients receiving this cannabinoid increased their caloric intake and reported improved quality of life versus the control group. They concluded, "Nabilone is an adequate and safe therapeutic option to aid in the treatment of patients diagnosed with anorexia."[10] A 2019 Israeli study, "The Effects of Dosage-Controlled Cannabis Capsules on Cancer-Related Cachexia and Anorexia Syndrome in Advanced Cancer Patients: Pilot Study," demonstrated comparable results, with a significant minority of these extremely ill patients gaining weight and also reporting "improvement in appetite and mood as well as a reduction in pain and fatigue."[11]

In my personal experience with cannabis, it makes me starving regardless of whether I am actually hungry or not. Give me one puff or a small edible, and once it hits I am ravenous, even if I've eaten a large meal in the previous few hours. I am almost just as starving if I have just finished Thanksgiving dinner as if I haven't eaten for twelve hours. For me, this is an unfortunate side effect, as I already eat too much, but it can be lifesaving for cachexic cancer patients.

When deciding whether to use cannabis for a patient, I ask not, "Is cannabis dangerous?" but, "Is cannabis less dangerous than whatever else I'd be using?" and, with cancer patients, often, "Is there anything besides cannabis that will do as good a job for this particular indication?" Often cannabis is the best option. That said, it is important to mention some of the risks that cancer patients might face if they decide to utilize medical cannabis.

If someone is highly immunocompromised, which can commonly occur from either the primary cancer or from the chemotherapy, they have to be careful when smoking or vaping cannabis, as serious fungal, and other, infections in the lungs or blood are a possibility.

There is also the question of whether cannabis can adversely affect some of the newer cancer treatments. Cancer patients are often on many different drugs. For example, there is a new type of treatment against certain types of cancer called "immunotherapy." The idea is to harness the power of our immune systems to fight the cancers. There is some data to suggest that cannabis might interfere with the efficacy of some aspects of this treatment. For example, in a 2019 study, "Cannabis Impacts Tumor Response Rate to Nivolumab in Patients with Advanced Malignancies," the use of cannabis reduced the response rate to an immunotherapy agent nivolumab, though it didn't affect progression-free survival or overall survival.[12]

A subsequent study, "Cannabis Consumption Used by Cancer Patients during Immunotherapy Correlates with Poor Clinical Outcome," also showed some results of concern:

> In this report, we provide the first indication of the impact of cannabis consumption during immune checkpoint inhibitors (ICI) immunotherapy cancer treatment and show it may be associated with worsening clinical outcomes. Cancer patients using cannabis showed a significant decrease in time to tumor progression (TTP) and decreased overall survival (OS) compared to nonusers.[13]

This particular study had some big methodological flaws, yet it urgently highlights the need for more study of these drug interactions and helps illuminate why it is critical that you inform your oncologist if you are using cannabinoids.

Cannabis can be quite expensive, as American health insurance doesn't yet cover it, and this presents a major and unjust obstacle to care for many people on a fixed income, such as many older patients or veterans. It solves one social justice issue but creates another if we legalize cannabis so that the arrests go away but make it so that only wealthy patients can afford to be treated with cannabis.

In rare cases, particularly at high doses, cannabis can make nausea and vomiting worse due to a paradoxical reaction called "cannabis hyperemesis syndrome." This might have to do with an overstimulation of the same receptors that ordinarily block nausea and vomiting with cannabis, leading them to act in the opposite fashion. Sometimes it can be difficult to distinguish this from a similar condition called "cyclic vomiting syndrome"—the only way to tell is to stop cannabis for three to six months.

Finally, there is the question of safe and legal access. Medical cannabis is not legal in all fifty states yet, as inhumane as that sounds. Some states have "legalization lite," with very limited medical cannabis programs that strictly restrict the level of THC allowed. This can severely undermine the care and comfort one can provide to a patient with medical cannabis in those states. It still isn't legal to fly with medical cannabis in the United States or internationally, or even to drive over the border between two legalized states, due to federal illegality.

Most hospitals believe they can't allow patients to bring cannabis on the premises without risking vast amounts of federal funding due to the conflict between state and federal laws. This situation leaves medical patients in the lurch, unable to access their cannabinoid medication when they are the sickest and need it most. All patients have a difficult enough time eating and sleeping in the hospital on a good day, so why would you exacerbate this by taking away their medical cannabis? Many patients bring it with them anyways, and this puts the hospital security staff in a horrible situation of potentially being instructed to confiscate cannabis from infirm patients. None of these staff members that I have chatted with are against medical marijuana, and the last thing they want to be doing is searching, harassing, and confiscating edibles and vapes from dying patients. Videos of staff and police doing exactly this have gone viral. It is a lose-lose situation for everyone and needs to change.

When our hospital met about this, I suggested "don't ask, don't tell," which they ostensibly rejected as not solving anything, but I suspect that's what they de facto adopted, along with most other hospitals. What other choice is there right now with federal illegality? "Don't ask, don't tell" quietly and unobtrusively makes all of these problems disappear, in lieu of a sensible legal solution. Patients can do their part by respectfully bringing in unmarked candies rather than belligerently insisting on being able to vape weed in hospitals, all of which are nonsmoking facilities.

Recently California passed a state law that allows cannabis possession in hospitals. Hopefully other states will follow suit, and ideally the feds will legalize cannabis before too long, which will make this cruel problem go away.

The answer to the question of whether cannabis can help *cure, treat, or slow* the actual cancer itself is complex and evolving. The conclusion of the 2017 NASEM report from six years ago simply states, "There is insufficient evidence to support or refute the conclusion that cannabinoids are an effective treatment for cancers, including glioma."[14] As we'll see, the glioma issue has evolved. There is "insufficient evidence" mostly because this hasn't been tested in humans yet, not because it has or hasn't worked. Cannabinoids are known to kill cancer cells—in the lab and in animal studies—in a variety of ways:

- They induce cell death or "apoptosis" in cancer cells.

- They can influence the immune response to cancers, which can provide a less (or at times more) favorable environment for the cancer to grow in.

- They interfere with the ability of cancers to grow new blood vessels, a process called "angiogenesis," which the cancers need to nourish themselves.

- They interfere with the spread or "metastasis" of cancers.

- Some cannabinoids, such as CBD, may facilitate the uptake of chemotherapeutic agents into tumor cells.

As summarized in a 2021 *Journal of the National Cancer Institute* monograph called "Cannabinoid Cancer Biology and Prevention," both THC and CBD have been shown to inhibit multiple processes involved in cancer progression (eg, inhibition of cancer cell proliferation, invasion, metastasis, and angiogenesis). In addition, both cannabinoids induce apoptosis and inhibit cancer stem cell maintenance and self-renewal. THC and CBD have also been shown to enhance the activity of multiple first-line therapies across cancers.[15]

Of the two, CBD is looking like the most promising alternative,

> Investigations across cancers show CBD targets many downstream genes involved in cancer, leading to inhibition of cancer cell proliferation, invasion, metastasis, and angiogenesis and induction of apoptosis as well as regulation of immune surveillance.[16]

The challenge has been translating the witnessed cancer-killing potential of these cannabinoids in cells into successful human studies that could demonstrate that cannabinoids play a role in helping actual people with cancer. At the time of this writing, you can count the published studies that can begin to answer this on one . . . finger.

In a small 2021 study called "A Phase 1b Randomised, Placebo-Controlled Trial of Nabiximols Cannabinoid Oromucosal Spray with Temozolomide in Patients with Recurrent Glioblastoma," researchers compared usual treatment for recurrent glioblastoma—a deadly brain tumor—with this treatment and a mixture of CBD and THC in a double-blinded, placebo-controlled study. This mixture was well tolerated. Survival at one year was 83 percent with the cannabinoid-augmented treatment group and 44 percent for the standard treatment group. Survival was also higher at two years, with 50 percent of the cannabinoid-augmented group still being alive versus 22 percent of the placebo group.[17] This is incredibly promising!

Keep in mind that one study, by itself, doesn't prove anything. Several other studies are ongoing but haven't been published yet, and research into this issue is being performed on a wide variety of levels. As such, we are, once again, in an intellectual twilight zone where there is scientific rationale saying that cannabis should be, or may likely be, an effective component of treatments for cancer, but we don't have much in the way of concrete proof that it is in fact effective in humans.

One recent, interesting study from 2021, "Scoping Review and Meta-Analysis Suggests That *Cannabis* Use May Reduce Cancer Risk in the

United States," showed a nonsignificant increase in the risk of testicular cancer with cannabis use, but *a decline in the rates of all other types of cancer*, especially head and neck cancers (which is surprising because so many people smoke cannabis). It concludes, "The data are consistent with a negative association between *Cannabis* use and nontesticular cancer," though in many cases the quality of the data was not robust.[18]

The idea that "cannabis cures cancer" is so appealing to a subset of cannabis advocates that some patients decide to forgo more conventional and highly proven treatments and instead opt to rely solely on cannabis preparations to treat their malignancies. An originally underground product called Rick Simpson Oil, or RSO, has gained a cultlike following for purportedly curing cancer, despite there being no hard scientific evidence that it prevents, treats, or cures cancer. RSO is comprised of very high dosage full-plant cannabis. I have no doubt it helps with some symptoms. It might be shown to help with the cancers themselves—we truly have no idea at this point.

I have friends and acquaintances who swear by RSO and believe that it is the only reason they are still living. Given that cannabinoids do prevent the progression of cancer cells, as we've *seen* them do quite effectively in the lab, it is *plausible* this preparation of very high-dose cannabinoid soup might hypothetically have an effect on the cancer cells in people. This needs to be studied. I strongly recommend that people use it solely as an adjunct to—and *not* a substitution for—their regular chemo if they wish to include it in their regimen.

I will not be surprised if, say, ten years from now, cannabinoids have become a standard part of many common chemotherapy regimens, at least as an adjunct. However, because there are still so many unanswered questions, this is far from certain, and we need to carefully investigate potential harms, such as interactions with immunotherapy. I suspect that cannabinoids are increasingly going to be the first-line treatments to counteract the effects of chemotherapy and many of the cancer-related symptoms. I also think cannabinoids are going to factor in much more centrally to care regimens, such as end-of-life care. This will help lower opioid-related problems while improving patient quality of life. And if it turns out that the "evil weed" that was maligned as causing cancer (it doesn't) for decades by Drug War propaganda has a significant role to play in treating cancer, all the better!

# CHAPTER EIGHTEEN
# CAN CANNABIS HELP AUTISM?
## Help on the Way

Autism spectrum disorder is one of the medical cannabis issues where there's a deep disconnect. On the one hand, there are countless parents who fervently believe they have seen drastic improvements not only in the disruptive and injurious behavior of their kids but also, not uncommonly, in cognition and social connection. On the other hand, there isn't much hard-core data suggesting it does or does not work—a reflection of our past funding priorities. A small but extremely capable cadre of cannabis providers are convinced that cannabis is a safe and effective medicine and appear to be having significant clinical success.

There's a taboo on testing THC on children because of fears that it may harm brain development (see chapter 13), so we have very few studies that include THC. We have a few more studies with cannabidiol (CBD) and other cannabinoids. Otherwise, we are left extrapolating from animal studies, which can be difficult to translate to humans, especially in something as socially complex involving subtle interpersonal connection, such as autism.

If we piece together what evidence we do have, starting with the mice, delving into some theory, and ending up with the human studies, we can see how far we can get. It was much further than I was expecting, and hopefully it is enough to kindle the curiosity, open-mindedness, and research dollars of the medical community.

Autism spectrum disorder (ASD) is broadly considered to have core and noncore symptoms. The core symptoms are deficits in communication and social connection as well as repetitive, restrictive patterns of behavior. There are no FDA-approved medications to treat the core symptoms of ASD.

The noncore symptoms of ASD can include irritability; self-injurious behaviors; aggression; headaches; anxiety; obsessive-compulsive disorder (OCD); tics; Tourette syndrome; depression; gastrointestinal symptoms such as heartburn, constipation, and diarrhea; impulsivity; and insomnia. Epilepsy is seen in up to one-fourth of patients with autism.

The current treatments for many of these symptoms are plagued by limited effectiveness, dubious safety profiles, and unpleasant side effects. For example, to control behavior, many kids are put on antipsychotics, which cause sedation and weight gain. Approximately two-thirds of children with ASD are on some type of psychotropic medications. For impulsivity they use methylphenidate (Ritalin, Concerta), and for insomnia they offer melatonin. With these lousy drugs, and with proliferating stories about the effectiveness of cannabis, it is not difficult to understand why people are turning to cannabinoids, out of some combination of hope and desperation.

Some of the questions that come up are:

- Which of the noncore symptoms do cannabinoids work for? For example, cannabinoids are quite effective for insomnia and anxiety in neurotypicals, but are they effective for insomnia and anxiety in patients with ASD? (Probably.)

- If CBD treats some types of epilepsy so well in children, and since epilepsy occurs in up to one-quarter of kids with ASD, is there some common underlying dysfunction or mechanism that can be or is treated with cannabinoids? (To be determined.)

- Are cannabinoids safe to give to kids? (This likely will come down to age of patient, dose and formulation of cannabinoids given, and a comparison with harms of alternative therapies.)

- Are cannabinoids safer or more effective than the heavy-duty pharmaceuticals that we are currently giving these kids, such as psychostimulants and antipsychotics? (That's the million-dollar question.)

- What is the ratio of CBD to THC that is most beneficial and least harmful? (This is currently under investigation, but some of the potential harms might not show up for a long time.)

- Finally, and critically, can cannabinoids help with the core symptoms of autism and improve the ability of people with autism to communicate and connect? (Hopefully!)

The concerns that many medical providers have in treating ASD with cannabinoids run along these lines:

> Our first job is to do no harm. THC is thought to harm brain development in children and adolescents. Cannabinoids could be harmful on a variety of levels. Many parents are using unregulated supplements with who knows what in them on their kids. Even if you know what you are getting with a cannabis product, we just don't know the long-term effects of THC, or many of the other constituents. We are less concerned about giving CBD, as there is more safety data, though we don't truly know the long-term effects.
>
> We know that families are desperate for a cure, but there hasn't been a "magic bullet" for autism yet—this seems "too good to be true." We have concerns that some of these cannabis providers in this underregulated industry are preying on the false hopes of the parents. The pursuit of cannabinoids siphons limited resources from established treatment with actual data to back them up, such as behavioral therapies, so that these children can learn to best manage these conditions. Using cannabis deviates from established standards of care and is another example of the cannabis industry trying to cash in. The use of cannabis can open the family up to legal risks, which they must be educated about (e.g., another provider reporting them to the Department of Social Services [DSS], or potentially getting in trouble when traveling in a locality where cannabinoids aren't legal). We are going to pass on this treatment until we have much better evidence that it works. Though, just as with Epidiolex (CBD) in refractory childhood epilepsy, we'd love to be pleasantly surprised and find out that it does work well and consequently receive FDA approval so that we can prescribe it. (And—we appear to have collective amnesia as to how vigorously and recently we opposed CBD treatment for epileptic kids as well, on similar grounds, as we are now opposing cannabinoids for ASD.)

The American Association of Pediatrics (AAP) opposes cannabinoids for children in general, but "the AAP endorses compassionate use of medical marijuana for those with a disease that is unresponsive to usual treatment."[1] In truth, it is not much of a stretch to include severe autism in that category. This doesn't mean that cannabis is effective but that it's reasonable to try it.

Even more unyielding, the American Academy of Child and Adolescent Psychiatry flat-out opposes all use of cannabis or isolated cannabinoids in ASD, stating that no evidence exists whatsoever (including, I suppose, the evidence that does exist . . . as you'll see in this chapter). They state that these agents are unacceptably harmful—including CBD, which is now an FDA-approved drug for children. Their position statement is from 2019, the latest I could find (and not all of the data presented below existed back then). They warn that "exposing children and adolescents with developmental disorders such as Autism Spectrum Disorder to marijuana or cannabinoids could further increase the prevalence or severity of psychiatric disorders and intellectual disability in this highly-vulnerable population"—as if our current ineffectual practice of blasting them with neuroleptics, psychostimulants, antipsychotics, and sedatives, none of which work *at all* for the core symptoms of autism, is actually known to be *better* for these kids. They recommend that "families should be educated about risks and discouraged from using marijuana and cannabinoids for Autism Spectrum Disorder."[2]

Slamming and holding a door shut that many people are walking through fosters polarization and diminishes credibility. I would not wish to witness what would happen if these sanctimonious shrinks walked into the headquarters of MAMMA (Mothers Advocating for Medical Marijuana for Autism) or any other parents' advocacy group and announced their blanketly and paternalistically dismissive attitude. The vehemence of this type of incurious and dogmatic response really makes one wonder if the "we don't want to be cut out of the loop" factor is playing a role as well. If you don't have to consult and pay us, we guarantee that it will never work.

This dismissive attitude also ignores the fact that the case for using cannabinoids for ASD has been steadily strengthening and complements the compelling anecdotal stories. Doctors were eventually led to accept CBD as a treatment for childhood epilepsy—after tremendous outcry from patients and numerous cases of witnessed benefit, over the frenzied objections of the pediatric psychiatric community. As we'll see, the current evidence base should be robust enough to, at the very least, spark curiosity and induce a sense of déjà vu and humility.

Why do we think autism has anything to do with the endocannabinoid system (ECS)? Generally speaking, the ECS is critically and fundamentally involved in the regulation of emotional responses, social interaction, and behavioral reactivity, which underlie the core symptoms of ASD. There is not one of the noncore symptoms that isn't mediated at least in part, if not mainly, by the ECS. It almost defies imagination that manipulating the ECS wouldn't have a role in addressing some of the symptoms of ASD. One is tempted to speculate that the reason we don't have any effective treatments for the core symptoms of ASD is because we have so thoroughly ignored the ECS—a clinical endocannabinoid deficiency.

Mice are pretty different from people, and autism is complex and poorly understood in humans. So I just don't know how much of these murine findings we will discuss truly pertain to humans. What they did find in mice is intriguing, though.

In mice, there are at least four different ways to induce models of autism in order for different potential treatments for autism to be studied. No matter which of the mouse models of autism you use, if you increase the levels of anandamide—a primary endocannabinoid found in all mammalian brains—you can improve or fully reverse the social deficits that were created by inducing autism. Imagine the implications for humans if even a fraction of this finding does translate. For example, administering CBD is a safe and easy way to increase anandamide in humans, but more on this later.

Given that so many different mouse models of autism were improved by boosting the same cannabinoid (anandamide), some of these researchers hypothesized that the ECS might be a *converging pathway*—the deficits caused by different variants of ASD might all be mediated by the ECS. The hormone oxytocin is a molecule that promotes social bonding and connection, the love hormone that comes out with hugs, emotional support, and orgasms. It has been shown, in mice, that the prosocial effects of the endocannabinoid anandamide are mediated by an interaction with oxytocin.

In a study called "Endocannabinoid Signaling Mediates Oxytocin-Driven Social Reward," as they put it, "an oxytocin-dependent endocannabinoid signal contributes to the regulation of social reward." This leads to the conclusion that "deficits in this signaling mechanism may contribute to social impairment in autism spectrum disorders and might offer an avenue to treat these conditions."[3] This is exactly what they found in these mice—you replace the endocannabinoid anandamide, and the social connectivity returns. You need both the oxytocin and anandamide for bonding to occur. Without significant amounts of either of these, the system by which we connect with others might not function. Could autism in part be mediated by a deficit in certain endocannabinoids?

What about in humans? It's great that we've found a way to help autistic mice to communicate and connect with each other—this will contribute to mouse happiness for generations to come. But is there any evidence that this approach will help our kids? The first question is whether there's evidence of any deficiency of the ECS in kids with ASD as there was found to be in mice.

When researchers looked at anandamide levels in the serum of kids with ASD and compared them with a sample of kids without ASD, the *anandamide levels were significantly lower in the ASD kids than they were in the neurotypical controls*.[4] In another study, they showed that not only anandamide, but also two other molecules that boost the ECS, PEA and OEA, were lower in the serum of kids with ASD.[5] These studies, along with other studies, strongly suggest that the ECS is a major player in autism in humans. Unfortunately, in this study, they didn't assess the levels, or try to correlate the levels, with the severity of the ASD, which would have been illuminating.

One of CBD's main mechanisms of action is to raise anandamide levels, which, as we have demonstrated (at least in mice), is vital for oxytocin to work properly in models of autism. Giving CBD is found to enhance oxytocin release during social activities. It is known that if you give oxytocin to patients with ASD, there is improvement in social memory, eye gazing, emotional recognition and interactions, and the processing of social information.[6]

To summarize so far: thousands of parents swear by cannabinoids for their autistic children, cannabinoids work to alleviate social deficits in mice, and there is a plausible biological mechanism by which they might work in humans, along with a demonstrated deficiency in humans that is consistent with this biological mechanism. Are there any studies that directly show that cannabinoids work to alleviate the symptoms of ASD in humans? Just a few currently, with many more in progress.

As of this writing, in May 2022, a study came out in the journal *Trends in Psychiatry and Psychotherapy* titled "Evaluation of the Efficacy and Safety of Cannabidiol-Rich Cannabis Extract in Children with Autism Spectrum Disorder: Randomized, Double-Blind and Controlled Placebo Clinical Trial." This study was a randomized, double-blind, placebo-controlled study, so it can't be easily dismissed by conservative doctors as the wrong type of evidence (see chapter 7). The researchers studied children ages five to eleven who were either given a CBD-rich preparation or placebo. The preparation was a 9:1 CBD:THC ratio, so there was included a nonnegligible but modest amount of THC. The findings were truly remarkable,

> Significant results were found for social interaction, anxiety, psychomotor agitation, number of meals a day and concentration, the latter being significant only in mild autism spectrum disorder.[7]

Improved social interaction! A lack of social interaction is a core symptom of autism, and in many ways the cruelest for family members. It is one of the holy grails of treatment. Moreover, this study confirms what parents have been saying, that *cannabis can help with social interaction*. This study urgently demands further exploration in this area.

To briefly summarize some of the other research: In a 2021 Turkish study, "CBD-Enriched Cannabis for Autism Spectrum Disorder: An Experience of a Single Center in Turkey and Reviews of the Literature," they treated kids (average age 7.7) for an average of more than six months with high-CBD/very-low-THC preparations, with the following results:

> A decrease in behavioral problems was reported (32.2%), an increase in expressive language was reported (22.5%), improved cognition was reported (12.9%), an increase in social interaction was reported (9.6%), and a decrease in stereotypes was reported in 1 patient (3.2%). The parents reported improvement in cognition among patients who adhered to CBD-enriched cannabis treatment for over two years.[8]

This was a small study, and the outcomes were determined as follows: "Parents were asked to evaluate the effectiveness of the CBD-enriched cannabis treatment,"[9] which wouldn't factor out expectancy or placebo effects. Still, it is suggestive.

From Brazil, a 2019 study, "Effects of CBD-Enriched Cannabis Sativa Extract on Autism Spectrum Disorder Symptoms: An Observational Study of 18 Participants Undergoing Compassionate Use," they cite "increasing data support for the hypothesis that non-epileptic autism shares underlying etiological mechanisms with epilepsy"[10] (some types of which are very well controlled with cannabinoids). They used a CBD:THC ratio of 75:1, meaning hardly any THC, which is likely safer. They found,

> After 6–9 months of treatment, most patients, including epileptic and non-epileptic, showed some level of improvement in more than one of the eight symptom categories evaluated: Attention Deficit/Hyperactivity Disorder; Behavioral Disorders; Motor Deficits; Autonomy Deficits; Communication and Social Interaction Deficits; Cognitive Deficits; Sleep Disorders and Seizures, with very infrequent and mild adverse effects. The strongest improvements were reported for Seizures, Attention Deficit/Hyperactivity Disorder, Sleep Disorders, and Communication and Social Interaction Deficits.[11]

Sixty percent of the patients "were able to keep the improvements even after reducing or withdrawing other medications."[12] This, too, was a small study.

Now, from Israel, in a 2019 study, "Real Life Experience of Medical Cannabis Treatment in Autism: Analysis of Safety and Efficacy," they treated 188 kids with ASD with a low-THC/high-CBD cannabis product and followed both their symptoms and a global wellness assessment for the next six months. At this end point, 30 percent of the patients had significant improvement, 54 percent had moderate improvement, 6 percent slight, and 9 percent had no improvement. A quarter of the patients had at least one side effect, most commonly restlessness. They concluded that "cannabis in ASD patients appears to be a well-tolerated, safe and effective option to relieve the symptoms associated with ASD."[13] This conclusion is fairly striking, though it is an observational study, not a randomized controlled trial.

Another 2019 Israeli study, "Brief Report: Cannabidiol-Rich Cannabis in Children with Autism Spectrum Disorder and Severe Behavioral Problems: A Retrospective Feasibility Study," similarly found benefit with high-CBD/low-THC preparations. In this case they were studying children with ASD and refractory disruptive behaviors. The good news is that, "following the cannabis treatment, the behavioral outbreaks were much improved or very much improved in 61% of patients."[14] A significant proportion of the kids were able to meaningfully cut down on their medication usage. The bad news was that one girl had a transient psychotic episode in response to a higher-THC preparation she was using that had to be treated with an antipsychotic. So, remember that THC is by no means without the possibility of harm, and be careful of the dosages you use!

There aren't that many more studies to discuss. A 2020 review article in *Seminars in Pediatric Neurology*, "Autism Spectrum Disorder and Medical Cannabis: Review and Clinical Experience," found that 60 percent of the autistic kids whom they treated with CBD for aggressiveness, including self-injurious behavior, reported improvement, and concluded that "the intervention has potential for therapeutic benefit amongst some persons with ASD and is overall well tolerated."[15] Another 2019 Israeli study, this time of the primary caregivers of kids with ASD, showed that among children with a median age of eleven who received CBD for an average of sixty-six days, 67 percent had an improvement in self-injury and rage attacks, 68 percent had an improvement in hyperactivity symptoms, 71 percent had an improvement in sleep problems, and 47 percent had an improvement in anxiety. The side effects were found to be mild and were mostly sleepiness and appetite changes.[16]

What is around the corner in this exciting new potential avenue for treatment of ASD? Not nearly as much as should be. As I reviewed these articles in order to write this chapter, I came away astounded that this level of smoke, along with some actual small fires, hasn't ignited the attention of the medical and pharma community. There are some studies percolating, but not nearly as many as one might expect given how hopeful and convincing a possibility there is that the ECS presents as an effective treatment target for ASD. At the very least, we can get these kids off of some of the awful medications they are taking, such as the antipsychotics. And possibly we can address some of the core symptoms that are so discouraging and limiting to the patients and their families alike.

CBD is considered to be neuroprotective because it is a potent inhibitor of neuroinflammation. Neuroinflammation is increasingly implicated in ASD. The acidic cannabinoids, such as THCa and CBDa (which are simply precursors to THC and CBD in the form that comes directly from the plant, before being "decarboxylated" by heat), have tremendous potential as anti-inflammatory agents. Providers are reporting clinical success with these agents as well. Other cannabinoids, such as cannabidivarin (CBDV), may work even better than CBD.[17] What is the role of THC? How can it be used safely? Do we even need it? There are a few studies ongoing at the time of this writing, but it's just a drop in the bucket compared to what needs to be done.

What if ASD *is* mediated by the ECS, but we (the medical establishment in this case) missed it due to the War on Cannabis and the fact that the ECS has been largely ignored by medical schools and doctors alike? That would be tragic beyond words. The pioneering doctors and nurses who do provide care with cannabinoids for kids with ASD say that the literature is far behind what they currently are able to do for their patients. Maybe Mothers Advocating for Medical Marijuana for Autism, Cannamoms, and Whole Plant Access 4 Autism have had it right all along. Doctors, pediatric psychiatrists in particular, could be a bit more humble about the fact that they don't know much about the ECS and could be a little more curious about the role it might play in ASD (especially given what recently transpired with the widespread acceptance of CBD as an effective treatment for childhood epilepsy syndromes).

We won't truly know until we study all of this with an open mind. We can't deny kids medicine that works due to a failed and failing War on Drugs. But we can't just treat kids with drugs when we don't truly know if they work, or if they cause harm. It's past time that we got our act together on this issue and invested in research. The millions of kids with ASD across the globe deserve no less from us.

## CHAPTER NINETEEN
# CANNABIS AND MENTAL HEALTH
## Planet of the Shrinks

Does cannabis help or hurt one's mental health? It depends on whom you ask. Most of the millions of patients who use cannabis for mental health issues, or for general wellness, believe that it is remarkably effective, particularly for anxiety. Veterans in particular are reporting outcomes for PTSD that far transcend what traditional medications are able to provide for them. Many people use cannabis to help control their ADHD, often without disclosing this because of stigma. Users and cannabis clinicians alike witness that cannabis commonly provides patients relief from the entire gamut of mental health conditions that has commonly eluded them through traditional modalities (except psychosis). There is an ethos in parts of the cannabis community that taking pharmaceuticals is analogous to eating junk food, while using cannabis is akin to eating fresh, natural organic food.

On the other hand, if you were to ask a composite elder representative of the American psychiatric community, they likely would contend that the cannabis is making all these conditions worse. For example, according to a heading-grabbing 2019 article in *JAMA Psychiatry*, which has more than one hundred thousand views, called "Association of Cannabis Use in Adolescence and Risk of Depression, Anxiety, and Suicidality in Young Adulthood: A Systematic Review and Meta-analysis,"

in this systematic review and meta-analysis of 11 studies and 23,317 individuals, adolescent cannabis consumption *was associated* with increased risk of developing depression and suicidal behavior later in life, even in the absence of a premorbid condition.[1] (emphasis added)

They warn,

> Preadolescents and adolescents should avoid using cannabis as use *is associated* with a significant increased risk of developing depression or suicidality in young adulthood. . . . The high prevalence of adolescents consuming cannabis generates a large number of young people who *could* develop depression and suicidality attributable to cannabis.[2]

Unless you remember our discussion that "associated with" in no way means "causes," you walk away with the overarching impression that cannabis use is causing all of this depression and suicidal behavior. It isn't until you read the "limitations" section, at the very bottom of the study, that you are informed that

> strong causal association cannot be made with respect to the relationship between cannabis and later depression, suicide, or anxiety. . . . Not all studies have adjusted for other drugs of abuse and cigarettes, or psychosocial factors (ie, school abandonment, drug abuse in peers) that may be linked to depression and early cannabis consumption. . . . The longitudinal studies included in our analysis used heterogeneous methods of detecting major depressive disorder. . . . It was also not possible to evaluate the exact quantity of cannabis consumed among adolescents in individual studies since they used measures of frequency of use rather than the precise quantity.[3]

The cannabis absolutely *could* be causing the depression and the suicidality later in life, and I'm not at all in favor of adolescents using cannabis (see chapter 13). But there are certainly enough caveats and alternative explanations. For example, perhaps troubled teens, who haven't been diagnosed with depression or anxiety yet, turn to cannabis for relief. They will eventually be diagnosed with depression and anxiety and are at higher risk of suicide because they have depression and anxiety—but the cannabis isn't "causing" any of this, and might be helping. It makes one truly wonder which way the directionality flows, and if, just possibly, cannabis is again being thrown under the bus as a hangover from our Drug War mentality.

It makes sense that cannabinoids could help—or worsen—psychiatric conditions given that the ECS is involved in regulating virtually every part of the brain that is involved in processing fear, memory, emotions, anxiety, reward, and stress. This entire area is also fraught with controversy concerning issues such as what role cannabis has in causing or worsening psychosis, and what role cannabis and various cannabinoids will come to play in treating various substance use disorders, such as opioid addiction and alcohol use disorder.

The "does cannabis help or hurt mental illness?" issue represents one of the areas where cannabis patients and addiction psychiatrists are furthest apart from each other.

The chicken-versus-egg problem here is so big it could fill an entire continent. Study after study has shown that anxiety, depression, and suicide *are* linked to cannabis use. Heavy cannabis use clearly is associated with worse outcomes. Psychiatrists interpret and explain this as meaning the cannabis is *causing* and worsening the mental health issues, even though, as each of the studies concede, we can't truly deduce this one way or another from a statistical association. It becomes a "where there's (cannabis) smoke there's fire" argument. Historically, the psychiatrists—who, it must be noted, overwhelmingly haven't treated and don't treat patients *with cannabis* for these issues—have used the mantle of "we are the expert doctors" to seize the intellectual high ground, to insist that their truth is reality and to dismiss the lived experience of the cannabis patients who feel they are deriving benefit. Many of these patients wholly ignore the psychiatrists, and we thus, once again, have a dangerous disconnect, with patients not even telling their psychiatrists about their cannabis use.

A recent review article came out in the *American Journal of Psychiatry* that stated, "The current evidence base is insufficient to support the prescription of cannabinoids for the treatment of psychiatric disorders."[4] The millions of patients who have experienced the long-term beneficial effects of cannabis on their mental illness, often after getting nowhere with a psychiatrist, but at great expense, might take offense at this blanket dismissal. They think the psychiatrists are the ones whose heads should be examined, at least on this issue.

To clinicians who are facile with prescribing cannabis and who routinely treat people with cannabis for these issues, reliably achieving good outcomes, there is an obvious alternative explanation: people who have more severe mental health issues, or who have failed with the remedies of traditional psychiatry, are the ones who are more likely to use cannabis to self-treat, so *of course* cannabis *is associated with* worse outcomes, such as severe depression and suicide. As an analogy, a more serious cancer diagnosis *is associated with* more intensive chemotherapy, but the chemotherapy obviously isn't causing or worsening the cancer; it is treating it. A common sentiment is, "We all know that correlation doesn't equate to causation, so why are you still bringing up this Drug War canard?"

I believe there is a legitimate hypothetical concern that cannabis may appear to alleviate depression in the short term because it causes relaxation and euphoria, but it could simultaneously be worsening these symptoms over time. If one uses a large amount of cannabis every day, the natural receptors by which cannabis works on the body "downregulate," or thin out, in response to chronic external stimulation. Hence, the phenomenon known as tolerance—you need more and more to get the same effect. When the external chemical is withdrawn after prolonged use, the body is left in the lurch and is forced to rely on natural stores of these chemicals, called "endocannabinoids," which have to fish around for less abundant receptors to do their job. Symptoms of this often include anxiety and depression. This makes sense as, without the external and large doses of cannabis to boost up this increasingly depleted system, one's baseline is more anxious and more depressed, as our natural endocannabinoids have fewer receptors to trigger. Fortunately, the receptors return to normal levels within weeks. Of course, people frequently have rebound depression and anxiety with almost all antidepressants, so cannabis is hardly unique in this manner. For example, people who stop their venlafaxine (Effexor) abruptly can attest to this—the rebound is vicious.

There's also the problem that people "learn to cope" with negative emotions by using cannabis rather than by natural means such as simply tolerating the emotion, exercising, or talking with a friend—this is of particular concern for teens, who are just learning how to get by in the world and are thought to be more vulnerable to all substance addictions than adults.

The American Psychiatric Association, in their 2019 statement, "Position Statement in Opposition to Cannabis as Medicine," states,

> There is no current scientific evidence that cannabis is in any way beneficial for the treatment of any psychiatric disorder. In contrast, current

evidence supports, at minimum, a strong association of cannabis use with the onset of psychiatric disorders. . . . Policy and practice surrounding cannabis-derived substances should not be altered until sufficient clinical evidence supports such changes. . . . Medical treatment should be evidence-based and determined by professional standards of care; it should not be authorized by ballot initiatives.[5]

The American Psychiatric Association has been highly supportive of the War on Drugs over the last five decades and—as expressed by their public opinions against legalization or decriminalization—seems to believe that arresting and possibly imprisoning people is better for their mental health than cannabis use, especially Black and brown people. They must think cannabis is pretty harmful! From the uncompromising nature of their statements, one can understand why some patients might not feel comfortable mentioning their cannabis use. (There is also a distressing lack of humility in their absolute antipathy to medical treatment "being authorized by ballot initiatives," as this presupposes that the doctors always have been, are now, and always will be correct about all medical issues, which clearly hasn't remotely been the case.)

A recent summary in the *American Journal of Psychiatry* titled "Risks and Benefits of Cannabis and Cannabinoids in Psychiatry" goes over this purported lack of evidence for the usage of cannabis for anxiety, depression, and PTSD in detail. However, "the authors outline the evidence [only] from randomized double-blind placebo-controlled trials."[6] This means that, by fiat, they decided to ignore all real-world evidence—the evidence that demonstrates what effects real cannabis users are actually experiencing, as they are actually using normal cannabis (i.e., not Moldy Mush from NIDA) (see chapter 7). Instead, they seem content to rely exclusively on the studies that were the funding priorities of the U.S. government's War on Drugs. As discussed, these priorities featured a massive search for harms and avoided funding the search for, or finding, any benefits of cannabis use. This is not to mention that many of these studies were done on cannabis that was still illegal and unregulated, without the guidance of a cannabis clinician or mental health provider. Further, they state, "articles that did not contain the terms 'clinical trial' or 'therapy' in the title or abstract were not reviewed."[7] You can't make this up! If you know anything about the cultural, social, or academic history of cannabis, this a priori rules out most articles that could show benefit. What a surprise that they didn't find any evidence for benefit! Better stick to the psychiatric drugs that the psychiatrists prescribe. They would counter that RCTs are the only reliable forms of evidence, but this notion was thoroughly debunked in chapter 7.

One starts to see why there is a trust gap.

They go on to state, "There are currently no psychiatric indications approved by the U.S. Food and Drug Administration (FDA) for cannabinoids."[8] However, we doctors use medications "off-label" all the time, so when they try to weaponize "no indications approved by the FDA," it is a red herring. For example, there are no FDA-approved medications for cannabis use disorder, but these same exact psychiatrists throw Ambien, gabapentin, and all other types of medicines at this condition. Why? Because they think it helps. Why is this practice valid in one context and not another? Further, this ignores the fact that the U.S. FDA has been less than neutral on cannabis and has no coherent pathway for approving a botanical drug with five hundred components.

Or, another example, from a 1998 paper by my dad and his longtime writing partner James "Jake" Bakalar: "An analogy is drawn between the status of cannabis today and that of lithium in the early 1950s, when its effect on mania had been discovered but there were no controlled studies."[9] Luckily, psychiatrists were courageous and open-minded enough to forge ahead, improving the lives of millions, and didn't say, "Sorry, no controlled studies, no lithium for you."

Recently I treated a twenty-five-year-old professional woman with cannabis for her anxiety and depression, which she has struggled with since her late teens, including a suicide attempt at age seventeen. She went from one psychiatric drug to another—none of them made her feel any less despondent. Eventually, after several years, she gave up on traditional medicine and discovered cannabis. Her anxiety and depression promptly resolved, and she was able to finish college. She is having no ill effects from the stable dose of cannabis that she is on and attributes to it the success she is increasingly having in all walks of life. She is now in a happy, stable relationship. This type of story is by no means rare.

My question is, do people like her not count? There's no RCT that could or would capture the nuanced way in which cannabis has alleviated her suffering and allowed her to thrive. She's not particularly vocal about her cannabis use because of the stigma, so stories like this are undercounted. She has never encountered a psychiatrist that she could openly discuss her cannabis use with. To the psychiatrists, this would be another case of "the anxiety and depression *is associated with* cannabis use." Wouldn't the thousands upon thousands (likely millions, actually) of cases like this at least stimulate some sense of wonder and curiosity. Like, "Hey, is it possible that we are missing something here?"

The authors go on to state, "There is considerable evidence that cannabinoids have a potential for harm in vulnerable populations such as . . . those with psychotic disorders." As discussed in chapter 8, there are sensible ways to be cautious around this, such as obtaining a good family history for schizophrenia and discouraging people with active psychosis, or a propensity toward psychosis, from using THC. They advise, "Prescribing clinicians should avoid initiating or recommending cannabinoid pharmacotherapy for most psychiatric patients." But, one must ask, *if none of these psychiatrists treat—or ever have treated—patients with cannabis, how would they have any idea if it does or doesn't work?* Surely not by putting blinders on and ignoring real-world evidence, or by ensconcing themselves in anti-cannabis echo chambers. And on what grounds do they dismiss the broad clinical successes that cannabis physicians are having? How do they dismiss the millions that are benefiting? Are patients just making it up?

Here's how. They warn, with a near-lethal dose of protective paternalism, and I'm drawing this straight from the article,

> These discussions [with patients about cannabis] must consider that many patients may feel that cannabis preparations have been helpful to them or people they know.[10]

I'm not trying to cause trouble. I'm just trying to illuminate the attitude that cannabis patients have dealt with for decades and to explain the breakdown in trust. This illustrates why patients often don't tell their shrinks about their cannabis use, which is the most dangerous of outcomes. The subtext in this is pretty clear: "Silly little patients who think they know what helps them and alleviates their symptoms . . . leave the adult decisions to us, *we know what is good for you*, and abandon all of this childish voodoo and mysticism."

In other words, the exact people who (mostly) haven't tried can-nabis themselves (or who won't publicly admit they have used it); who participated (often indirectly) in the Drug War effort to focus solely on the harms in research and education while ignoring or curating evidence of the benefits; who never treat, or have treated, patients with cannabis for *any* of these indications; and who have never even considered the possibility that cannabis *might* be an effective treatment are somehow *the* experts on this? When searching for explanations, it is difficult not to marvel at the coincidence that these particular professionals also happen to lose business when people treat themselves with cannabis instead of psychiatrist-prescribed psychotropics.

As my Yiddish-speaking ancestors would say, oy vey.

I particularly take issue with the trivialization of the lived experience of patients. For example, I was part of a small team which included several addiction psychiatrists and one other internist for the Physician Health Program. We were discussing cases in our usual collegial manner when one of the addiction psychiatrists, who is an astute clinician, said, "One of my patients says his anxiety is controlled by a type of marijuana called 'Purple Haze.'" They all started laughing in a derisive, "what a simple, superstitious patient who just wants to get high and pretend it's medicine" type of way. I was shocked at this utter dismissal of medical cannabis. Purple Haze is a fairly good strain for anxiety. It is a moderate THC strain with the calming terpene myrcene in it. I tried to explain why and how it might work for anxiety to this group of addiction experts, but there was no interest, no curiosity, and no wiggle room in their belief system. I gave up after a few minutes.

This group later vetoed my push to allow medical cannabis for physi-cians who are in the Physician Health Program receiving care and monitor-ing. They said that they wanted to follow Colorado's example. The law in Colorado said, at that point, that medical cannabis is for debilitating condi-tions. Therefore, anyone, including doctors, who uses cannabis medically is "debilitated." Therefore, they are, as such, unfit for practice because they are debilitated. Therefore, we can't allow doctors to use medical cannabis.

This type of reasoning wasn't taught in my logic classes at Swarth-more. It was taught in ancient philosophy as sophistry, which is defined as "the use of fallacious arguments, especially with the intent of deceiving."[11] I tried to point out how arbitrary and irrational I thought this was, but the decision had already been made before it was even brought up to the group.

Most anxiety and depression is treated by primary care doctors, not by psychiatrists. According to a 2010 study, "some research has suggested that the number of mental health patients treated in primary care may be as high as 70% and that as many as 66–75% of all depression cases are treated by PCPs instead of by mental health providers."[12] So, it is not as if primary care doctors do not have experience treating anxiety and depression. It makes up a large and increasing part of every primary care clinic. I can assure you, through decades of clinical experience—mine and that of other colleagues with whom I am frequently in contact—that many patients do well on cannabis, particularly for anxiety. Others do well with SSRIs and other conventional antidepressants. Many improve with therapy alone, or just with the passage of time and the adoption of healthier habits. There is no "one size fits all" in treating mental health. It is the height of hubris, and a grave disservice to patients, to entirely discount so much lived experience or to blanketly dismiss an entire line of treatment—especially if you don't know much about the endocannabinoid system or the practicalities of medical cannabis.

There's also the question of autonomy, which is integral to mental health. One wonders why people shouldn't be allowed to opt for a natural, plant-based treatment if they feel it resolves their symptoms.

What does NASEM say? NASEM also didn't include much real-world evidence, but at least it made a good-faith effort to be objective. For anxiety, it "did not identify any good-quality primary literature that reported on medical cannabis as an effective treatment for the improvement of anxiety symptoms." They did cite one study where taking a single dose of CBD helped people suffering from social anxiety disorder during a simulated public speaking test (see chapter 20). NASEM also references benefits of cannabinoids for anxiety associated with chronic pain, which makes sense under the "cannabis works on several symptoms at once" theory: anxiety, pain, sleep.

According to a summary by Dr. Staci Gruber and Kelly Sagar from the MIND Institute at Harvard's McLean Hospital, the conclusions from NASEM are nuanced:

> The report concluded that cannabis use does not appear to increase the likelihood of developing depression, anxiety (with the exception of social anxiety disorder), or posttraumatic stress disorder but noted that cannabis use may exacerbate symptoms in those already diagnosed with mood/anxiety disorders and that heavy cannabis users are more likely to report thoughts of suicide than non-users. . . . Importantly, however, the studies that met NASEM's rigorous criteria for review were predominantly focused on the impact of THC. Newer research focused on specific cannabinoids vs. the impact of "cannabis" use in general will ultimately allow for more thoughtfully crafted, informed policies designed to protect the mental health of all Americans.[13]

Critically, they continue,

> It is also important to note that the continued criminalization of cannabis in some jurisdictions across the US has a measurable impact on Americans' mental health. According to the Federal Bureau of Investigations Uniform Crime Report, just over 350,150 Americans were arrested for cannabis-related crimes in 2020, with 91% of arrests for possession only. The negative impact on mental health associated with interactions with the criminal justice system is well established.[14]

One might question why the American Psychiatric Association hasn't concerned itself with this type of harm, which has harmed millions of Americans?

One interesting 2018 study, from the *Journal of Affective Disorders*, called "A Naturalistic Examination of the Perceived Effects of Cannabis on Negative Affect," provides some evidence for both sides of the dispute over efficacy. Note the word "naturalistic" in the title—this is based on real-world evidence and might, as such, be invisible to the psychiatrists. In this study, the researchers used an app to track the mood of thousands of cannabis sessions in medical cannabis patients. Their stated goal was to fill a large gap in our knowledge base by "tracking the perceived efficacy of inhaled cannabis in coping with feelings of negative affect in medical cannabis users' naturalistic environment." They tracked a total of almost twelve thousand cannabis sessions. They found the following:

1. Cannabis significantly reduced ratings of depression, anxiety, and stress.

2. Women reported larger reductions in anxiety as a function of cannabis than did men.

3. Low-THC/high-CBD cannabis was best for reducing perceived symptoms of depression.

4. High-THC/high-CBD cannabis was best for reducing perceived symptoms of stress.

And, importantly,

5. Use of cannabis to treat depression appears to exacerbate depression over time.[15]

Notably, the same was not found to be true for anxiety. The authors point out that these results are similar to how people respond to conventional antidepressants: "Similar to more conventional pharmacological treatments, cannabis may temporarily mask symptoms of negative affect but may not effectively reduce these symptoms in the long-term."[16]

In this context, it is important to remember that the long-term data for SSRIs and the other medications that we dispense for depression isn't overwhelmingly impressive either. These medications have some scary side effects as well, including a black-box warning about increased suicidality for younger patients. SSRIs can be incredibly difficult to get off of. It has not been established whether they are safer or more effective than judiciously prescribed cannabinoids for the treatment of anxiety—the two haven't been compared. Certainly, cannabis is safer than the tranquilizers used, such as Valium and other benzodiazepines.

As a clinician, I can say that the actual effect of cannabis on anxiety is nuanced. Generally, THC tends to lower anxiety at low doses and can heighten anxiety at high doses—it is "biphasic." CBD, to the extent that it does anything as it is commonly consumed (see chapter 20), lowers anxiety at all dosages. If someone takes too large a dose of cannabis, such as a cannabis newbie eating a huge dose of edibles in the tradition of Maureen Dowd as memorialized in her 2014 *New York Times* column, it can cause a massive panic attack. If the first time you tried alcohol you drank an entire quart of tequila, you'd get sick. It's about education and common sense. This is why cannabis clinicians go to great lengths to drill into patients the need to "start low and go slow." I am proud to say that I have never had a patient "freak out" from taking too high a dose.

Many of the studies of cannabis and anxiety have been done under highly artificial laboratory conditions, and they are done with oral (or, God forbid, intravenous) cannabinoids, both of which tend to be more anxiety provoking than smoked cannabis. If you ask me, just the thought of taking an oral cannabinoid in a lab, or getting injected with it, and then being analyzed by judgmental, cannabis-dismissing psychiatrists—who are strictly trying to find harms—monitoring and prodding me, as one would do a lab animal, would be enough to *cause* a full-blown anxiety attack, even without the cannabis. Then, it's like, "Aha—cannabis causes anxiety; let's define that as a 'psychotic' symptom and say cannabis causes psychosis."

As all cannabis users know, "set and setting"—meaning both one's mind-set at the time and one's external environment—are a critical component of how relaxed or anxious one feels during any particular episode of cannabis use. That is why "naturalistic" studies are vital.

PTSD is another hotly contested indication for cannabis. Veterans, and other patients, including many of my patients, say it greatly helps them, and, in general, psychiatrists say it makes them much worse off. The veterans feel devalued, ignored, and misunderstood when psychiatrists—most of whom haven't treated a single patient with cannabis—like a Greek chorus, tell the vets that cannabis doesn't work and is, in fact, harming them.

When you speak with veterans, many of them will readily tell you how profoundly grateful they are to have discovered cannabis, especially for PTSD. They will also tell you how relieved they are to be done with cocktail after cocktail of opiates, sedatives, muscle relaxers, sleeping pills, and antidepressants that tone-deaf clinicians at the veterans' hospitals foist on them, or the alchemy of alcohol and illegal drugs such as heroin and cocaine they were using to self-treat their emotional and physical pain before finding their way to cannabis. They also express quite a bit of anger that the Veterans Administration currently prohibits their doctors from recommending or certifying medical cannabis. Until recently, they weren't even allowed to discuss cannabis with patients. They also complain about the price of cannabis, which is extremely difficult to afford on the modest fixed income that our government awards disabled veterans.

There aren't any medications that work particularly well for PTSD, so it's a big deal for the psychiatrists to continue to advocate for prohibiting vets and others from having access to cannabis. "We don't have much to offer you, yet we're going to block you from using what you think/know/feel helps you." This doesn't always go over well, as all people want their autonomy respected, especially those who risked their lives to protect ours.

Vets who believe in cannabis are obviously going to use it anyway. I can't understand why we would allow them to get arrested, or to lose their service benefits for this, even if we are among those who think it doesn't work. I also don't understand why the psychiatrists wouldn't at least meet the vets halfway and explore with them how they think they are being benefited.

The 2019 position statement of the American Psychiatric Association says cannabis "should not be authorized by ballot initiatives"[17] or, in other words, should stay illegal until someone like Donald Trump or Joe Biden—two Einsteins when it comes to cannabis—or our fractious congresspeople decide to legalize it. This is like waiting for the Great Pumpkin. They also put medical marijuana in quotes: "Physicians who recommend use of cannabis for 'medical' purposes should be fully aware of the risks and liabilities inherent in doing so." This attitude all but ensures that patients, particularly vets, won't discuss their cannabis use with their psychiatrists. I always encourage them to do so, to keep trying, as it is safer and more coherent for everyone to know what medicines a patient is taking, but countless patients have said, "When I brought it up, he or she looked so displeased, I never brought it up again," or something along those lines.

I have used cannabis to treat hundreds of patients with PTSD—many of whom bring this up in primary care clinic after having failed miserably with their VAH psychiatrist, or without even having tried to discuss it with them. I have mostly had positive results, in many cases strikingly so. A few can't use it because it makes them more anxious.

One middle-aged Vietnam vet whom I treat was so troubled by his flashbacks and anxiety—caused by a nasty tour of duty in Vietnam—that he was drinking six shots of vodka twice a day to quell them. He was miserable, hiding out in his home, increasingly isolated, bloated, and suicidal. We switched him to taking a puff (on his dry herb vaporizer) of medium-potency cannabis (with some CBD) twice a day. His mood has now been stable—and vastly improved across the board—on this regimen for years. No problems, no side effects, no dose escalation. He now leaves his house (without driving!), hangs out with his buddies during the day, and even goes fishing again—without being troubled by flashbacks and intrusive thoughts, as long as he has his trusty vaporizer nearby. His liver tests have also come back to normal, free from the beating that the alcohol was giving his liver.

He had gotten nowhere with his VAH psychiatrist, who looked disdainful when he brought cannabis up, wouldn't discuss it with him, and who kept trying to load him up on sedatives. He never went back.

What does the research say about cannabis and PTSD? It is contradictory. A 2019 review article, "The Effectiveness of Cannabinoids in the Treatment of Posttraumatic Stress Disorder (PTSD): A Systematic Review," sums up the situation well,

> Most studies to date are small and of low quality, with significant limitations to the study designs precluding any clinical recommendations about its use in routine clinical practice. Evidence that cannabinoids may help reduce global PTSD symptoms, sleep disturbances, and nightmares indicates that future well-controlled, randomized, double-blind clinical trials are highly warranted.[18]

People who have experienced a traumatic event often report that cannabis is particularly helpful for sleep. A 2014 study, "Using Cannabis to Help You Sleep: Heightened Frequency of Medical Cannabis Use among Those with PTSD," found that sleep improvement was a prime motivator for cannabis use in patients with high PTSD scores.[19] This coincides with what I see in clinic. Many vets are tired of the tranquilizers that the Veterans Administration dumps on them and are delighted to have discovered a good night's sleep with cannabis instead, which enables them to wake up feeling refreshed, not drugged.

There is evidence that the synthetic THC analogue nabilone may be effective in the management of nightmares among individuals with PTSD and may also help patients get off of more dangerous meds. In a 2014 study, "Use of a Synthetic Cannabinoid in a Correctional Population for Posttraumatic Stress Disorder–Related Insomnia and Nightmares, Chronic Pain, Harm Reduction, and Other Indications," patients with PTSD were given nabilone.

> Results indicated significant improvement in PTSD-associated insomnia, nightmares, PTSD symptoms, and Global Assessment of Functioning and subjective improvement in chronic pain. Medications associated with greater risk for adverse effects or abuse than nabilone were often able to be discontinued with the initiation of nabilone, most often antipsychotics and sedative/hypnotics.[20]

This is exactly what all the vets are saying! We could simply listen to them.

In a 2009 study, "The Use of a Synthetic Cannabinoid in the Management of Treatment-Resistant Nightmares in Posttraumatic Stress Disorder (PTSD)," "the majority of patients (72%) receiving nabilone experienced either cessation of nightmares or a significant reduction in nightmare intensity."[21]

A very thorough 2021 study, "Cannabis in the Management of PTSD: A Systematic Review," demonstrates the contradictory nature of some of the research:

> A single RCT showed that nabilone [synthetic THC] was significantly associated with a reduction in overall PTSD symptoms. Four observational studies reported that cannabis significantly reduced PTSD symptoms, whereas one observational study reported an insignificant effect of cannabis on PTSD symptoms. In two studies cannabis use exacerbated PTSD symptoms.[22]

In summary, the study concluded, "Cannabis was associated with a reduction in overall PTSD symptoms and improved QOL [quality of life]."[23]

This is not inconsistent with NASEM, which concludes, "The committee did not identify a good- or fair-quality systematic review that reported on medical cannabis as an effective treatment for PTSD symptoms."[24] They do cite one study of Canadian male military personnel treated with nabilone which shows that "nightmares, global clinical state, and general well-being were improved more with nabilone treatment than with the placebo treatment." NASEM concludes, "There is limited evidence (a single, small fair-quality trial) that nabilone is effective for improving symptoms of posttraumatic stress disorder."[25] NASEM references a study that was pending at the time of the writing, which has since been published, "Cannabinoids as Therapeutic for PTSD,"

> CBD and THC+CBD may be capable of modulating fear memory in PTSD by blocking reconsolidation and facilitating extinction learning. Research suggests that CBD may also have acute positive effects on anxiety and anhedonia, though the cross applicability of these findings to humans is unknown. Finally, preliminary data suggests that THC may have an effect on the reduction of nightmares, while THC+CBD may be important to further examine in terms of therapeutic potential for insomnia and sleep problems in PTSD.[26]

One longitudinal study of veterans, "Marijuana Use Is Associated with Worse Outcomes in Symptom Severity and Violent Behavior in Patients with Posttraumatic Stress Disorder," studied veterans who were in a specialty treatment program for PTSD. They compared the outcomes of vets who never used cannabis, started using cannabis, continued using cannabis, and stopped using cannabis. They found that cannabis

> starters and continuing users had significantly higher measures of PTSD symptom severity at follow-up compared to never-users and stoppers.[27]

The cannabis was also associated with more violent behavior. However, as is the problem with many of these studies,

> this study cannot exclude the possibility that PTSD patients refractory to treatment are more likely to use marijuana in an attempt to self-medicate.[28]

Egg, meet chicken. They included some interesting speculation on how to reconcile the perceived benefits of PTSD for vets and the data showing worse outcomes:

> Another possible interpretation of these data is that marijuana use in patients with PTSD provides transient relief but that subsequent periods

of withdrawal contribute to a worsening of baseline symptoms. Hence, *while patients may feel that marijuana improves their PTSD, it may contribute to an overall worsening of the disorder.*[29] (emphasis added)

This is similar to the theory of depression getting transiently better with cannabis, but worse as time progresses. This theory certainly needs to be further investigated, but I don't think many vets would be convinced by this. The ones I know medically (and socially for that matter) paint an extremely different picture of having been given too many opioids and sedatives before, but now experiencing greatly improved stability and mood with cannabis.

A large 2020 naturalistic study, "Short and Long-Term Effects of Cannabis on Symptoms of Post-Traumatic Stress Disorder," which tracked more than four hundred vets who use cannabis for PTSD over time and evaluated their symptoms with an app that was used to track PTSD-related symptoms (intrusive thoughts, flashbacks, irritability, and anxiety) right before and after using cannabis. There were almost twelve thousand data points. Their results are telling:

*All symptoms were reduced by more than 50% immediately after cannabis use.* Time predicted larger decreases in intrusions and irritability, with later cannabis use sessions predicting greater symptom relief than earlier sessions. Higher doses of cannabis predicted larger reductions in intrusions and anxiety, and dose used to treat anxiety increased over time. *Baseline severity of all symptoms remained constant across time.*[30] (emphasis added)

Cannabis did provide symptom relief, but it didn't improve (or worsen) the symptoms over time. This is a win, as treating symptoms is half the battle, especially for PTSD where there aren't any curative treatments (though MDMA is an interesting possibility). The dosage needed to alleviate symptoms increased over time, which isn't necessarily sustainable but could be addressed with carefully monitored tolerance breaks.

A 2020 study by star cannabis researcher Dr. Stephanie Lake, "Does Cannabis Use Modify the Effect of Post-traumatic Stress Disorder on Severe Depression and Suicidal Ideation? Evidence from a Population-Based Cross-Sectional Study of Canadians," looked at twenty-four thousand charts of a nationally representative sample of Canadians.

Twenty-eight percent of people with PTSD reported past-year cannabis use versus 11 percent of those without PTSD. They found that

> post-traumatic stress disorder was significantly associated with recent major depressive episode (seven times increased risk) and suicidal ideation (almost five times increased risk) *among cannabis non-users.* Post-traumatic stress disorder *was not associated with either outcome among cannabis-using respondents.*[31] (emphasis added)

This paper concurs with the vets and others with PTSD who maintain that cannabis is beneficial and protective.

Another recent study, which is a prospective study, "The Long-Term, Prospective, Therapeutic Impact of Cannabis on Post-Traumatic Stress Disorder," assessed PTSD symptoms and functioning over time and compared groups that were using dispensary weed versus a group that didn't use cannabis. They found that,

> over the course of 1 year, the cannabis users reported a greater decrease in PTSD symptom severity over time compared to controls. Participants who used cannabis were 2.57 times more likely to no longer meet DSM-5 criteria for PTSD at the end of the study observation period compared to participants who did not use cannabis.[32]

Notably, they are using high-quality dispensary weed, not the Moldy Mush strain that NIDA forced everyone to use in their research.

It is difficult to reconcile the studies represented above, as well as the virtually unanimous opinion of veterans, with recent pronouncements from the psychiatrists: "The current evidence base is insufficient to support the prescription of cannabinoids for the treatment of psychiatric disorders."[33] While the jury is, to a certain extent, still out with cannabis and PTSD in terms of the long-term outcomes, it seems pretty clear that cannabis alleviates symptoms, which, again, is *really important if you have PTSD*, especially if it doesn't worsen your disease over time. Further, cannabis replaces many of the other more dangerous meds the vets are using. A cynical interpretation is that the psychiatrists don't want to be cut out of the process, either intellectually or financially, as vets can treat themselves with cannabis (as, sadly, they have been doing due to the utter dismissal on this issue of their feelings and beliefs by the psychiatrists, who appear to be fixating on gloomy observational studies rather than talking to, and studying, their patients over time).

Cannabis should clearly, in my opinion, be legally available to all veterans, as the least we can do to thank them for their service, as we continue to study its long-term effects. It should be paid for by our government to save the vets from worrying about how to afford it. The Canadian government supplies cannabis to their vets—there's no reason for them to continue to put us to shame on this issue.

My final thought on PTSD relates to Michael Pollan's brilliant book *The Botany of Desire*. He points out that cannabis helps us forget, and that forgetting is a critical function. Many others have brought up this point, including the Israeli cannabis researcher Raphael Mechoulam, the psychologist William James, and the philosopher Friedrich Nietzsche. If we remembered every detail, every face on the bus, every menu item from the diner in the morning—our brains would get overloaded and would soon shut down. Cannabis and the ECS help us to forget; a short-term side effect of cannabis, so our brains can continue to function. This forgetting function may be part of how and why cannabis alleviates symptoms in PTSD. We know from animal studies that

> administering THC or CBD before extinction learning trials in rats and mice reduces cue-elicited fear, blocks reconsolidation of fear memory, and facilitates faster extinction of fear memory in animal models of PTSD.[34]

Perhaps forgetting our pain, and our fears, is part of the key to treating PTSD, so that we can heal. For that matter, perhaps this is part of the key to being human.

People with ADHD are more likely to use cannabis. I don't think many doctors realize how many people are using cannabis to *alleviate* their ADHD symptoms as opposed to escaping from them. They don't ask, and many patients don't volunteer this information due to fear of condescension and criticism. I personally know dozens of people who use, or who have used, cannabis to mitigate the symptoms of their ADHD, and have treated many more. When it works, it is surprisingly effective. I can't tell you how many times I've heard, "It's the only thing that got me through college." Cannabis can clearly make ADHD symptoms worse in other people.

People with ADHD who use cannabis describe its effect as a slowing down of the overwhelming and incessant flood of ideas in their brains. This enables them to focus on specific ideas so that they aren't paralyzed in thought. It clears their heads from the clutter. It can also affect them differently than it does the rest of us. Just as a person with ADHD might find psychostimulants calming, whereas the rest of us tend to get wired and experience them as "uppers," many people with ADHD find that low doses of cannabis are focusing and energizing. They don't seem to get particularly stoned. Cannabis enables them to function at a higher level.

A 2022 case series, "Cannabis for the Treatment of Attention Deficit Hyperactivity Disorder: A Report of 3 Cases," features three cases where they were able to corroborate the claimed improvement in ADHD symptoms on validated rating scales. Across the board, improvements in anxiety, depression, regulation, and inattention were seen. They demonstrated that the measured effect was temporally related to cannabis by checking blood levels. The cannabis, in these cases, was an adjunct treatment, not the sole treatment, and it was clearly helpful.[35]

This case series echoes what was found in a 2015 study from Germany, "Successful Authorised Therapy of Treatment Resistant Adult ADHD with Cannabis: Experience from a Medical Practice with 30 Patients." These were all patients who failed conventional treatment with psychostimulants. The results are impressive:

> Under Monotherapy with Cannabis, 73% of patients reached an ADHD-symptom level that allowed them to participate in working and social life. In 47% of cases, an improvement of concentration abilities were mentioned explicitly. Especially helpful appeared the reduction of agitation and impulsiveness.[36]

If your traditional medication isn't working for adult ADHD, this study suggests trying cannabis. I agree (utilizing the expertise of a cannabis specialist) and would add that cannabis can work as an adjunct to psychostimulants and can also help with side effects from the psychostimulants, such as anorexia and insomnia.

It's not clear how exactly cannabis might improve ADHD. I saw one piece that cited "a hypothesis that cannabis might address frontal dysregulation, which is more typical in combined type ADHD that includes hyperactive-impulsive symptoms."[37] This is a little vague.

A 2020 Israeli study, "Cannabinoid and Terpenoid Doses Are Associated with Adult ADHD Status of Medical Cannabis Patients," had an unexpected wrinkle in it. What they showed was that "higher-dose consumption of MC (medical cannabis) components (phyto-cannabinoids and terpenes) is associated with ADHD medication reduction."[38] Given how dangerous psychostimulants like Adderall are, any dose reduction is welcome news. What was particularly interesting is that they demonstrated that "high dosage of CBN was associated with a lower [ADHD] score." What on earth is CBN? CBN, or cannabinol, is a cannabinoid present in trace amounts in the cannabis plant. CBN is marketed for its sedative and sleep-inducing qualities. Marijuana that has been sitting around for too long has a reputation for becoming "sleepy old marijuana" because the THC naturally degrades to CBN with exposure to time and light. Why would CBN help with ADHD? We don't know, but CBN may turn out to be a nonintoxicating alternative or adjunct to psychostimulants.

It's interesting that even some of those studies that seemed to be interested in discrediting cannabis as a therapy had a difficult time proving that cannabis worsened ADHD. One study had its expectations overturned:

> To our knowledge, this is the first study investigating the combined effects of ADHD and cannabis use on Executive Function (EF). *We predicted childhood-diagnosed ADHD and cannabis use would be related to worse EF.* Instead, for almost all tasks we observed a clear effect for ADHD but *not for cannabis use, either contemporaneous or historical.* The strongest negative effects of ADHD were on impulsivity, working memory, and verbal memory. Although we also expected individuals with a childhood history of ADHD who used cannabis regularly would demonstrate particularly poor EF performance, we found no significant ADHD by cannabis use interactions.[39] (emphasis added)

Imagine what we might find when we start looking for benefits rather than merely trying to prove harms.

The one RCT that exists on cannabis and ADHD, "Cannabinoids in Attention-Deficit/Hyperactivity Disorder: A Randomised-Controlled Trial," randomized one group to cannabis and another group to placebo. The results had relatively low statistical power due to the small sample size. They found that

Sativex [a medical preparation of THC and CBD] was associated with a nominally significant improvement in hyperactivity/impulsivity and a cognitive measure of inhibition, and a trend towards improvement for inattention and EL (emotional lability). *Adults with ADHD may represent a subgroup of individuals who experience a reduction of symptoms and no cognitive impairments following cannabinoid use.*[40]

The final study I'll mention is a large 2022 survey with more than seventeen hundred participants, "Self-Reported Effects of Cannabis on ADHD Symptoms, ADHD Medication Side Effects, and ADHD-Related Executive Dysfunction," which found that

participants with ADHD who have used cannabis reported that cannabis has acute beneficial effects on many symptoms of ADHD (e.g., hyperactivity, impulsivity). Further, they perceived cannabis to improve most of their medication side effects (e.g., irritability, anxiety).[41]

Surveys aren't always the most objective way to measure treatment effects. People who are using cannabis for ADHD obviously think it works for ADHD or they wouldn't be using it. This can produce an "expectancy effect" where expectations become a placebo-like reality. Overall, the evidence that cannabis can alleviate ADHD symptoms is quite suggestive, especially if you've witnessed it in person as I have (see afterword). It is astounding. Clearly, this issue is crying out for further study.

The studies on the effects of cannabis on bipolar disorder are about as contradictory as they are for PTSD. According to Dr. Gruber,

some studies assessing cannabis use among patients with BPD note reduced compliance, higher illness severity, and exacerbation of manic symptoms, while other data indicate that patients with BPD frequently report subjective clinical improvements as a result of cannabis use, underscoring the need for more work in this area.[42]

We need a neutral evaluation of this issue as well.

One final point, and I strongly agree with the psychiatrists here. If we are having a difficult time diagnosing someone, the presence of a lot of cannabis use (or other drugs or alcohol) can make it much more difficult to come to an accurate diagnosis. What is helped by the cannabis? What is worsened by the cannabis? Are these withdrawal symptoms? Often, to figure out what's ailing a person, ideally, you have to take them off all psychoactive substances to see where they are at baseline. It can be difficult to do this if the patient is addicted or is convinced that the cannabis is helping. People, especially young people, may think it's medical when it could be part of the problem.

# CHAPTER TWENTY
# CBD
## Gourmet Placebo or Wonder Drug?

Recently, the popularity of the nonintoxicating cannabinoid CBD, or cannabidiol, has exploded like an H-bomb, with seismic ripples of curiosity and interest reverberating around the globe, and with the fallout of enthusiasm infecting hundreds of millions of people. Just ten years ago, few people would have even heard of CBD, and now one in seven Americans is taking some form of it. One in three Americans has tried it. Is this spectacular rise in the popularity of CBD due to the unparalleled healing properties of CBD or to faddish thinking and clever marketing? The answer is . . . yes.

CBD can now be found in burgers and pizzas, and in the toothpicks you can use to clean your teeth after eating these burgers and pizzas. One group even spliced a CBD gene into a potato so that the fries you eat with your burger could have CBD in them as well. It can be found in the lattes and cappuccinos you drink to wake up after stuffing yourself with so much fat. It can be found impregnated into the workout clothing you wear when working off this meal, and in the soaps, lotions, or bath bomb you use to relax and wash up after your workout. As you rest at night after all of this, you can use a CBD pillowcase to get that extra expensive rest. Is this giving you a headache yet? If so, I know exactly what you can take for it.

More traditionally, people find CBD in the massive, unregulated, and often unreliable supplement industry in the form of pills, oils, vapes, creams, tinctures, hemp cigarettes, and gummies. This industry has a major problem with quality control, and study after study has sampled random products off the shelf only to find them either entirely lacking in any CBD, or having wildly low (or sometimes high) levels of CBD compared to how much the label states they have. Also, not infrequently, they have unwelcome and unexpected ingredients such as THC. As a medical cannabis doctor, I am not against THC, but *you can't have THC when you aren't expecting it,* as you might be driving home or, who knows, in charge of your neighbor's screaming toddler for a few hours. (Actually, THC might help prevent a headache from the toddler's howling in this situation . . . just kidding.)

The CBD industry tries to compensate for this across-the-board lack of regulation by doing its own independent laboratory testing. One should always ask for a COA, which stands for "certificate of analysis," when purchasing CBD, as this denotes that an independent lab has sampled and verified the claims that are on the labels (unless they have fabricated the lab testing as well . . . not likely).

There are three general categories of CBD:

1. Isolate: chemical CBD, usually made in a lab; tends to be pure but without any of the other molecules that cause the "entourage effect" and without contaminants.

2. Broad-spectrum is a botanical formula containing all the molecules that would be in cannabis/hemp, except no THC; it's ideal if you believe in the "entourage effect" so you want all of the minor cannabinoids, yet you need to pass a drug test for cannabis/THC (assuming this sample is of good quality and there really isn't any THC).

3. Full-spectrum CBD, which is just like broad-spectrum but it *does* contain THC in trace quantities (be careful not to flunk that drug test!).

CBD can also be found in medications. The FDA has approved one medication, named Epidiolex, that is CBD based for several different types of childhood epilepsy. The very existence of this medication might lead one to question the basic sanity of the U.S. government, which still maintains, via the Controlled Substance Act, that cannabis is a Schedule I substance that has "no medical benefit," given that CBD is quite obviously a significant component of cannabis. Sanity on cannabis (or any drug for that matter) has never been our government's strong suit. CBD is one of two major components (the other being THC) in a popular cannabis-based medication called nabiximols (Sativex), which is currently approved in many different countries including Canada, England, and France, and which is used for pain and spasticity. Nabiximols is not approved by the FDA despite ample evidence of safety and efficacy—another manifestation of our painful, ongoing Drug War hangover.

Increasingly, CBD can now be found again in cannabis. CBD used to be present in higher levels in cannabis before prohibition. The financial pressures put on smugglers during the War on Drugs were such that it was most economical to breed up the THC at the expense of the other cannabinoids. In this sense, cannabis became less "medicinal," at least in chemical composition, during prohibition. Now, with legalization or decriminalization spreading, there is more market pressure to breed back up not only the CBD, but also the other medicinal cannabinoids like CBG, THVC, and CBN, which can help with conditions such as inflammation, anxiety, weight loss, and sleep.

What exactly is so medicinal about CBD that it has captured so many people's imaginations and pocketbooks? In the same way that cannabis, with its hundreds of different components, has multiple different molecular targets and mechanisms of action, CBD, even though it is only one molecule, is considered to be "promiscuous" in that it has an extraordinary number of different receptors it interacts with. This, in theory, allows it to be helpful in a wide variety of disease states. We are still figuring out exactly which receptors and pathways it interacts with, though this currently numbers in the dozens. Ironically, some of the only receptors it seems to not have a close affinity for are the cannabinoid receptors. It even inhibits the ability of THC to bind to the CB1 receptor by subtly changing its shape. However, CBD does increase our "endocannabinoid tone" in an indirect fashion, by inhibiting the enzyme named fatty acid amine hydrolase, or FAAH, that breaks down our major endogenous cannabinoid, anandamide. This leads to higher anandamide levels in the brain and more pro-cannabinoid-like activity.

CBD interacts with serotonin receptors, which might explain how it helps with anxiety and mood. It works on the capsaicin receptors, which might explain how it helps with pain. CBD also has strong effects on our immune system and inflammatory systems. Specifically, CBD is a powerful anti-inflammatory agent, especially in our brains, and thus is thought to have potential to be helpful in neurodegenerative conditions. A 2022 study, "Cannabinoids in the Management of Behavioral, Psychological, and Motor Symptoms of Neurocognitive Disorders: A Mixed Studies Systematic Review," notes "an apparent association between cannabidiol-based products and relief from motor symptoms in HD [Huntington's disease] and PD [Parkinson's disease]."[1] Other disease states such as multiple sclerosis and Alzheimer's are under active investigation. It is speculated that CBD has the potential to be highly neuroprotective in cases of traumatic brain injury.

It can, at times, be difficult to discern whether the perceived benefits of CBD for conditions like pain, anxiety and insomnia are due to the actual CBD or due to the placebo effect, particularly an "expectancy effect," or expectation/belief that the treatment will be beneficial. Some people half-jokingly respond, "Who cares?" As long as people are feeling better, isn't that a win? As I understand it, doctors are no longer allowed to treat patients with placebo pills, as this is considered misleading and unethical (except in research where patients know they might be getting a placebo).

Another problem with the current usage of CBD is that many of the animal studies that have demonstrated the efficacy of CBD were done on animals with doses that were much higher than what humans are typically using. In animal studies, the doses range from twenty to thirty milligrams per kilogram. This would translate, in an average seventy-kilogram-weighing human, into a dose of 1,400 to 2,100 milligrams. The gummies that people tend to buy are in the thirty-milligram range, so this isn't even close. It is likely the case that people are vastly underdosing their CBD. Worse, when taken orally, only 6–20 percent of the CBD is absorbed. Six percent of a thirty-milligram gummy is 1.8 milligrams.[2] So, instead of 1,400 milligrams, people are effectively taking 1.8 milligrams—no wonder people complain, "Doc, I tried CBD, it was expensive and nothing happened. Great recommendation!"

Under-the-tongue drops are likely more effective, but in any case, the dosages almost certainly need to be higher, possibly by an order of magnitude.

What are the likely benefits of CBD? Childhood epilepsy syndromes are the least controversial, as the data for this indication was so compelling that the U.S. FDA approved Epidiolex, a CBD-based medication. Autism is looking like an increasingly promising indication for CBD (see chapter 18), as are some preliminary cancer-based indications, mostly for symptoms (see chapter 17).

The most common conditions that people use CBD for—why the bulk of the one in seven Americans who uses some sort of CBD product is using it—is to alleviate pain, anxiety, and insomnia. Most of the data for these indications is based on animal data, though human studies are increasingly being completed and published. As with most things cannabis related, the data is years behind the clinical usage due to the (misplaced) funding priorities during the War on Drugs.

An interesting Canadian study came out in 2021 in the *Journal of Cannabis Research* called "Cannabidiol Use and Effectiveness: Real-World Evidence from a Canadian Medical Cannabis Clinic," where they evaluated 279 patients who were given CBD-predominant treatment at baseline, three months, and six months. This CBD-rich treatment showed a significant effect on patients suffering from pain, anxiety, and depression, as well as a measured improvement in their overall well-being. These results were only seen in patients who had moderate to severe symptoms. There was no observed effect on patients with mild symptoms. Interestingly, "the addition of delta-9-tetrahydrocannabinol (THC) during the first follow-up had no effect on symptom changes."[3] So, in this sample at least, it was the CBD doing the healing, independent of any need for THC.

This dovetails nicely with a 2022 Canadian real-world evidence study that came out in the journal *Drugs and Aging* called "Medical Cannabis Use among Older Adults in Canada: Self-Reported Data on Types and Amount Used, and Perceived Effects," in which they evaluated the use patterns of almost ten thousand older Canadian medical cannabis patients. Patients were mostly using CBD, "compositions containing only or mostly cannabidiol (CBD) had been used by 84%." This CBD-rich treatment was quite effective: "The majority of older adults reported improvements in pain (72%), sleep (64%), and mood (58%), with 35% reporting reduced dose of opioids and 20% reduced dose of benzodiazepines."[4] Fewer opioids and benzos means lives saved.

As for more traditional human studies demonstrating that CBD works for anxiety, pain, and sleep, there aren't a lot of them. I'll mention a few. I'm surprised that more people haven't paid attention to a 2011 placebo-controlled, double-blinded study of people with social anxiety disorder which has practical implications. In this study, "Cannabidiol Reduces the Anxiety Induced by Simulated Public Speaking in Treatment-Naïve Social Phobia Patients," they subjected experimental volunteers to what many find to be the most stressful conceivable activity: public speaking. To people with social anxiety, this must be about as upsetting as the rat facemask was to Winston Smith in the classic book *1984*. One group was given a placebo, and another group was given a largish dose of CBD, six hundred milligrams. According to the study,

> pretreatment with CBD significantly reduced anxiety, cognitive impairment and discomfort in their speech performance, and significantly decreased alert in their anticipatory speech. The placebo group presented higher anxiety, cognitive impairment, discomfort, and alert levels when compared with the control group.[5]

I know it's just one study, but if I had anxiety before public speaking, I'd certainly consider taking CBD over a beta blocker, which can make you unpredictably drowsy and dull. Of course, I wouldn't try the CBD for the first time right before my talk, in case there might be any side effects.

A 2019 double-blinded, placebo-controlled study of Japanese teenagers suffering from social anxiety disorder, "Anxiolytic Effects of Repeated Cannabidiol Treatment in Teenagers with Social Anxiety Disorders," demonstrated that those consuming three hundred milligrams of CBD daily for four weeks showed statistically significant improvements as gauged by several different scales of social anxiety and social interaction.[6]

As for pain, in a 2020 study from New Zealand demonstrating the efficacy of CBD for pain control in humans, called "Cannabidiol Prescription in Clinical Practice: An Audit on the First 400 Patients in New Zealand," hundreds of patients—real-world evidence here—were treated with CBD oil and were then queried about their pain and their mental health. The report found that "patients with non-cancer pain and mental-health symptoms achieved improvements to patient-reported pain and depression and anxiety symptoms. There were no major adverse effects. Positive side effects included improved sleep and appetite."[7]

Another interesting study on pain done in 2021, called "The Effects of Cannabidiol and Analgesic Expectancies on Experimental Pain Reactivity in Healthy Adults: A Balanced Placebo Design Trial," first tested the important question of whether having an expectation of receiving CBD by itself would lower the pain. They tested this by misleading the patients about whether they had taken CBD and, in fact, found that expectancies did have an effect on pain. They also found that the CBD itself had an effect on lowering the pain, regardless of the expectancies.[8]

As for a third common usage of CBD, insomnia, one 2019 case series called "Cannabidiol in Anxiety and Sleep: A Large Case Series" found that CBD was well tolerated and that, while CBD did work well for anxiety and these results were sustained throughout the entire three-month study period, the sleep results were less robust. The sleep measurements did improve in about two-thirds of people at first, but, importantly, the improvements in sleep were not sustained.[9] Of course, if CBD helps with anxiety and pain, it should help with sleep, as other studies have shown.

What other things might CBD help cure? The evidence for CBD as an adjunct treatment for addiction is piling up. These range from animal studies to human studies and run the gamut of misused substances, from tobacco and alcohol, to uppers like meth and cocaine, to cannabis and opioids.

One of my favorite studies was done by top-notch cannabis researcher Dr. Yasmin Hurd and colleagues and is called "Cannabidiol for the Reduction of Cue-Induced Craving and Anxiety in Drug-Abstinent Individuals with Heroin Use Disorder: A Double-Blind Randomized Placebo-Controlled Trial." In this study, they assessed whether CBD was able to impact cue-induced cravings in patients with heroin use disorder who are newly abstinent. As someone who is in long-term recovery from opioid addiction, I can tell you that cravings can present an incredibly powerful impetus to restart one's use despite one's best intentions, especially in early recovery, and cues or triggers can make the cravings much worse. They can become almost unbearable. Hurd's group gave their test subjects either four hundred or eight hundred milligrams of CBD once daily for three consecutive days and demonstrated that, in both groups, the CBD "significantly reduced both craving and anxiety induced by the presentation of salient drug cues compared with neutral cues."[10] This effect lasted for seven days even though they gave the CBD for only three days. In addition, there was objective proof of a response: "CBD reduced the drug cue–induced physiological measures of heart rate and salivary cortisol levels."[11] The CBD was well tolerated.

This certainly doesn't put CBD up on the level of buprenorphine or methadone as replacement medications, but it is suggestive. A more recent study by Hurd and colleagues, "Adjunctive Management of Opioid Withdrawal with the Nonopioid Medication Cannabidiol," was more of a literature search to see how much evidence there is that CBD can play a role in treating opioid use disorder. They conclude,

> Growing evidence suggests that CBD could potentially be added to the standard opioid detoxification regimen to mitigate acute or protracted opioid withdrawal-related symptoms. However, most existing findings are either based on preclinical studies and/or small clinical trials. Well-designed, prospective, randomized-controlled studies evaluating the effect of CBD on managing opioid withdrawal symptoms are warranted.[12]

As I suggested in chapter 15, CBD (and I believe full cannabis as well) will have a growing role as an *adjunct* treatment for people suffering from opioid addiction.

Can CBD help with tobacco? In a 2018 study called "Cannabidiol Reverses Attentional Bias to Cigarette Cues in a Human Experimental Model of Tobacco Withdrawal," they found that "a single 800-mg oral dose of cannabidiol reduced the salience and pleasantness of cigarette cues, compared with placebo, after overnight cigarette abstinence in dependent smokers."[13] Hmm, we've moved on from heroin to tobacco, but CBD had the same effect on cues and cravings. Now that is interesting. What about changes in actual number of cigarettes smoked? In a 2013 study, "Cannabidiol Reduces Cigarette Consumption in Tobacco Smokers: Preliminary Findings," smokers were randomized to a CBD inhaler versus a placebo inhaler and told to inhale when they felt the urge to smoke. The placebo group showed no difference in numbers of cigarettes smoked, yet "those treated with CBD significantly reduced the number of cigarettes smoked by ~40% during treatment. Results also indicated some maintenance of this effect at follow-up."[14] As a doctor who spends a good deal of his time trying to get people to quit cigarettes, I can only wonder why on earth this hasn't been studied more aggressively, given its obvious potential.

Finally, does CBD help with cannabis addiction? I always chuckle to myself when clinicians say, "Hey, look, nabiximols (Sativex) works for cannabis use disorder" because nabiximols is made up of THC and CBD, which essentially *is* cannabis, with an extra side of CBD included. "Hey, look, vodka works for alcohol use disorder—the patient stops withdrawing, and if they drink this, they stop craving alcohol for several hours at a time!" I guess one might argue that this is a controlled substitution effect analogous to buprenorphine (Suboxone) or methadone, but I don't think there's similar data of benefit to patients, such as fewer overdoses and deaths (which don't happen with cannabis . . . so it would be difficult to prove a benefit), just short-term evidence of less cannabis use. There's clear benefit for the company selling Sativex.

What about CBD? Can it play the same role it plays with other drugs in diminishing cravings and helping with cannabis addiction? The data is scarce, but a 2020 study from *Lancet Psychiatry* (which has been about as neutral about cannabis as *JAMA Psychiatry*—faithfully keeping the cannabis barbarians at the gate!) called "Cannabidiol for the Treatment of Cannabis Use Disorder: A Phase IIa, Double-Blind, Placebo-Controlled, Randomized, Adaptive Bayesian Dose-Finding Trial" found that both the four hundred milligram and the eight hundred milligram dosages of CBD lowered the number of days of using cannabis per week (somewhat, by a fraction) as well as the cannabis metabolites in the urine.[15] The results were modest and need to be confirmed, but they did seem to show that CBD was potentially efficacious. I've had some clinical success transitioning patients off of cannabis with CBD when they need to but can't quit.

CBD also shows other emerging treatment potential as an adjunctive antipsychotic and as an antimicrobial, as well as many potential dermatological applications, based on its anti-inflammatory qualities. An entire industry of wellness has grown up around CBD that involves spas, massages, skin products, soaks, and many other things that allow mostly well-off people to escape the perceived stresses of their lives.

There is a certain yin-yang quality to CBD and THC, as they can complement each other, but they can also work antagonistically. THC can be pro-addictive, while CBD can work against addiction. THC can pro-mote psychosis or psychosis-like symptoms under certain circumstances, whereas CBD can help mitigate these symptoms. On a superficial level, these opposing effects are in part explained by the fact that CBD partially inhibits the binding of THC onto cannabinoid receptors by changing their conformation, but given how multifaceted the endocannabinoid sys-tem is and how "promiscuous" CBD is, the molecular interplay is vastly more complicated.

Critically, CBD helps mitigate or limit some of the negative effects associated with THC. CBD is thought to have potential in limiting the anxiety and paranoia symptoms that some people experience with canna-bis. CBD is often suggested as a remedy to cannabis-induced anxiety at-tacks, along with some less palatable options like chewing on peppercorns. (Yuck. Maybe you'd be so traumatized and grossed out by having a mouth-ful of peppercorns that you'd forget your anxiety attack). The theory is that peppercorns contain a lot of one terpene called beta caryophyllene—which is also a cannabinoid—that stimulates the CB2 receptor and thus promotes the antianxiety aspects of THC.

CBD has also been shown to counteract some of the THC-dependent memory impairments, under experimental circumstances, if given to subjects before they are given intravenous THC. More "naturalistic" studies—defined as more likely to represent the human creature in its natural habitat—have demonstrated that there is less cognitive impair-ment when cannabis users smoke high-CBD strains of cannabis. For example, one 2018 study called "Impact of Cannabidiol on the Acute Memory and Psychotomimetic Effects of Smoked Cannabis: Naturalistic Study" evaluated two groups of cannabis smokers. The THC content was the same for both groups, but the CBD content was markedly different. The study flat-out concluded, "Unlike the marked impairment in prose recall of individuals who smoked cannabis low in cannabidiol, participants smoking cannabis high in cannabidiol showed no memory impairment."[16]

CBD doesn't work as absolutely to reverse the memory impairments as this study implies, but it is thought to help mitigate them. Higher CBD levels is one of the hypotheses for why Dr. Staci Gruber and her team found that cognitive performance improved with medical cannabis users vis-à-vis recreational cannabis users (see chapter 10). Medicinal preparations ideally should have much higher levels of CBD and less of the focus on THC über alles that plagues the American cannabis industry.

One can hope that CBD has a prominent role to play in harm reduction for our society-wide reimplementation of legalized cannabis. A 2022 study that came out in *Addiction Biology* makes exactly this point. This naturalistic study, "Effects of Cannabidiol in Cannabis Flower: Implications for Harm Reduction," randomly assigned participants, ad libitum, to high-THC/low-CBD cannabis and to cannabis that was equal parts THC and CBD. They found that "the THC + CBD chemovar was associated with similar levels of positive subjective effects, but significantly less paranoia and anxiety, as compared to the THC-dominant chemovar."[17] If this bears out with other studies, why *wouldn't* you add in some CBD? I'm not sure these results will fully hold up, as some patients report that the CBD eats away at the intensity and quality of the "high" that they get from THC-predominant cannabis. There's even a 2021 study that shows this, "Opposite Roles for Cannabidiol and δ-9-Tetrahydrocannabinol in Psychotomimetic Effects of Cannabis Extracts: A Naturalistic Controlled Study," where they compared cannabis users from a social club and found that "participants under the effects of THC + CBD showed lower psychotomimetic scores in subjective scales when compared with THC alone."[18] In other words, CBD does modify the buzz to a certain extent, but it protects your brain. Seems a small price to pay.

In summary, or in case you've already forgotten because you use cannabis without CBD, CBD might dull the high a little, but it wards off anxiety and protects your memory. It is ideal for harm reduction, but cannabis users will have to buy into the compromise—a potentially (slightly) less intense and interesting experience in exchange for brain health and a lower chance of having your experience derailed by paranoia. Also, CBD adds to the expense. Whether people accept the concurrent use of CBD will probably come down to why they are using cannabis in the first place. If it is for pain control, the CBD will likely enhance this. If it is for mental sharpness and energy, I'm not sure the CBD will be an easy sell. It would also be good to further characterize how the high is changed. In my experience, it does feel a little muddier and less electrifying, but that could have been the expectancy effect after reading these studies and, again, is a small price to pay. It would help if more dispensaries offered higher CBD chemovars for people to consume.

The use of CBD in clinical practice appears to have encountered much less resistance among doctors than cannabis has, despite a similar lack of RCT-based clinical evidence. One might speculate why this is the case. My guess is that many doctors feel they have to approve of *something* in the face of patient queries about and requests for medical cannabis. CBD is a safe way to simultaneously not be accused of reefer madness or intransigence, but to not fully cede the culture of medicine to the smoky vagueness of Woodstock. Maybe it's the general harmlessness of CBD that disarms them, though I know that there is widespread (legitimate) concern expressed about the quality and consistency of the CBD products their patients are taking. Maybe it is because they believe that cannabinoids might truly work for pain and insomnia, and CBD is a noncontroversial way to dip their foot into the water.

Most doctors don't appear to be up to speed on the benefits and pitfalls of CBD. For example, in a 2018 survey, "Knowledge, Attitudes, and Perceptions of Cannabinoids in the Dermatology Community," 86 percent of dermatologists thought that cannabis should be legal for medical treatment, but "64% of respondents did not know that cannabidiol is not psychoactive and 29% did not know that tetrahydrocannabinol is psychoactive."[19] How does one get through high school, let alone medical school, without knowing that THC is psychoactive? We urgently need to teach the ECS in medical schools!

CBD, like all medications, is not without side effects or potential downsides. With all medications, there is no free lunch, meaning that they all have pitfalls. It is all about balancing benefits with risks and toxicities— what is the least dangerous path forward? That said, CBD is relatively harmless compared to a lot of the other stuff we give people for epilepsy, insomnia, chronic pain, anxiety, autism, addiction, and many of the other indications that CBD is starting to become established for.

Assuming that you have found a way to obtain a safe and reliable source of CBD (e.g., getting it from a company that has independent laboratory testing), the second concern is that your wallet or pocketbook will become quite aggrieved at the cost. Many of the dosages of CBD that people take are minuscule compared to what they likely need, though you wouldn't know this from the price. Thirty-milligram gummies can cost a dollar or two each. What if the dose you need is six or eight hundred milligrams per day? Are you going to spend $10,000 per year on CBD? For many people, that price range is prohibitive, even if you can get some better pricing with bulk purchasing. Medical insurance currently doesn't reimburse a penny of this cost, even though they profit when patients substitute and use CBD instead of the medications they do have to pay for. The last thing our society needs is another treatment that only the rich can benefit from.

In terms of medical effects to watch out for, drug interactions are the first thing that come to mind. CBD works in the same way that grapefruit juice does in that it competes with other medications for the same liver enzymes to degrade it. This means that CBD can raise the concentration in the blood of the other medications a person is taking. This can be a particularly big deal if they are taking a medication that needs to have stable blood levels within a certain range, such as a blood thinner, an anti-epileptic, or an immunosuppressant. This is why it *is critical for all patients to tell their doctors when they start CBD.* You likely won't get the same dismissive, judgmental attitude as you do with cannabis, as CBD is more accepted. CBD can also cause liver inflammation in high doses, so these numbers may occasionally need to be monitored. Other side effects are pretty mild, including diarrhea, GI upset, and sleepiness.

We are entering a brave new world with CBD, but brace yourself! This is the very beginning. One in seven Americans taking CBD? CBD toothpicks and bras? These times will be remembered fondly as the early days, *before* the cannabinoid takeover was complete. There are greater than a hundred cannabinoids in cannabis, and more are being discovered. As they become better characterized, distributed, marketed, and sold, we will be bombarded by claims of benefit. Just as with CBD, some of these claims will be true, while others will soar above the evidence, propelled with a punt in the rear by overzealous marketing departments, far beyond our current scientific knowledge base.

Recently we have been hearing more about CBG for inflammation, CBN for sleep, THCV for weight loss—all of which are quite exciting, but just as with CBD, these are already being marketed as cure-alls without great controls on the quality of their production. They are also being actively studied by scientists, but the marketing claims travel more rapidly, fueled by a mixture of company profit motive and patient desperation. We are also hearing about some of the new cannabinoids that have been discovered, or rediscovered, since the 2018 Farm Bill made it legal to sell hemp products, such as THC-8, the miraculous cannabinoid with all the benefits of regular THC but no anxiety! But what the heck does THC-8 do to us? Its safety hasn't been studied. Now there is also THC-10 and THC-0, all as opposed to good old, natural THC-9, which we have been consuming harmoniously for five thousand years.

I read an interesting article claiming that THC-0 takes twenty to thirty minutes to kick in as it is a "pro-drug" that needs to be metabolized by our bodies before it works. As a scientist, I felt that it was my sacred duty to try this molecule. Of course, by the next day, when I was ready to try it, I promptly forgot that it doesn't take effect right away. I thought my vape pen was broken as I took puff after puff after puff. My wife was like, "Cut it out, we're going to be late for the play." Thirty minutes later, just as the curtain went up, it was as if an atomic bomb of pure stonedness exploded in my brain. I was at a play at the American Repertory Theater (not driving, no work the next day), and while I appreciated the play immensely—it certainly seemed far more colorful and philosophical than it usually would—I was glad that I wasn't in a social situation such as a party or a dinner. Fortunately, by the end of the play, I was functional again! I can confidently report that there is nothing special about THC-0, except for the delay in effect, which, as with edibles, is a true menace in terms of accidental overconsumption and will cause problems.

If you are going to be a user, medical or otherwise, stick to the plant!

# Part IV
# ENHANCEMENT

## CHAPTER TWENTY-ONE

# CANNABIS FOR WELLNESS AND LIFESTYLE

**B**eyond the obvious medical reasons, why do people use cannabis? Why have people risked so much to consume this substance? Obviously, people don't like their liberties needlessly infringed upon, but if you live in, say, Oklahoma in the late 1960s and face up to five years in prison and a lifetime of being branded as a felon for smoking a joint, how is this worth it? More broadly, why has cannabis been along with us, our steady companion, for our journey as modern humans for the last five thousand years? What is its appeal? What other things does it do for us?

If you strictly want to feel pure euphoric, I can tell you, as someone in long-standing recovery from opioid addiction, opioids are vastly more effective (though, in truth, the euphoria from cannabis is less selfish and more "connected" and communal than that from opioids; you are together, not alone). People say cocaine is euphorigenic as well, though it never had any effect on me, maybe because I'm naturally hypomanic. If you want to feel relaxed, benzodiazepines and barbiturates accomplish this far more readily. If you are looking to dull the pain and monotony of a long workday, alcohol is universally available and has been socially acceptable, with fewer penalties. For insight into ourselves and into the nature of the universe, we have psychedelics. What is it about cannabis?

The answer to this question is much more nuanced than one might suspect. I don't want to be in the position of appearing to advocate for the use of cannabis; that is not the point of this chapter, though I do advocate for *the right* of responsible adults to be able to use cannabis without criminal consequences, as long as they don't harm others. I feel that it is critically important that the full truth about the benefits of cannabis be discussed so that we can have an informed and honest discussion of the risks *and* benefits, a complete discussion. How can anyone make an informed decision without hearing *both* sides of the issue? An open discussion has, historically, been quite difficult, because most discussion of the benefits has been discouraged, if not outright censored, in hundreds of different ways.

Why have the upsides of cannabis, especially the extramedical or wellness components, been willfully ignored or actively hidden? One reason is that the goals and means of our War on Drugs necessitated painting an intentionally misleading negative picture of cannabis. Without this, the whole propaganda edifice was liable to crumble (which we are currently fortunate enough to be witnessing). The U.S. government, working with corporate nonprofits like Partnership for a Drug-Free America and the Ad Council, and various large for-profit corporations, deliberately created negative, misleading images of cannabis and censored all positive references.

Our public health strategy to keep teens, and others, off pot has seemingly been to follow a strategy of "maintaining negative perceptions of cannabis" at all costs, even if that involved flat-out lying, such as with the catastrophic DARE program. Talking about any positives of cannabis use became viewed as tantamount to encouraging its use and was highly discouraged. This proscription distorted the discourse right from the start. It only succeeded in dividing people into hostile camps and making them distrust the messengers.

We wouldn't mislead people by telling them that ice cream is poisonous to address the obesity epidemic. We wouldn't censor people from discussing their enjoyment of ice cream for fear of having dieting patients lose their "negative perceptions" about ice cream. We reasonably concede that it is delicious, but suggest eating it in moderation; using harm reduction products like froyo; or, if you have diabetes, trying to avoid it entirely. This is the approach we should have been using all along with cannabis. The experiences of tens of millions of cannabis users filter through, especially in (more or less) free societies. All that is accomplished by curating the narrative, and criminalizing its use, is to transform cannabis into an idealized forbidden fruit, so a counternarrative develops, with its positives exaggerated and the negatives discounted.

It's time that doctors, nurses, and other professionals were unmuzzled and allowed to say truthful, experienced-based things about the upsides of cannabis use, as well as harms. Instead of selectively omitting part of the truth—a "big lie" of omission about cannabis—let's educate people on all wellness aspects of the plant, beyond solely the medical uses. By doing so, we will help countless people make truly *informed* decisions about cannabis, about whether the harms (discussed in detail in earlier chapters) are worth it. We have to evolve beyond NIDA's Drug War compulsion to lower cannabis use universally, as if it is an unequivocal harm like tobacco. It isn't. There are countless ways that it improves people's lives. We have to evolve different strategies, beyond pretending that cannabis doesn't have positives—this will be more effective in our shared goal of preventing teenagers from using it. The current strategy doesn't work at all and gravely insults their intelligence to boot.

Cannabis fulfills many different roles, at different times, in different contexts, depending on the person, their age, their experiences with it, and their goals of using it. It enhances the color and texture in people's lives by expanding and disinhibiting their thoughts, feelings, and sensations. It helps people find meaning in the world by providing insights and perceptions that they wouldn't ordinarily come by. It helps us to connect with others in a direct, genuine way by unblocking us emotionally and by anchoring us in the here and now. It can transform experiences of music, art, and nature into immensely powerful and beautiful "peak experiences." It helps users to slow down and to mindfully inhabit the present moment, and to truly feel alive—something that is increasingly difficult to do in our frenetic, fractured society. It provides joy and laughter and allows adults to reconnect and to play, with that excited, youthful energy that we all felt when we were younger and freer. It reminds us of who we are and what is important to us.

Cannabis lets people engage with their feelings on a more elemental level, undistracted by all the static and the noise that rattles around our heads. It puts us more directly in touch with our bodies in a healthy and deep way, sometimes so intensely that it is as if you can feel every nerve ending, such as during intimate physical contact. Intimate relations are indescribably more pleasurable, and orgasms are so intense they are at heart attack level.

When used wisely and judiciously, cannabis can be an immensely powerful social, creative, and intellectual lubricant. It can open up parts of our minds that we can't otherwise enter, whole vistas of intellectual and artistic potential that are, ordinarily, not accessible to us. This has been invaluable to artists, sages, musicians, writers, and religious leaders for millennia. It can turn everyday activities that are ordinarily torturous drudgery into fun, meditative activities, such as raking leaves, exercising, or shoveling snow. It truly helps you get into a flow state. Before you know it, the task is done. The most mundane food tastes gourmet. Gourmet food approaches a religious experience.

This isn't addiction; rather, it is enhancement. At modest dosages, there is little to no hangover the next day. Cannabis is not fattening like alcohol (unless you go to something like a Chinese food buffet; then it might be like that scene in the Simpsons where the buffet collapsed under the weight of Homer's appetite).

According to a close friend of mine who is a well-respected attorney, "modern life can be very trying, and many have found that cannabis provides some space and perspective that helps them to make sense of things and identify their own priorities, rather than those of their employer or other authorities."

Many people find cannabis to be helpful and enjoyable. If used in moderation, it is not known to be harmful. The head of NIDA, Dr. Nora Volkow, recently said, "There's no evidence to my knowledge that occasional [adult] marijuana use has harmful effects. I don't know of any scientific evidence of that."[1] This begs the question of why doctors, who are dropping like flies, burned out from dealing with exploitative and broken systems, are forced to be secretive about their cannabis use. This is one remedy that could truly help breathe joy and meaning back into (some of) our lives. The hypocrisy is astounding. Doctors are allowed to guzzle alcohol in their spare time; take Ambien or any other highly impairing sleep medication; use muscle relaxants or nerve pain agents like gabapentin (Neurontin), which turn you into a potted plant; and chill out on Valium—all as long as it doesn't noticeably affect performance. Traditionally, the minute the medical boards get wind of any cannabis use, they often view it as a red flag or have an all-out conniption fit. This is based on stigma, not science, a holdover from the War on Drugs, and needs to end.

As cannabis legalization is becoming the norm, this needlessly selective and punitive policy is starting to change. The same medical board members don't seem particularly opposed to psychedelics, which are recently in vogue but equally illegal. Doctors should have the same right to alleviate their discomforts and to pursue wellness with medical marijuana—during their spare time, away from work—as everyone else does. Doctors have one of the highest suicide rates of any profession—we could use the gentle relaxation, fellowship, and joy that cannabis provides.

Of course, no one should use cannabis before taking on any activity where extreme professional competence is required, such as if you are the on-call doctor fielding phone calls or the night before a long neurosurgery. This holds for alcohol and other intoxicants as well. It wouldn't be particularly helpful if you called your doctor and they were inebriated or stoned out of their minds. If we are adult enough to be doctors, to make life-or-death decisions over patients every day, and to manage the use of alcohol and all of these other medications, one might suppose that we are adult enough to manage cannabis.

This chapter is about fully explaining the positive side of cannabis use so that our discussions of pros and cons can become more nuanced and more representative of the reality of actual cannabis users. This will help people with their decision analysis—trying to decide whether to use cannabis based on an accurate tally and comparison of the pros and cons.

Imagine little kids pretending what it's like to be drunk. They stumble around and slur their words, and they capture, with an exaggerated and cartoon-like essence, a tiny part, without, obviously, having a deeper understanding of the experience of alcohol intoxication. Many people in the cannabis community feel that is the level of understanding of the cannabis experience by many of the cannabis "experts" funded by the federal government or by groups who have opposed legalization, such as rehab and law enforcement, the "prohibition for profit" industries. It is felt that these experts criticize and pathologize but haven't had the inclination or curiosity to ask "why" or to try to characterize, acknowledge, or research the benefits, except for a recent, grudging acceptance of the "medical" uses of cannabinoids. This bias is borne out by evidence. A recent analysis of cannabis funding showed that between the years 2000 and 2018, the vast majority of funding in the United States, the UK, and Canada went toward funding studies of the harms of cannabis, not into investigating benefits.[2]

The benefits they do study are almost exclusively medical benefits, such as CBD's efficacy with addiction. There has been scant attention paid to most of the benefits related to lifestyle and wellness enhancements, which I have cited above, and which tens of millions of Americans are currently enjoying.

One just has to look at the morbid history of cannabis experimentation to uncover this zeal to establish and magnify only the negative aspects of the cannabis experience. Remember, set and setting are critical for anyone's experience of drug use. In one group of experiments intended to demonstrate that cannabis causes psychosis-like symptoms, which they defined very broadly, including "anxiety," researchers injected people with very large intravenous dosages of THC in a laboratory. They injected the equivalent to about a forty- to eighty-milligram edible. For reference, if I were to take a fifteen-milligram edible, I'd be high for a day. Injecting is a completely artificial and harsh way to introduce cannabis. Further, this is about as far as you can get from the naturalistic setting of a relaxed community of friends sharing a joint in the woods—unless you decided to do the experiment on Pluto, in space suits, with blinders and earplugs, and a failing supply of oxygen. No wonder the test subjects experienced anxiety and disorientation. No one uses THC or cannabis intravenously; it's not heroin. I'm not clear why this delivery method was picked, if not to magnify the results. Next, let's try shooting alcohol enemas into the rectums of test subjects and say, "Hey, alcohol causes inebriation and rectal irritation."

For cannabis, many addiction clinicians impose the paradigm that they use for other drugs: intoxicated versus nonintoxicated. With cannabis, this is relevant if we are talking about driving or operating heavy machinery, or other areas where impaired psychomotor coordination, which cannabis can cause, may lead to harm. But if someone is using it to self-treat their ADHD, for example, or if a writer or painter is using it to help facilitate their creative process, they often become, *with respect to what they are trying to accomplish*, less intoxicated and more capable. The fact that cannabis, to many, can be a performance enhancer has never been acknowledged, studied, accepted, or even alluded to by mainstream medicine.

One issue to ponder is why (most) psychiatrists, particularly addiction psychiatrists, have been so fervently and aggressively anti-cannabis for the last five decades but are so readily and easily accepting of psychedelics. A recent study shows that three-quarters of addiction specialists support legalized psychedelics.[3] This is amazing because, with cannabis, there has always been a moral panic, "Oh no, golly, it's illegal; it's not FDA approved; we can't use *that* as a medicine! Let's pathologize it and stigmatize people who use it." Yet, with LSD, or shrooms, or molly, it's like, "Hey man, it's all good. Why don't you drop some acid or eat some shrooms and we can chill out and do some therapy . . . Who cares about the Man! It's all about the healing and the default mode network. Groovy!" Having watched these two issues my entire life—remember, my dad wrote a book, *Psychedelic Drugs Reconsidered*, calling from the rooftops for the use of psychedelics in psychiatry in 1979, when I was thirteen, and got the frostiest possible reception from Harvard and from the psychiatric community—I have been mystified.

I put forward the following theories:

1. Pot paved the way for acceptance of psychedelics by breaking down cultural barriers.

2. They might believe that there is more concrete clinical evidence that psychedelics are beneficial, as there are some RCTs.

3. As explained to me by a very smart physician leader, psychedelics are thought to be potentially *curative*, whereas cannabis is thought to be more like Valium—a drug you have to continue giving and dependently taking for relief.

4. Cannabis takes business and control away from psychiatrists (as people can self-treat anxiety, depression, and PTSD with cannabis without a shrink prescribing meds for them), whereas psychiatrists will be able to control and charge a fortune for psychedelic therapy—this is the cynical explanation.

5. Dr. Carl Hart's theory that psychedelics are drugs by and for white people so they are more acceptable, due to implicit bias (or maybe not so implicit in some cases) against cannabis.

I bet that all of the five contribute to some extent, and would be interested in other thoughts.

As an interesting aside, one of the most admired and accomplished groups advocating for legal psychedelics in the world is MAPS, which stands for the Multidisciplinary Association for Psychedelic Studies. They have a more progressive view of marijuana than most of our society. They are widely credited with destigmatizing psychedelic medicine (and cannabis) by conducting rigorous clinical trials and by extensive education over the last several decades. They have also fought for the right of scientists to do cannabis research. Much of this was done following the several-decades-long plan of their visionary and tireless leader, Rick Doblin, who was friends with my dad. They are as respectable and as credible as it gets.

Recently, MAPS came out with a cannabis use policy that is ahead of its time and which I predict will be emulated by other workplaces in the not-too-distant future, as legalization progresses. MAPS' new policy states,

> We do have a detailed employment manual and . . . one of the details is about a concept called "smokable tasks." These are work tasks, different for each staff person, that they think, and their manager agrees, they do better while under the influence of marijuana, such as working on complicated spreadsheets. For me [Rick Doblin], smokable tasks primarily include strategizing, protocol design, and editing of regulatory submissions.[4]

In other words, they realize that some people perform some tasks more efficiently under the influence of cannabis and are therefore allowing their employees to do so, if it is helpful. The choice of "complicated spreadsheets" is interesting, as I know people whose "math brains" get totally unleashed by cannabis. Personally, I'd agree with editing and might add writing and brainstorming.

How solid is the barrier between medical use and "recreational" (or "adult") use of cannabis? This is somewhat of a false dichotomy that evolved, in part, due to the haphazard way in which cannabis has been being legalized in this country. There has always been more support for, and less stigma toward, medical cannabis use than recreational use. As such, medical use generally becomes legalized first, causing some prohibitionists to call foul, as "medical" cannabis was seen by them as a Trojan stoner. A few states more recently didn't follow that pattern, such as South Dakota, which directly legalized recreational use by a 54–46 margin in 2020 (until it was overturned by a hyperpartisan state court system for contrived reasons—shameful!).

Some cannabis advocates say there is no difference between medical and recreational use and claim that "all use is medical use." I would not go nearly this far. For example, if I were to take a few puffs of Durban Poison from a vape pen with a gang of my cousins before an outdoor Who concert at Fenway Park, how is that in any way medical? It would be, in fact, extremely fun, magical, and almost transcendent, as it would amplify all of the senses. This is all (relatively harmless) fun and good for the spirit, but it isn't per se medical unless you define the word "medical" so broadly as to render it meaningless.

On the other hand, many uses are clearly medical, such as a dying cancer patient trying to hold down food, as was the case with my brother Danny. I consult with people in this situation frequently, and believe me, it is not "recreational" in any sense of the word. There are clearly purely medical and purely recreational uses.

However, there is a large gray zone where it would be awkward to force a particular type of use strictly into one category or the other. Many of the patients I see fall into that category. When a person takes a puff from their dry herb vaporizer at the end of a grueling, frustrating day of work to calm their nerves or soothe their sore muscles and enable them to be in a present, grounded state of mind at home, is this not both recreational and medical? Or what about a construction worker, tasked with lifting heavy objects all day, who takes a few puffs from her vaporizer when she gets home to alleviate the muscle strains and spasms that accompany her job? The cannabis energizes her and makes her feel rejuvenated enough to participate in her favorite hobby, which is ice hockey. She has a practice that evening, and the cannabis is what enables her to participate rather than stay home and watch TV. Is this medical or recreational? Both.

There are studies that bear out the overlapping nature of "medical" and "recreational" cannabis use. According to cannabis researcher Dr. Kevin Boehnke, "My colleagues and I have shown that patients using medical cannabis often use cannabis for combined medical and recreational purposes."[5] Their work involves several studies that evaluate the impact of cannabis on chronic pain, demonstrate a drop in opioid and benzo use, and document that—wait for it!—many medical patients also use cannabis recreationally. Is this bad? It depends, I suppose, on how responsibly they use it, and how one feels about the use of cannabis that was obtained under medical auspices being used recreationally (or, relatedly, how one feels about it having been illegal in the first place).

A 2019 study, "Use of Cannabis to Relieve Pain and Promote Sleep by Customers at an Adult Use Dispensary," surveyed one thousand customers at recreational or "adult use" cannabis stores in Colorado. They specifically excluded medical cannabis patients. Among these "recreational" users, 65 percent reported using cannabis to help control chronic pain, and 74 percent reported using it to promote sleep.[6] Again, these were strictly "recreational" patients, at least on paper, demonstrating what is, largely, an artificial dichotomy between medical and recreational use.

A few studies of the benefits of recreational cannabis did manage to squeak through before the Iron Drug War Curtain fell. In 1970 in the journal *Nature*, in a study called, "Marijuana Intoxication: Common Experiences," a researcher named Charles Tart did what one might consider to be the absolute antithesis of injecting IV THC into subjects in a cold laboratory setting. His philosophy was as follows:

> The traditional "neutral" setting of the laboratory . . . can provide a very limited configuration of determining variables: thus many potential effects will not show up in the laboratory situation, so that the picture of marijuana intoxication obtained there may be only partial. Indeed, *it has been argued that the laboratory setting positively inhibits many important human manifestations*.[7] (emphasis added)

Well stated! This goes back to distinguished cannabis researcher Norman Zinberg's pioneering work on "set and setting." Unless you are encouraged by your funding sources, your personal biases, or the immediate culture you are working for to conclude only negative things about cannabis, or unless you have absolute logistical constraints, why wouldn't a researcher opt for a "naturalistic" setting? One can argue that it is impossible to study something as complex and as socially oriented as cannabis—which has evolved with us as social creatures for millennia—without meeting cannabis users where they are, or where they unself-consciously interact. Unsurprisingly, Tart's work on cannabis was criticized at the time for being "unscientific," meaning "don't find anything positive about cannabis during Nixon's reign."

Tart came up with an incredibly detailed questionnaire, which was distributed to experienced marijuana users, to try to get an accurate description of what the marijuana-using experience was like. What a concept! Ask the drug users themselves, without bias or agenda, what their drug experience is like, in their natural setting. Ask about the good, the bad, and the ugly. *See what you find without any preconceived findings or political agenda that you want to get at or conclude with.* The study's results were as follows:

> The chief experiential effects of marijuana have been elucidated with the help of a detailed questionnaire given to seasoned marijuana users whose experiences, it seems, are almost entirely pleasant.[8]

More specifically, this study found that visual effects were enhanced (e.g., "I can see new colors or more subtle shades of color"); auditory effects were enhanced (e.g., "The notes of music are purer and more distinct"); touch effects were deepened (e.g., "My sense of touch is more exciting, more sensual"); taste effects were enhanced (e.g., "Taste sensations take on new qualities. . . . I crave sweet things to eat, like chocolate"); space-time perception was changed ("Time passes very slowly"); body perception was changed ("I feel a lot of pleasant warmth inside my body"); interpersonal experiences were changed ("I empathize tremendously with others; I feel what they feel; I have a tremendous intuitive understanding of what they are feeling"); sexual experiences were affected ("Sexual orgasm has new qualities, pleasurable qualities; when making love, I feel like I'm in much closer mental contact with my partner; it's much more of a union of souls as well as bodies"); and thought processes were changed (too many examples of this to cite, but to name a few, "I give little or no thought to the future; I am completely in the here-and-now," "The ideas that come to my mind are much more original," "If I deliberately work on it, I can have important insights about myself, my personality, the games

I play," and "I have more imagery than usual when I'm reading; images of the scene I'm reading about just pop up vividly").

I can tell you, from personal experience, that most of Tart's findings powerfully resonated with me and with what I know about and have learned of other cannabis users' experiences. Now that, increasingly, people have a real choice whether to consume alcohol or cannabis, it mystifies me why anyone would use alcohol—though, it's true that I've never had a good reaction to alcohol, and I understand that many people enjoy it. Cannabis is less unhealthy, less costly, less fattening, and I've always found it so much more interesting and enjoyable, but to each their own. Tart points out the great deal of agreement among the different respondents regarding their descriptions of their marijuana experiences and notes that "nearly all other common effects seem either emotionally pleasing or cognitively interesting."

One of the last statements is, "This research was supported in part by the US Public Health Service." This was 1970, a year before Nixon's War on Drugs started. By God, this type of study—one that neutrally evaluated the attractions of cannabis—wasn't going to happen again, with U.S. government funding, for a very long time! We are still waiting.

One objection that is commonly raised is that "today's marijuana is so much stronger. It isn't your parents' weed." While there has been strong hashish around for centuries, it is true that there has never been this much ready access to extremely potent concentrates—shatter, wax, crumble, etc.—with such astronomical levels of THC. I am not necessarily a fan of these concentrates, as I agree that some of the harms from cannabis do come from an overemphasis on super-high dosages of THC rather than on quality of experience and judicious mixtures of cannabinoids (including CBD) and terpenes. Also, the cannabis flower is much stronger, up toward 20 or even 30 percent THC, when it used to be less than 4 percent in the 1970s.

In some ways, paradoxically, the stronger flower is safer, as one needs to consume less of it to achieve the desired level of intoxication/relief. An argument *against* legalization when I was growing up was that if one smoked an entire joint to get high, that was bad for the lungs. Now the prohibitionists point to how *little* one has to smoke as a harm. The plant can't win!

A very real risk is that it is easier to overconsume and suffer from unwanted anxiety now that the cannabis is so much stronger. One hears many stories of boomers taking three or four hits, like they used to, after not using cannabis for several decades. They can have an awful experience because they didn't remember to factor in that the weed is five times stronger, not to mention they are older, they are on other medications, and they don't have any tolerance. I've had to deal with the consequences of this on several occasions, such as at parties where someone is in a panic or they are greening out (i.e., throwing up from overconsumption), and it is not fun—for them or for me! (I was once at a New Year's party at a rabbi's house, and a cousin ran in and said, "Pete, you're the only doctor here who isn't stoned—come quickly." A seventy-year-old woman had thrown up and was repeating, "I'm going to die." I was like, "True, but not right now." Then she passed out. Then her husband, who saw her pass out, passed out. Why did I become a doctor? [Scary, but they were fine.] *Please, if you haven't used cannabis recently, just take one puff and wait a few minutes!*)

That said, experienced users tend to be adept at titrating to their own desired effect. It can be quite unpleasant and anxiety provoking to be more stoned than one wishes. This doesn't tend to happen to the same user more than once or twice, unless they are utterly incapable of learning from their previous mistakes or are gluttons for punishment. Users also learn how to deal with being too high in a way that is not a freak-out. Having overcome it before, they are familiar with this state, so it is less frightening. You aren't going to die. People often develop habits and mechanisms to cope if needed, like listening to music or deep breathing, or sitting quietly with a friend, until they come down.

Overall, I think that the "this isn't your parents' weed" argument is overblown. If you overregulate or ban the concentrates, they just pop up in the illicit market and are far more dangerous. If you set potency limits on the flower, users will have to spend and consume twice as much—it doubles the expense for medical patients and harms the lungs. The best approach to this issue is to educate people on risks and proper consumption, and to offer and encourage (but not legislate) lower THC, higher CBD preparations.

All of this brings us to the most brilliant person I have ever met by a long shot: the astronomer Carl Sagan. He and my dad became fast friends when they met at a dinner party given by social activist Dr. Jack Fine (father of Dr. Jonathan Fine, who founded Physicians for Human Rights)in 1966, in Brookline, Massachusetts. They bonded over their early opposition to the Vietnam War. My dad invited Carl over for dinner when my mom was eight months pregnant with me and my twin. My mom tells me that she was lying on the floor of the living room after dinner, and Carl was full of curiosity about us, with questions like, "Do they sleep at the same time?" I was too young to answer for myself.

Carl was a fixture of my childhood. He was a positive cannabis role model, becoming even more eloquent and brilliant after a puff or two. He wasn't a bad intellectual role model either. He consumed information like the rest of us consume our favorite foods when we are starving. I've never seen anyone devour a book like he did, like an alligator swallowing a small, yappy dog in one satisfied bite. He contributed a profoundly interesting chapter to my dad's book, *Marihuana Reconsidered*, in 1971 under the name Mr. X. After Carl's death in 1996, it was revealed that he was Mr. X. The chapter is a must-read for every human being. It's easy to find online.

He waxes eloquently about his beautiful visual experiences on cannabis, about how it increased his appreciation for art and music: "Cannabis enables nonmusicians to know a little about what it is like to be a musician, and nonartists to grasp the joys of art." And sex:

> Cannabis also enhances the enjoyment of sex—on the one hand it gives an exquisite sensitivity, but on the other hand it postpones orgasm: in part by distracting me with the profusion of images passing before my eyes. The actual duration of orgasm seems to lengthen greatly, but this may be the usual experience of time expansion which comes with cannabis smoking.[9]

Moving from sex to existentialism, I particularly relate to this description:

> I do not consider myself a religious person in the usual sense, but there is a religious aspect to some highs. The heightened sensitivity in all areas gives me a feeling of communion with my surroundings, both animate and inanimate. Sometimes a kind of existential perception of the absurd comes over me and I see with awful certainty the hypocrisies and posturing of myself and my fellow men.[10]

It truly does give one perspective! He also discusses insight:

There is a myth about such highs: the user has an illusion of great insight, but it does not survive scrutiny in the morning. *I am convinced that this is an error, and that the devastating insights achieved when high are real insights; the main problem is putting these insights in a form acceptable to the quite different self that we are when we're down the next day.*[11] (emphasis added)

Amen to that. Almost every important insight I've ever had has been under the influence of cannabis. This is echoed by some writings of my dad that I cite in the afterword. Carl concludes,

The illegality of cannabis is outrageous, an impediment to full utilization of a drug which helps produce the serenity and insight, sensitivity and fellowship so desperately needed in this increasingly mad and dangerous world.[12]

In his masterpiece (one of many) *Dragons of Eden*, which won the Pulitzer Prize, Sagan speculates on how, essentially, "stoned thinking" comes about:

Our awareness of right hemisphere function is a little like our ability to see stars in the daytime. The sun is so bright that the stars are invisible, despite the fact that they are just as present as they are in the daytime as at night. When the sun sets, we are able to perceive the stars. In the same way, the brilliance of our most recent evolutionary accretion, the verbal abilities of the left hemisphere, obscures our awareness of the functions of the intuitive right hemisphere, which in our ancestors must have been the principal means of perceiving the world. . . . Marijuana is often described as improving our appreciation of and abilities in music, dance, art, pattern and sign recognition and our sensitivity to nonverbal communication. To the best of my knowledge, it is never reported as improving our ability to read and comprehend Ludwig Wittgenstein or Immanuel Kant; to calculate the stresses of bridges; or to compute Laplace transformation. . . . I wonder if, rather than enhancing anything, the cannabinols (the active ingredient in marijuana) simply suppress the left hemisphere and permit the stars to come out.[13]

Whenever I suggest that, if those addiction psychiatrists and cannabis researchers in the Reefer Pessimism camp, as well as other prohibitionists, were ever to actually try cannabis, they would have a much broader, balanced, and more nuanced view of it, I get rebuffed with extreme prejudice. The retort runs along the lines, "You don't have to overdose on heroin to write about the opioid epidemic." This misses the point because cannabis is relatively harmless to try and has genuine upsides and benefits that have been hidden. There is no substitute for lived experience, especially when the science has been curated and the information and public messaging has been censored and deliberately distorted. Of course, no one is going to suggest an opioid addiction or a fentanyl overdose for pedagogic purposes!

My argument is that they would certainly garner some insight into how it helps people, and why people are so committed to using it in the first place. They would better understand and *contextualize* some of the side effects that they describe so frighteningly. It would also inform treatment. It is fully legal (on the state level) in at least nineteen states, and there really aren't many barriers to trying it, discreetly, under responsible conditions, at the start of a vacation or a long weekend. This has evolved into a Catch-22 where they have convinced themselves that cannabis is so dangerous and scary that they won't try it in order to understand that it isn't as dangerous or scary as they state it is. I suspect that, for some, the actual fact of experiencing the effects of cannabis (with an open mind) would provide an essential context for its effects in a way that would force a rather drastic reevaluation of some of their past opinions on its dangerousness, its utility, and the overall balance of harms and benefits. This would be a surefire way to narrow the gap between the two sides of the cannabis debate.

As a related side note, my dad told me that he and several of his classmates at his psychiatry training program at Harvard Medical tried the antipsychotic Thorazine so they knew what patients would be experiencing on this medication. This spirit of curiosity, empathy, and discovery always struck me as something that was missing in our modern medical training. My dad said it was an awful, if illuminating, experience and that he always kept this in mind when he was prescribing these meds—which he would prescribe judiciously, understanding the side effects involved. It is no coincidence that someone this thoughtful wrote a groundbreaking book on schizophrenia.

In September 2019, while simultaneously pondering these issues and procrastinating on Twitter, I conducted a twitter poll with the question, "If you are a cannabis user, and you find benefits beyond merely enjoying it recreationally, or its intended medical indication, which is the most important to you?" and, with 1,666 responses, out of four choices given, the results were as follows: increase human connection, 34 percent; deepen creativity, 30 percent; enhance spirituality, 20 percent; and improve sex life, 17 percent.

To me, these results are telling on a number of levels. I didn't anticipate so many responses; it was as if people were eager for an outlet to communicate the underdiscussed extramedical benefits of cannabis. The top vote getter, "increase human connection," resonated with me because, as a primary care doctor, I see people who are literally dying from loneliness every day, especially some of the older patients, who, during the pandemic, would make appointments just to have someone to talk to. Cannabis is uniquely suited to facilitating human connection. Perhaps that's why it's been with us for so much of our journey, helping us get along with each other.

Our humble narrator cannot truthfully deny that he has taken a puff or two in his time. This section is written in the present for the sake of narrative fluidity, but the author only admits to past use of any and all drugs and medicines.

For me, cannabis has always helped with my personal efficacy and with navigating some of life's thorniest issues. Cannabis enables me to organize my time more efficiently by helping me to prioritize my activities. After consuming, I often get a self-corrective injection of insight, which I write down or record. Later, when the weed wears off, I use this insight to help me to more efficiently and meaningfully execute my work and life priorities.

The same goes for writing an essay, blog, speech, or paper. I can write a coherent and grammatical piece without cannabis, as I have for many long stretches in my life during periods of abstinence. However, after one puff, a much more interesting and creative structure will come to me in a flash. I scribble the main ideas down, or record them on my phone, and then implement them later. These are insights that categorically don't come to me without cannabis. With cannabis, it is as if I transiently have access to an extra, dormant part of my brain, the most creative part. This has been true since I was writing papers in high school, through college, and in medical school. I also write more fluidly, creatively, and eloquently—and with humor. For me, cannabis is essential to writing material that's funny. It can also help me get started, transitioning me from a dense writer's block to a completely immersed flow state within minutes.

In my experience, to harness the creative power of cannabis absolutely requires the right conditions, the right "set and setting." First, I can't be too mentally or physically fatigued, or the electrifying free-associational supercharge to my thoughts that cannabis ignites just doesn't happen. It's like flicking a lighter that's out of butane. I might become happy and relaxed and enjoy the sensory enhancements, but my thoughts are no less muddy and sluggish than before I consumed. I get nothing done. After a ten-hour day in primary care clinic, speaking English and Spanish, trying to solve problems that have no solutions, and fighting with the electronic medical record system and the insurance companies, even with cannabis, it is useless to try to think about or accomplish anything. Second, the dosage must be within the right range: too little, nothing happens; too much, and I am a space shot, which can be perceptually entertaining, especially when I close my eyes and see all the colors and shapes dance by, but it isn't particularly productive. Third, I have to be in the right setting, such as peaceably typing on my computer in front of the fire, out in the serenity of nature, or quietly conversing with friends. It's difficult to think if one is at a loud party or concert.

When the stars align, it is nothing less than magical, with a free flow of thoughts and ideas—better thoughts and ideas than I usually have—that seem to come out of a now-awakened part of my brain. It is always a race against time to get them down before they vanish, analogous to trying to remember a dream.

What the magic of "stoned thinking" consists of is what I'd describe as an exuberant, insight-based, free-form, creativity-infused generation of ideas. The quality of the ideas is different—better but inconsistent—from ideas that one might get if not stoned. Some of them are fanciful, to be rejected the next day. It might be something that's true and that's hitting you in a new and deep way in the stoned moment, but that doesn't translate well in the sober light of the next day's reality. Something like, "People are so subsumed by their own problems that they rarely truly listen to others." I might look at my notes and wonder, "What was I thinking? What's the hell's so deep about that?" However, there are other ideas that I never would have had otherwise, which retain every iota of their importance the next day. These remain among the most creative and helpful ideas that I can lay claim to.

Most importantly, I find using cannabis is also like checking in with my true self. Being "stoned" can be, in essence, a state of deep mindfulness, as time slows down and the present moment attains a profound intimacy. This is mixed in with heightened sensations, feelings of benevolence toward others, subtle euphoria, and interesting thoughts.

Cannabis has a self-corrective function as it forces me back in touch with my authentic self, even if this isn't always pleasant. It is like a truth serum. It is an antidote to the narcissistic, lazy, or selfish parts of my personality—the parts that get in the way of everything else that's important to me. *It allows me to reconnect with who I want to be* and to understand the ways in which I have been acting out of fear, insecurity, or egoism. It gives me clarity into my goals, whether they are interpersonal, professional, or existential. The first puff is like the moment one puts on 3-D glasses at the start of a movie: my entire perspective changes, and I can often better discern what about myself, and others, is sincere versus what is false and trivial.

Cannabis sparks my motivation to exercise, makes me less oblivious about what needs to be done around the house, makes me nicer and less judgmental, and gives me insight into the things I did wrong or—at least—might have done better. When I use cannabis, I think about work/life balance and whether I'm doing enough to help the people around me. I replay interactions and conversations I've had—could I have handled a particular situation with more empathy? Cannabis can help me process the experiences, interactions, and emotions of the day. It fosters humility.

There's no question that cannabis can temporarily somewhat fuzzify one's immediate short-term memory, so I am always careful to write down or record my thoughts, which I learned to do from watching Carl Sagan, who carried a little voice recorder with him. I remember being out at a Chinese restaurant in Washington, DC. He and my dad shared a joint before dinner, and they, as usual, were discussing something phenomenally interesting, and my teenage self would be straining to think of an intelligent and appropriate way to contribute to the conversation. From time to time, Carl would say, "Excuse me," whip out his recording device, and start quietly speaking into it. He'd say something like, "Life might evolve on other planets, though it might not necessarily be carbon based," or something else that wouldn't make any sense out of the context of the immediate conversation, but which would blow my mind to shreds.

I'm too modest to discuss, in detail, the ways in which cannabis improves sex. It's almost as if you haven't had relations if you haven't had them while high on marijuana. It's that much better.

Not all the effects of cannabis are reliably good. Sometimes I go straight for the junk food. When I'm in this mode, you do not want to get between me and the chips. Once you start eating, it is hard to stop—everything tastes a thousand times better. If I am too sleepy, none of the good effects of cannabis work—it just makes me groggy. It can make me anxious if I take it in the wrong setting or, particularly, if I take too big of a dose (which is rare because I know my limits). I'm a true believer in low doses. And, sometimes, it just makes me feel dull, like if I'm trying to read a book or something, and I'm like, "Why did I do this—I was doing just fine before."

I should note that there are big differences among people in how cannabis affects them. It's not for everyone. Some find it more focusing, and others find it makes them distractible. There is also a difference between different strains or chemovars of cannabis—one type can make you feel very different than another type, and there are hundreds of active ingredients in each type. Some promote relaxing sleepiness, while others are quite stimulating. Dosing is critical as well. At low doses, I am usually quite functional (though I wouldn't work or drive), yet at high doses, it can be incapacitating. When you close your eyes, you see beautiful colors, patterns, and designs, and it can be extremely euphoric and relaxing. Cannabis can definitely act as a psychedelic drug at high doses—not always in a good way—which is why education and careful dosing are key!

Perhaps, to a certain extent, it is a question of definitions and perspective. What some anti-cannabis researchers might label "psychotic symptoms," cannabis users might call interesting, out-of-the-box thinking and thrillingly enhanced perceptions.

This insight-generating component of cannabis is nothing short of miraculous. It astounds me that we (mostly) haven't been harnessing this in psychotherapy. I've used it in therapy (as a patient), and my fairly straitlaced psychiatrist agreed it was helpful. It is absolutely tragic that psychiatry has, in my humble opinion, so needlessly positioned itself as the anti-cannabis voice. They could have been using this insight-generating quality over the last fifty years to treat people, just as they are now excited to use psilocybin and MDMA, instead of carrying water for the U.S. government's War on Drugs. Instead of helping people to understand and heal themselves and others, they've helped to put dark-skinned people in prison and to discredit those who do find benefit with cannabis.

One theory my dad had was that cannabis is an "enhancer," in that it can make motivated people more motivated and less motivated people less motivated, though much of this might just come down to privilege and opportunity. In this sense, you can find what you are looking for with cannabis; so if you are absolutely determined to find only negative things, that is possible. In any case, it has been a tremendous disservice to the millions of cannabis users who have been dismissed, pathologized, discredited, and arrested over the decades, instead of supported, understood, and, as necessary, treated. This attitude has set the science back by decades. All for what? What have we accomplished, beyond earning a few bucks for the prohibition-related industries and ruining lives?

In the end, it's about wellness, which cannabis, despite its potential harms, can powerfully facilitate if used responsibly. Many people are aided by that certain something at the end of the day, when they are exhausted and drained and achy, or when they are feeling closer to the end of their rope. In a perfect world, we'd all do yoga, eat tofu, and meditate, but the world isn't perfect, and we certainly aren't perfect either. All of the psychopharmacological options except alcohol were either criminalized or heavily controlled and regulated. Now that cannabis is opening up as an option, it is easy to see why people are opting to use it, given the wide array of lifestyle enhancements it offers, as well as its limited toxicity and its ability to rejuvenate and refresh. Cannabis can be an important part of the wellness equation that many are looking for. Is it a shortcut? That's complicated. Is it harmless? No. Does it work for people? A resounding yes!

## CHAPTER TWENTY-TWO
# THE ONCE AND FUTURE PLANT

As we reconsider what is and isn't true about cannabis, and as we attain a longitudinal yet modern understanding of the plant, hopefully we can bridge, or at least narrow, the divide between the Reefer Pessimists and the Cannatopians. One of the most powerful actions of cannabis, both helpful and inconvenient, is that it helps us forget. Forgetting is going to be a large piece of this reconciliation between the dueling parties about the nature of cannabis. Both sides have to do their share, with or without the use of cannabis.

Now that cannabis is being re-legalized and normalized, the Cannatopians need to let go of their anger and distrust of both the U.S. government and, at times, science in general. Yes, science was distorted by the Drug War. To date, the U.S. government—as a whole—has almost certainly told many more lies than truths about cannabis. However, times are changing, policies are lightening up, and, increasingly, better people are in charge. Cannatopians need to trust the scientific process and look at each study on its own merits, no matter whether it claims harm or benefit. It is just as important to know about harms as it is to understand benefits so that cannabis can be used safely and effectively. Any cannabis user should want to know about both, including the concerning environmental effects of cannabis production with its massive usage of resources.

The Reefer Pessimists must forget, or at least contextualize, much of what they have learned because so much of this knowledge was manufactured with an agenda, leading to overly negative beliefs. The cynicism regarding cannabis from the War on Drugs created an echo chamber of presumed harm and dismissiveness that artifactually distorted and obscured the true nature of cannabis. Skeptics can work with the rest of us to advocate for safe practices, many of which most of us can agree upon, such as avoiding cannabis during pregnancy and breastfeeding (except under certain very narrow circumstances), before driving, and during adolescence. We do better when we work together. It is time to support balanced research and to forgo all the myths and superstitions of the past. For the Cannatopians, no more reflexive belief in cannabis as a miracle cure, such as for cancer (until it is actually proven). And for the Pessimists, no more adding air quotes when you mention the words "medical marijuana."

What we must not forget is the cruel, pointless, and destructive criminalization—over the last eight decades—that forced millions to suffer, to resist, and to carry us to where we are today. We are just beginning to discuss rebuilding the communities that have been harmed by the War on Cannabis. The battles over legalization, expungements, reparations, and the future direction of the cannabis industry are far from over.

Cannabis is being destigmatized and reintegrated into human society at a rapid but uneven pace across the globe. This is long overdue, as its criminalization and demonization has caused infinitely more suffering than benefit. Cannabis is a complex drug, which we are, in some senses, extremely familiar with from thousands of years of use as well as thousands of studies. At the same time, there seem to be a growing number of unanswered questions as we learn more about the intricacy and complexity of the endocannabinoid system. The more we learn, the less we seem to know. Certainly, in researching and writing this book, after reading everything I could find, I feel on less solid ground than I did when I started. It's a lesson in humility.

Cannabis is becoming renormalized in our society, and it's long past time that we renormalize our thinking about it, as well as our policies. The more we can work together collegially, compromise on the issues we disagree on, and respectfully listen to each other, the better these policies will be. We should neither idealize nor needlessly restrict its use.

What lessons have we learned from our eight-decade-battle over cannabis? How can we apply this to the future so that our society can derive maximum gain and minimum harm from cannabis, and so that this issue ceases to provide further fodder for the culture wars?

## Finding a Way Forward

We need to get doctors and patients on the same page about cannabis. Physicians don't need to be in absolute agreement, or even support its use, but there needs to be open, nonjudgmental, two-way communication. No more dismissiveness or criticism. In this way, harms and risks, such as drug interactions, can be communicated and minimized. Doctors can help emphasize harm reduction practices like incorporating CBD to mitigate cognitive effects and using a dry herb vaporizer instead of smoking to spare the lungs. This will create an opportunity to emphasize basic safety issues like safe storage (so kids, teens, and pets don't get into it), avoiding driving after use, safe dosage ("start low and go slow"), and integrating cannabis with the rest of the patient's care. Patients will feel heard, can express thoughts and ideas, can get help if needed, and can help educate their doctors about the rudiments of cannabis medicine.

A critical component of this is educating doctors on the endocannabinoid system and on the practical basics of cannabis medicine. Physicians from a century ago knew much more about the use of cannabis than do contemporary physicians—it is unfortunate that this part of the art of medicine, utilized by great physicians throughout history, such as Sir William Osler, has been lost to all but the minority who take an active interest in cannabis medicine.

From what I've seen, cannabis is rarely, sparsely, and very poorly covered in the continuing medical education in my field, internal medicine, even at the most "prestigious" conferences associated with top medical schools. We aren't going to get anywhere if we keep going at this pace. Mainstream medical conferences either ignore it, pay lip service to it, or echo nonsense from the past. The evolution of physician knowledge is glacial; the best you can say is that at least now they occasionally mention the words "medical marijuana" instead of fully ignoring it. At the same time, there are separate medical cannabis conferences, for cannabis supporters, that, to a certain extent, "preach to the converted," because if you are there, you have an interest and probably some facility with medical cannabis. This subject needs to be taken seriously, by our entire profession, as seriously as patients take it, if doctors wish to be viewed as legitimate partners and reliable sources of information. Doctors can't simultaneously know hardly anything about cannabis and complain that budtenders are advising patients.

It would be wonderful if we could create some type of objective, independent council, made up of collaborative, experienced experts from across the cannabis spectrum, to evaluate and interpret new evidence (including real-world evidence) about benefits and harms. If we choose the right participants—all without conflicts of interests—this process could have enough credibility with most people across the spectrum. This would shield us from the twin corrosive influences of government propaganda and corporate manipulation. It could help decode the plethora of biases that are out there: academic, historical, fishing, publication, confirmation, and all the others. It would also help address the harms of the War on Cannabis, particularly to communities of color, and the best ways to redress these.

Having a group that could neutrally arbitrate all of these different preconceptions and agendas, factor them in, and help us assess information in a neutral fashion would help us in a myriad of ways. For example, we could sensibly and coherently respond to timely issues such as "Can cannabis help with COVID?" which came up weeks into the pandemic. With one voice, or with a few, in a collegial point-counterpoint kind of way, we could counter the incoherent chorus of opposed opinions that we all had to suffer through. This process would include scientists, cannabis clinicians, addiction psychiatrists, harm reductionists, and cannabis patients with lived experience, all working together. It would not include the tobacco, cannabis, or alcohol industries, the rehab industry, or a representation from law enforcement.

This is a vision for the—hopefully near—future. At present this goal is aspirational, as we are still in a Tower of Babel with many cannabis "experts" and users with impossibly conflicting views. I'm looking forward to seeing us move past this phase, toward a world where we can agree on harms and benefits, can research earnestly and without agenda, and can work together to make restitutions for the War on Drugs. In the process, we can mend fences, build bridges, and help make the world a more reasonable, hopeful, and equitable place.

As we legalize, we need to regulate in a sensible way. Legal cannabis doesn't have to be a commercialized free-for-all, devoid of any limits or restrictions. There are practical, painless ways to simultaneously increase knowledge, permit usage, and reduce harm, such as:

- Limiting or banning advertising for cannabis, at the same time as we ban it for tobacco, alcohol, and Big Pharma too. None of these ads are helpful to society.

- Educating people about the higher risks that likely pertain to specific populations, such as teens; those with, or predisposed to, certain psychiatric conditions; and pregnant/breastfeeding women.

- Not taxing cannabis at such a high rate, which only fosters the less regulated, and less safe, illicit market.

- Figure out, once and for all, how to detect (if possible) and discourage stoned driving (without getting people who aren't impaired in trouble).

- Stop making cannabis into tasty edibles, chocolates, or candies that any small child (or pet) would happily overconsume.

- Provide neutral education on harms that are credible and believable, given without judgment, exaggeration, or stigma.

- Pursue research that isn't based on any corporate or political agenda and which isn't biased in either direction.

- Address whether any limits on potency of flower or concentrates make sense—and how to do this without either inadvertently pushing consumers into the illicit market (if even possible) or making medical cannabis even more expensive for patients on fixed incomes.

- Regulate CBD and other minor/new cannabinoids in a coherent and helpful way, not like we are currently doing. We need to regulate the production of these products, not permit them as "supplements" without any control over their manufacturing or safety/benefit claims.

- Destigmatize all aspects of cannabis so people who need it medically aren't intimidated/ashamed and so that people who

344

find themselves addicted to it can ask for help and can freely discuss their use with their doctors.

- Legalize federally so that regulation, safety standards, labeling, and commerce can be coherent and consistent, throughout the United States and, ideally, the entire world.

- Come up with standardized dosages to help make research and clinical care more consistent, for each type of consumption method.

- Better define "cannabis addiction" beyond the deeply flawed concept of "cannabis use disorder," which ropes in many of the medical marijuana patients. I suspect we are going to need a new category for some patients—"addicted but also deriving benefit"—for cannabis; sometimes both are occurring simultaneously.

- Allow hospitals to allow inpatients to use medical cannabis so they don't have to either withdraw from cannabis in the hospital, use it surreptitiously, or interrupt their care regimens. (This doesn't mean smoking or vaping in a hospital.)

- Use legalization as an opportunity to redress as many harms of the War on Cannabis as possible: let all nonviolent cannabis prisoners out, expunge all records for nonviolent cannabis offenses, and find a way to help the families and communities that have been harmed heal their traumas and regain financial stability.

Some of these are being addressed, but we have a massive amount of work to do.

There are debates in the Cannatopian activist groups about whether to support legalization initiatives that are disconnected from, or which inadequately address, social justice issues. An example is "safe banking" bills, which force the government to allow cannabis transactions to go through the traditional banking system so that everything doesn't have to be done in cash (which is an invitation to violent crime against dispensary workers).

Major banks are currently afraid that the feds could go after them, given the federal illegality of cannabis, with charges such as money laundering, and need some protections before they open their doors (wires? computers?) to the cannabis industry.

On the one hand, of course we need safe banking, so this seems like an obvious issue to support, a way to dismantle yet another brick in the edifice of prohibition. It makes everything safer. However, many cannabis activists are leery of "piecemeal" legalization measures, some of which primarily assist the cannabis industry. They worry that equity provisions will never be addressed in the future if we don't accomplish everything at once while there is such tremendous momentum for change. For example, a 2021 headline in *Marijuana Moment*, involving one of the most passionate and sincere voices for legalization in the Senate, stated, "Cory Booker Vows to Block Marijuana Banking until Senate Passes Comprehensive Legalization," for these exact reasons. This makes for complicated politics of who's supporting what.

I feel that it is critical to integrate medical cannabis into all branches of medicine, but particularly into primary care and oncology. It would be much better if we, rather than cannabis specialists, were the ones doing most of the certifying for cannabis. We could then rely on cannabis specialists for complex cases (as we do with other specialties). The PCP, or the primary oncologist, is often connected to the patient, their families, and to their other caregivers by years of shared experiences and history, in addition to the computerized medical record and the staff. We know their meds, preferences, and habits and what has or hasn't worked for them previously. We can obviously do a better job of integrating their medical cannabis care into the rest of their care—as a whole—than even an extremely talented cannabis specialist. These other providers have often just met the patient, don't have much time with them, see them infrequently, don't deal with their other problems, and are usually unknown to the other caregivers and practitioners because they aren't part of the same medical system. To make things worse, the medical records usually don't connect with each other, so outside practitioners are flying blind.

This is borne out by research. In a 2020 study of oncology patients, "Cancer Patients' Experiences with Medicinal Cannabis-Related Care," patients were surveyed about their experiences with trying to access medical cannabis. What they found is what I often observe as well, regardless of why they are seeking out medical cannabis:

> Patients with cancer used Medical Cannabis with minimal medical oversight. Most received Medical Cannabis certifications through brief meetings with unfamiliar professionals. Participants desired but were often unable to access high-quality clinical information about Medical Cannabis from their established medical teams. Because many patients are committed to using Medical Cannabis, a product sustained by a growing industry, medical providers should familiarize themselves with the existing data for Medical Marijuana and its limitations to address a poorly met clinical need.[1]

The only solution to this problem is for physicians to educate themselves so that patients can "access high-quality clinical information about Medical Cannabis from their established medical teams." No more outsourcing! This may seem like yet another burden being dumped on primary doctors. In truth, being able to offer medical cannabis to my patients makes my life much easier as a PCP by giving me a relatively nontoxic, plant-based option to address some of the most common and difficult-to-treat ailments that PCPs see, such as chronic pain and insomnia. Like most other things in medicine, the basics of it aren't rocket science, but it can become complex and uncertain, and that's why there are experts to consult with.

Locating cannabis medicine in primary care (and oncology) would *integrate* the care. Doctors would know what other meds their patients are on so as to watch out for interactions. The computer could back this process up and let us know about any potential medication conflicts. Just this one intervention could save lives. We could input into the computer "medical cannabis patient," "CBD," and other cannabinoids as they become available to patients, such as CBG and THCV, and connect with the vast data systems that look for dangerous drug interactions. If you are taking CBD and I try to give you the blood thinner Coumadin, an alert would pop up and say, "Alert: Medicine Interaction." This could be linked with information that enables us to address this particular concern. This is where legalization, integration, and open communication will greatly help with safety.

If you are a cannabis clinician seeing a patient without access to their medical records, you often rely solely on the memory of patients, who don't always accurately recall their medications, past drug allergies, or bad reactions. None of us do; that's why we, ideally, have an integrated medical system. Not infrequently, in my clinic, I hear, "I take a yellow pill, two blue pills, and the red pill—you know the red pill; *you* prescribed it a couple of visits ago." I'd be lost without the computer. It adds an avoidable component of risk to have the cannabis care split off.

If integrated into primary care, patients would have someone they know, and who knows them, to ask questions and guide them about the interplay of cannabinoids with other treatments. Primary care doctors also have access to specialists if the question is complicated, such as a patient with an arrhythmia or on an immunosuppressant who wishes to start cannabis (assuming the specialist knows something about cannabis). Further, inpatient hospital teams would have someone they can identify who knows the patient, to contact about the cannabis use or interactions with any newly prescribed medications, or any concerns, such as cannabis hyperemesis or addiction, when the patient is hospitalized. There would be continuity of care.

Moreover, this integration would make cannabis more affordable, as patients wouldn't have to pay a separate fee for a cannabis doctor, which typically isn't reimbursed by insurance. It also removes a dangerous conflict of interest. I believe that some doctors find it difficult to decline to certify a medical cannabis patient if they are being paid specifically to do this. If you think they aren't a good candidate, that is an awkward situation. Do you return their money for your consult (which you spent time and expertise on)? Or charge them and have them go away empty-handed and upset? According to one acquaintance who has been through this experience,

> Honestly, the three times I got certified for MMJ, there was no way the doctor was going to turn me, or anyone, down. I was paying them to give me an MMJ card (which I would use for recreational, medical, whatever use), and they went through enough motions so that if I was from the DEA, I couldn't say they weren't acting like a doctor, but it was understood that they weren't going to turn you down. It wasn't really a question whether they were going to decline you. Which was what people wanted—why they went to see this doctor.

As a PCP, who isn't being paid for certifying patients, I can tell you, it is much easier to say no to someone you think wouldn't do well with cannabis. The "no" is in the context of a lot of noes and yesses—not just that one issue—and there's no fee at stake.

Yet we do need clinical cannabis specialists. There is so much being discovered in this field, and so much more on the horizon, that we need to establish a separate discipline to accommodate this ascendant area of medicine. I suspect we are going to go from not teaching the endocannabinoid system at most medical schools to having it be a major feature of our canon. The ECS has the potential to bridge and link so many other areas of medicine. Some candidates for a name for this specialty are, according to my dad, cannabinopathic medicine, or endocannabinology. My vote is for, simply, "cannabinoid medicine," along the lines of "psychedelic medicine"—descriptive and concise.

The basics of benefits and harms, as well as the mechanics of utilizing cannabis clinically for common conditions, can readily and safely be adopted by primary care doctors (and oncologists) with less than ten hours of education. It will take even less time when they start teaching the ECS in med schools. Cannabis is less dangerous and complex than many of the other medications we manage. You can't kill someone with cannabis as you can quite easily do with a blood thinner, or the wrong dose of insulin, or even an antibiotic for that matter. Practicing medical cannabis is not that hard as long as you start slowly with the THC, screen for and educate patients about harms and interactions, have good follow-up, and communicate with all providers.

As with all specialties—and cannabis is no different—things can quickly get more nuanced or time consuming than a PCP has bandwidth for. There is such a tremendous volume of research and discovery within cannabinoid medicine, and it would be beyond the ability of PCPs, who are also in charge of everything else and are generally quite overtaxed, to assimilate this much new information. There is no way that most PCPs will be able to keep up with the latest trials, reports, formulations, and minor cannabinoids that are being discovered, marketed, and popularized, let alone discoveries pertaining to the ECS. We hardly have time to keep up with vaccine schedules, learn the names of all the new medications that come out, and order or perform mammograms, colonoscopies, vaccinations, blood pressure screenings, and screenings for diabetes or lung cancer—as well as whatever problems and complaints our patients walk into our office with.

We also need cannabis specialists for complex scenarios such as cannabis allergies, refractory cases, and more specific recommendations for less commonly used cannabinoids or for people with cannabis hyperemesis syndrome who wish to continue cannabinoids. Or for cases where a more detailed analysis of potential drug interactions or contraindications to using cannabis are needed. I suspect that cannabinoid specialists will be treating more cannabis addiction in the future, as they have much more facility with the cannabinoid system, and the clinical use of cannabis, than other doctors do.

One can make a strong argument that the academic and intellectual control of cannabis shouldn't be solely in the hands of those doctors, such as psychiatrists, who, collectively, have very little, if any, experience treating patients with cannabis, and who (generally) only focus on, and believe in, harms. The analogy with the blind men and the elephant comes to mind. If your hands remain stuck in the elephant's rear end, you'd never know that they are beautiful, intelligent, and graceful creatures. To be credible and effective, you have to view cannabis from a broader and more diverse lens—benefits as well as harms—and some consideration of *why* people use cannabis, not this bland, dichotomous focus on intoxicated versus not intoxicated. Patients will open up and engage more if they feel they have a capable physician partner in their journey.

Health insurance must pay for medical cannabis. This likely won't happen substantially until we achieve federal legalization, the lack of which gives avaricious health insurance companies an excuse to hide behind. They also hide behind "it hasn't been proven" and "it hasn't been approved by the FDA," knowing full well that there currently isn't the infrastructure to obtain the kind of evidence that the FDA would need, such as unfettered research or a workable pathway to approve botanical medicines. At the rate that we're going, psychedelics might get health insurance coverage before cannabis.

Cannabis can't be a medicine only for the well-to-do. In my primary care clinic, I've had numerous patients who were able to switch to cannabis from opioids, or benzodiazepines, yet who had to switch back because the unreimbursed medical cannabis was prohibitively expensive for them. "I felt much better off of the Percocets, but the cannabis costs me one hundred bucks a month, and I only have a dollar co-pay with MassHealth for the Percs."

The insurance companies are saving a fortune from the fact that so many patients are treating themselves with cannabis instead of with expensive pills, injections, and other therapies. A 2016 study in *Health Affairs*, after Colorado legalized, found that

> the use of prescription drugs for which marijuana could serve as a clinical alternative fell significantly, once a medical marijuana law was implemented. National overall reductions in Medicare program and enrollee spending when states implemented medical marijuana laws were estimated to be $165.2 million per year in 2013.[2]

The savings would be orders of magnitude greater today than as were reported in this study, as many more states have passed medical and adult-use cannabis laws, more patients are enrolled, and there is a spreading awareness of what conditions medical cannabis can alleviate. As more doctors become cannabis savvy and start incorporating it into their practices, the savings will further multiply.

There is absolutely no reason why health insurance companies shouldn't reimburse for medical cannabis in the same way that they (are hypothetically supposed to) pay for other medications and therapies.

Our research must become less tethered to political agendas and feature more balanced exploration. There is much that we don't understand that needs to be researched, such as the long-term effects of using cannabis as treatments for diseases such as insomnia and depression. This needs to be approached neutrally, not with an a priori agenda of finding harm or benefit.

We need to reassess the existing canon of cannabis-related studies and determine how to factor in the biases and agendas that have informed so many of the studies. Are any of the studies that were funded by the War on Drugs fully valid? Are most of them? Ideally, we would start with a blank slate. More realistically, we need a way to contextualize them so that we can extract what is true and helpful while exposing the distortions that have been tilting the findings toward the negative for half a century.

The problem with research is not just whether it has been conducted in a neutral fashion but how it is received, interpreted, and communicated. We need to disengage the cognitive filters that have been installed into both sides, which cause Cannatopians to automatically discount negative news about cannabis and which similarly insulate Reefer Pessimists from any evidence of benefit from "medical cannabis." This will come with time as this issue becomes less polarized. One thing that is helping to tamp down the polarization is that, with legalization, there is a lot more visibility of people using cannabis. People are seeing that towns with marijuana dispensaries are not descending into criminal hippie ghettos; rather, they are enjoying the tax revenues. Medical cannabis is around and visible, and users are just normal patients, so it is being seen as less exotic and scary and can therefore no longer be as easily demonized. Almost everyone, by this point, knows someone who has benefited from medical cannabis.

Each study needs to be evaluated based on the science, not on how expedient the results are or how the results are portrayed in the conclusions by the authors. For example, a recent study of cannabis, done at an institution that will remain unnamed, reported "no significant improvement in pain, anxiety, or depressive symptoms, but improved *self-reported* sleep quality" (emphasis added). Now, obviously the pain, anxiety, and depressive symptoms were "self-reported" too—it wasn't your third cousin, or a space alien, that is informing the researchers about these symptoms—so why put "self-reported" just before the positive finding, except to make it sound less solid and valid?

There are many government agencies and subagencies, such as SAM-HSA (Substance Abuse and Mental Health Services Administration) and the ONDCP (Office of National Drug Control Policy), that just need to be fully reprogrammed about cannabis. On Twitter, whenever you click on the hashtag #marijuana, an advertisement from SAMHSA offering you addiction treatment comes up. This doesn't occur with alcohol and couldn't possibly be more insulting or degrading to the millions who use cannabis for medicine or wellness.

We also need to find a way to address media biases. For example, the "publication bias" distorts knowledge in all directions. When the media just broadcasts positive findings, of harm or of benefit, but doesn't report on the studies that don't show harm or benefit, it distorts the findings by presenting them out of context. For example, if there is a study that shows an increase in pediatric emergency room visits for a particular year due to kids eating edibles, but the media doesn't report on or mention all the years that there *wasn't* an increase in ED visits for cannabis, it artificially magnifies the problem. (This is just an example; pediatric ED visits for cannabis *are* a problem, and it is why I am against making edibles into candies that appeal to kids.) In the same vein, a study that shows cannabis is effective for MS is a lot more interesting than a study that doesn't show any positive results—but both need to be part of our collective knowledge base.

Or, just as commonly, the media takes the summary of the study hook, line, and sinker, as intended by the researchers, in line with their agendas—"Medical Marijuana May Trigger Substance Misuse"—rather than critically understanding things such as, in the case of one recent study, the fact that you can't, by definition, develop "cannabis use disorder" in two weeks, and you don't have "tolerance" to cannabis if you are a new medical patient titrating up your dosage. The media is increasingly polarizing an already-polarized issue by not being sufficiently educated or skeptical on these issues. It they amplify nonsense about cannabis, the Utopians will continue to distrust the science. If they overly hype benefits, the Pessimists will just reject them all. It would help if news outlets had reporters dedicated to the cannabis beat who are familiar with the literature and are less likely to "fall for" these things.

Also, we can promote media literacy by educating people to be more critical (and less gullible) with their news and social media consumption. This would have been extremely helpful in getting patients vaccinated with the COVID vaccine and might have avoided many time-consuming conversations about Bill Gates, George Soros, 5G, the devil's chip, mind control, becoming magnetic, genetic mutations, location tracking, secret government plots to control and poison us all, etc.

As cannabis increasingly becomes mainstream for medicinal uses, or for whichever wellness and lifestyle enhancement people enjoy, it is critical to educate cannabis users about how to use cannabis safely. Understanding that everyone's needs and habits are different, here are some general principles:

1. Keep dosages of THC as low as possible. As with all drugs and medicines, the lower the (effective) dose, the less harmful. We fetishize high THC in the United States at the expense of other components. Periodic tolerance breaks help keep the dosage down.

2. Use CBD along with your THC. Get cannabis that has both CBD and THC in it or take the CBD separately—current research suggests this will protect your brain.

3. Don't smoke! (Unless you are a *very* occasional user). There's no reason to expose yourself to combustion products, such as tar, benzene, polycyclic aromatic hydrocarbons, etc. (Even though cannabis has never been shown to cause lung cancer or COPD, there's no reason to inhale all of this crap.) If you prefer to use cannabis inhalationally, use a dry herb vaporizer, which doesn't combust the cannabis but produces a less irritating vapor. Or explore edibles, tinctures, inhalers, oils, suppositories, patches, and lotions—there are lots of options these days.

4. Don't use cannabis, even medicinally, if you might have to drive. Not only is this dangerous and irresponsible; it is also extremely stressful and unpleasant, as well as unethical, as it puts others at risk.

5. Watch the dosage on edibles. It is very easy to take too much. Don't make the classic mistake of "Hey, nothing is happening" after twenty minutes and then take five more, as they can take up to two hours to kick in. Don't be like my friends who visited Amsterdam during college, did exactly this with Space Cakes, and then were so scared they hid in the closet of their hotel room for an entire day.

6. If you have a particularly good or bad reaction to a particular strain or chemovar, write it down. Journaling is good practice in any case—dosage, benefits, side effects, formulations, and delivery mechanism.

7. If you are smoking (or vaping), you don't have to hold your breath for more than a few seconds—it is a misconception that holding the smoke in longer gets you higher. It just irritates your lungs.

8. Use caution if you have any history of addiction or any history or family history of mental illness, particularly psychosis or schizophrenia. Speak with your doctor (or a doctor that is able to be helpful, if your doctor isn't) and exercise caution before starting cannabis. The use of cannabis, or any drug, can also make mental illnesses more difficult to diagnose and treat.

9. Use with great caution as well if you have a history of coronary disease or an arrhythmia; involve your medical providers and keep the dosages very low.

10. If your use is escalating and you find yourself craving cannabis frequently, or if you have trouble cutting down, ask for help. Addiction is a disease of isolation; be open and honest—especially with yourself. If people don't take you seriously because it's "just a weed addiction," seek help elsewhere. Any addiction—and people do get addicted to cannabis—should be responded to with empathy and competent treatment.

11. Ask your doctor, or a cannabis specialist, about any potential reactions there may be between THC, CBD, and any medications you are taking. This is particularly true if you are on blood thinners or other medications that need to be kept within a narrow range (e.g., antiepileptics, immunosuppressants, chemotherapeutic agents). Also, if you use cannabis frequently, make sure the anesthesiologist knows, before surgery, as you might have higher anesthesia requirements.

12. Know the relevant laws in your area, and don't get tangled up with law enforcement. You can't (yet) legally fly with cannabis. Other states where the legality is different might not accept your medical cannabis card and could even arrest you if they don't (yet) have legal medical cannabis.

13. Make sure that the product you are using is safe. This is best accomplished by going through the legal market if available (as these products are carefully monitored and regulated), growing your own, or knowing your grower.

14. Do not use during pregnancy or breastfeeding, if feasible, until we understand this area much better. If you are using, please let your care teams know. Care teams, on their end, must respond with compassion, not stigma and punitiveness.

15. Avoid using cannabis with other sedating drugs, particularly alcohol, or medications such as opioids or benzodiazepines, as the impairment can be additive.

16. Be careful with concentrates (wax, shatter, crumble, bubble hash, rosin, etc.), as we haven't really studied these for safety, and also it's easy to accidentally get way too high when using them, which is not pleasant and can be dangerous.

17. Learn how to read the labels on the cannabis so you know exactly what you are consuming and can better decide what works for you.

18. Learn enough about cannabis so that you can be your own advocate; this will help you speak with doctors and budtenders alike.

We must acknowledge all who needlessly suffered under the criminalization of cannabis, and those who fought to change this. It is an extraordinary tale of how ordinary people stood up, over several generations, to stigma and repression and faced down the combined forces of the government, corporations, and, unfortunately, much of the medical profession. Many paid a steep price, including arrests, loss of assets, jail time, and criminal records.

Critically, we need to right past wrongs, most immediately by freeing those still in prison for nonviolent drug offenses, and by expunging the records of all who have been harmed by the War on Cannabis. Groups such as the Last Prisoner Project are working on this. We need to ensure that reparations are made to individuals and communities that have been disproportionately harmed by the War on Cannabis. As the new cannabis industry grows, social equity must be at the forefront as a way to help undo the brunt of the poverty and dislocation that was engendered by the War on Drugs.

Stigma against cannabis users—all drug users for that matter—is a corrosive force in our society that we all must confront and reject.

## Lessons Learned

What lessons can we learn from the eighty-year fiasco of cannabis prohibition that might be applied to other societal issues?

To start, as Dr. Andrew Weil points out in the introduction, the ways that both sides strayed from objectivity about cannabis are instructive. Some major flaws of the medical establishment were exposed. They were too often narrow-minded, disrespectful of patients' stories and experiences, and closed off to new information that went against mainstream opinion. To an uncomfortable degree, many of the medical societies have been unduly influenced by the economic interests of Big Pharma and the political interests of NIDA and various other organs of the War on Drugs, such as the rehab industry and law enforcement. By being on the wrong side of the War on Drugs, our profession violated the dictate to "do no harm" and demonstrated a remarkable willingness to be accessories to the stigmatizing "your brain on drugs" culture war, rather than to think for ourselves, learn the nuances of the cannabis issue, and advocate on behalf of patients.

As for the cannabis activists, I'm reminded of an aphorism from Nietzsche which I can only paraphrase: "If you automatically react against something, you are just as controlled by it as if you comply." Confronted with relentless negative, and at times dubious, information about cannabis from the U.S. government and from anti-cannabis researchers, cannabis advocates have counterreacted and reflexively dismissed concerns about potential harms. Many of these studies are valid and important, or at least hypothesis generating, with major implications for health and harm reduction.

Cannabis consumers have had their rights trampled on so thoroughly for so long that now they unreasonably, in my opinion, won't make some basic concessions to safety, like not making edibles into tasty candies. I was recently speaking to a group of several dozen addiction doctors at a medical cannabis dispensary in the Boston area, and I noted that they sold a chocolate bar with 1,100 milligrams of THC in it—enough THC to give Godzilla a full-blown panic attack (and he's destructive enough when sober). That's like two hundred puffs worth of strong cannabis—profoundly dangerous! Each of the ten pieces had 110 milligrams. If I were to take a twenty-milligram edible, I'd be too high, and the entire bar is fifty-five times stronger than this. Imagine if a kid ate this, or if someone accidentally ate it before driving.

Some cannabis proponents have also been very quick to romanticize and seize on stories of miracle cures, such as the early "cannabis cures COVID" bandwagon, without doing enough "due diligence" to see if the weed they are so fond of in other contexts is truly helpful in this regard. Ideally, the same level of skepticism would be applied to positive claims as to negative claims. There is a tendency toward reflexive rejection of science in some parts of the cannabis community. Numerous people have said to me, "Why would I trust the government about a COVID vaccine if they lied about cannabis?" This represents an inaccurate attribution of traits from one department of government during one epoch to an entirely different part of government at a different time period. It also assumes that "government" is a homogenous entity. Science is science—we can't just reject it. As Neil deGrasse Tyson points out, science is true whether you believe it or not.

This attitude of scientific rejectionism leads to more alienation from the mainstream medical establishment, which then uses these unscientific attitudes on the part of cannabis advocates as further justification for their patronizing dismissal of cannabinoid medicine. It is a feedback loop that we need to reverse.

Again with Nietzsche, I wouldn't go as far as saying "there are no facts, only interpretations." But I do feel that science can be like a loaded gun, and its realization has to be ethical, meaning that it is free of politics, assumptions, and agendas. If used in the wrong way, science can have devastating consequences, as we've already seen in the drug realm. One example is the stigmatization of "crack babies," who essentially turned out to be fine—or, if not fine, they were damaged because of poverty and racism, not because of parental cocaine use. Another example is putting pregnant moms in jail or separating them from their children if they test positive for cannabis—under the assumption that this is child abuse because the drugs are potentially harming the fetus. All this accomplishes is destroying families. Science must be used for the good of humanity, not for the advancement of political, ideological, religious, financial, or corporate agendas.

In our increasingly posttruth world, science must never be used to mislead the population, as it was about cannabis from the moment that Nixon declared his War on Drugs, ignoring his own Shafer Report, which concluded that cannabis was not the menace he was claiming it was. These abuses ultimately caused a counterreaction that resulted in a breathtaking example of democracy in action, and democracy in medicine. Brave citizens advocated for, and achieved access to, cannabis medicine against a dismissive and paternalistic medical establishment, a hostile government, and antagonistic corporate interests. To do this, citizens and activists have been teaching themselves the science, such as how to read scientific papers, so that they are educated enough to debunk the mistruths and exaggerations about cannabis. A recent article on the cannabis site Weedmaps was titled "How to Read Cannabis Research Papers." If people implicitly trusted the cannabis research, they probably wouldn't be spending their spare time reading about how to read research papers. At least some good is coming out of all of this: improved scientific literacy.

At the same time, now that there is corporate backing for cannabis and an increasingly powerful cannabis industry, we can't repeat the mistakes we made with the alcohol and tobacco industries and let the corporate drivers of cannabis influence or distort the research.

Assumptions and stigma matter. If you assume cannabis is a scourge, it is likely that your subsequent interpretations and suggestions will be anti-cannabis. Some policy makers in the cannabis field appear to assume that the use of cannabis is inherently bad and thus propose regulatory structures to minimize its use, analogous to alcohol and tobacco. Take, for example, Jonathan Caulkins, who is an American drug policy researcher (not to single anyone out—I know him from being on a panel with him, he is a nice person who clearly means well). In a somewhat misleading and alarmist 2016 piece in *National Affairs*, "The Real Dangers of Marijuana," Caulkins stated,

With the exception of the Drug Enforcement Administration, most opposition comes not from government but from non-profit groups. . . . The governmental heavyweight, the National Institute on Drug Abuse, is quick to point out marijuana's dangers but even quicker to disavow having any official position on policy questions like legalization or decriminalization.[3]

NIDA is agnostic on legalization! They have done everything they legally can to taint public opinion against legalization since their inception in 1974, with Dr. Robert DuPont at the helm. Caulkins goes on to opine,

It is clear we would all be better off if marijuana did not exist. Given the abundance of alternative sources of intoxication and fun, the harm suffered by abusers probably outweighs the pleasure derived by its controlled users.[4]

This wasn't a verbal miscue, or a Freudian slip, like when Dr. Nora Volkow said, "Cannabis harms your humanity," when on stage in Boston.[5] Everyone is entitled to their opinions, but how would someone with this categorically dismissive an attitude interpret a new study that shows a benefit of cannabis? His entire piece is a cherry-picked rhetorical distillation of anti-cannabis thinking. Another example:

Part of the difference may be that most people who use marijuana do so with the express purpose of getting intoxicated, whereas many people drink occasionally just to quench their thirst or to complement their dinner.[6]

Anyone who uses cannabis is now likely deeply perplexed and offended at this phenomenal misunderstanding. The word "intoxication" captures such a tiny fraction of the cannabis experience. It is so profoundly more nuanced than that (see chapter 21).

This is not someone who is able to be neutral about the pros and cons of cannabis. In the same way, if one assumes that cannabis is a cure-all, then that can be equally blinding, especially if you have a financial interest. For example, early into the COVID pandemic, an ex-NFL player named Kyle Turley, who sells CBD, was claiming on his website and on social media that CBD cures COVID. There was no evidence at that point for this claim; it just seemed to stem from some magical thinking about the powers of cannabis, combined with the profit motive. I explained this to him, but he literally couldn't care less, and he started boasting on Twitter about his bravado in sticking with these claims. Very shortly afterward, he got into some hot water for this, as documented in *Marijuana Moment*, "FDA Warns Former NFL Player to Stop Claiming CBD Can Cure Coronavirus." I agreed with the FDA; in fact, I was the one who reported him, as he was harming people.

These persistent assumptions show why people are talking past each other on cannabis. They nourish the cognitive filters that people have on both sides. It's time to let them go and to approach this entire issue with an open mind and a clear slate.

## Cannabis Unites

Opinion on cannabis, particularly medical cannabis, is broadly positive. Ninety-four percent of Americans are in favor of legal access to medical marijuana. Can you name any other issue about which 94 percent of Americans agree? Can you even imagine it? I'm not sure that 94 percent of Americans believe the earth is round, that we actually landed on the moon, or that the sky is blue.

I remember a sort of playful protest at Trump's inauguration where cannabis proponents were passing out thousands of joints. One of the papers showed a photo of a group of young Trump supporters counterprotesting with signs, yet asking the anti-Trump protestors if they could share some weed. It was a humanizing moment. We have recently seen full legalization of cannabis in some of the more conservative states like Montana, Alaska, and South Dakota (until it was sabotaged by the courts). As of this writing, Republicans have a competing legalization bill in the U.S. House of Representatives, led by Representative Nancy Mace, who just won reelection and was quite educated and up to date on cannabis issues when I spoke with her. More than 50 percent of Republicans believe in full legalization. Cannabis unites.

When I spent six months living on a farm in rural North Carolina before medical school, almost everyone seemed to use cannabis regardless of whether they were hippies or rednecks. The similarities between these two groups are an example of convergent evolution. Cannabis was such an equalizer that smoothed out other differences: we're all just human beings getting high together in the beautiful outdoors, under the moonlight, as we've been doing for thousands of years. I've often wondered if perhaps the main difference between the Pessimists and the Utopians is lived experience. It makes obvious sense that the Utopians are much more inclined to use cannabis than the Pessimists are. If both groups can do the research and follow the science, it seems that the group which *also* has abundant lived experience might have an advantage in terms of knowledge about its effects.

In some ways, the debate is portrayed as being more divisive than it is in reality. The appearance of this "bothsiderism" comes from two causes. First, the "anti-" side includes many corporate and governmental organs of power, like those medical societies who can't seem to evolve their thinking on cannabis; agencies of the U.S. government such as NIDA, SAMHSA, and the ONDCP, which need to fully reprogram their anti-cannabis ideologies; the rehab industry; and law enforcement groups (and the pseudo-advocacy groups they fund). These entities, which collectively hold a lot of sway and have a disproportionate voice in the media and in policy, can give an impression that this issue is more contested than it is. Further, if 69 percent of Americans support fully legalizing cannabis, for medical and recreational use, simple math dictates that a quarter (94 – 69 = 25 percent) of people seem to want medical legal but recreational illegal. As people realize how thin the line is between medical and recreational use, as discussed in chapter 21, the rates of approval for full legalization will continue to climb, as they have been doing steadily since the 1980s.

The reality of the situation is that people across the globe, including most Americans, are waking up to the fact that they have been sold a bill of goods on cannabis. Many people want "something" after a long day at work, to soothe sore muscles and frayed nerves, and now that cannabis is increasingly a legal, available option, I predict that many will start choosing cannabis over alcohol. While not harm free, it is healthier, safer, less fattening (provided you don't eat your way through the kitchen after consuming), and, for many, more interesting and more productive. It is more conducive, in my opinion, to genuinely connecting to other people, which is particularly important given how isolated and lonely a great number of people are feeling these days.

Cannabis unites people in so many ways. It unites them when they use it together, it unites as a shared cultural practice and belief system, and it unites them politically over concerns about social justice. We are seeing examples of former influential Republicans, like John Boehner, and members of law enforcement "switching sides" and joining the cannabis train. The days of illegality of cannabis are numbered as, defying the organs of power, Americans are saying "just say legalize" to cannabis. This movement is spreading around the world too, with many countries liberating cannabis laws. Perhaps the United States, which has for so long been internationally influential in a corrosive way, by demanding that other countries march in step with our War on Drugs, could even help lead the world into a new, more enlightened phase in this area of policy. Currently, Canada, Uruguay, and Israel are the ones leading the way.

Are there any lessons from the cannabis story that might apply to the broader War on Drugs? If the illegality of cannabis was such a social and financial disaster for millions of people—with absolutely nothing of benefit to show for it—why prohibit the use of other drugs? Is the criminalization of meth, opioids, and cocaine any more sensible or productive than that of cannabis? Is prohibition really the best way to protect people from the harms of these drugs? Or is it time for this policy to be broadly reconsidered as well? On the one hand, cannabis is less dangerous, and less rewarding, than these other drugs, so it is easier to contemplate legalization. On the other hand, many of the dangers of criminalization—tainted supply, needless arrests for nonviolent crimes, wasted resources, racially biased arrests—apply just as much to these more dangerous drugs. The "tainted supply" problem, in particular, relates to opioids more than any other drug right now, with 108,000 overdose deaths in the last twelve months of this writing, mostly from fentanyl and other adulterants.

In my opinion, the issue of drugs lands somewhere between a medical issue, an economic issue, an ethical issue, and a social justice issue. People should be freely allowed to change their consciousness, as long as it doesn't harm or inconvenience other people. If people get addicted or have any medical consequences of their drug use, they ought to have unfettered access to medical attention, and to compassion. When people become addicted, it is often due to unresolved trauma, a medical issue, or socioeconomic problems such as homelessness or poverty—addiction is a "disease of despair." The last people who should be involved are law enforcement. Why are we punishing people for being addicted, or for just wanting something to help them get by? Again, as long as it doesn't hurt other people, it should be legal. And by legalizing, we make the supply chain safer, with no adulterants, and more ethical as well—no more cartels.

If people drive when impaired or act in a violent or antisocial way, such as they might do under the influence of alcohol, that reasonably becomes a law enforcement issue. One could argue that treatment is always more productive than punishment (which doesn't at all help people with the disease of addiction), although intoxicated drivers do need to be taken off the roads. Otherwise, the harms of being involved with law enforcement and the court system, including the carceral system, are often worse than the harms of the drug use itself, to individuals, their families, and their communities. The very involvement of law enforcement deters people from admitting they are struggling and from seeking help. Ideally, we could make our criminal justice system more rehabilitative and less needlessly punitive, like it is in many European countries.

I am convinced that if opioids were legal, no one would be dying of fentanyl overdoses. The supply would be regulated, monitored, and safe; the drug use wouldn't be underground; and we'd have safe injection sites everywhere they are needed. There wouldn't be legal and social barriers to asking for help. We'd also have billions of dollars freed up from law enforcement to use for addiction treatment, jobs training, and the basics that humans deserve and require, such as food, health care, and housing. I'm not saying "defund the police," just "defund the War on Drugs."

Portugal is an example of a country that has decriminalized drugs. They also redirected a large portion of their funding away from law enforcement to housing, job training, and addiction treatment. Their rates of addiction, HIV, and hep C plummeted. The only casualty was the bloated budgets of the different law enforcement agencies. Portugal defunded the War on Drugs and the results have been spectacular.

We can, and must, do the same thing here. The only way to win the War on Drugs is to surrender, retreat, apologize, expunge, make reparations, and reframe our entire attitude about drug use and addiction. The main obstacle to doing so in the United States is that we have a much more entrenched, enriched, and entitled law enforcement bureaucracy, which is used to funding itself with "asset forfeiture" and unlimited Drug War dollars. The War on Drugs is also a mechanism of racial oppression, which is destructive beyond words. We need to empty out our prisons of nonviolent drug offenders and get them the help they need to get back on their feet. I predict that some combination of decriminalization and legalization will be a major component of how we will solve the addiction crisis in this country. Legalization is a glowing success for cannabis, and I predict it will be so for most of the other drugs, within the decade.

# AFTERWORD
## From Danny to Lester: The Family Herb

Cannabis has done as much to benefit my family as any other medicine. It has always been uncomfortable for me to see it misrepresented, its harm exaggerated, and its benefits dismissed (or inflated). It boggles the mind that people are still getting arrested, or in any way punished, or stigmatized, for using this fascinating and useful plant which, as I've described through the experiences of millions, can be vitally helpful for a myriad of conditions. Even if it weren't helpful, people shouldn't get arrested for using it—as long as they aren't harming others. Like all other medicines or drugs, cannabis needs to be used with care and respect, thoughtfully, in moderation. It's not a cure-all, but the control or regulation of it should have little to nothing to do with law enforcement.

When my brother Danny was dying, cannabis enabled him to hold food down, weather the ravages of chemotherapy, engage with his family, and participate in life that much more fully during the short time he had left. Instead of being confined to bed, miserable and incapacitated, he'd be playing his guitar, doing art projects, and inventing board games with his little twin brothers. I cherish these memories, some of which were only possible due to the relief that cannabis provided, allowing Danny more joy and comfort during the last year of his life. I forgive him for trying to asphyxiate me with that first puff when I was seven years old—he was just a teenager being a teenager, and I'm glad he had somewhat of a chance to be a teenager.

It represents an utter failure in our entire approach to cannabis in society that my parents had to break the law and risk their careers to provide this medicine for him. Millions of families face the same dilemma. Some families haven't been as lucky as mine and are saddled with criminal records, or debt, or have members languishing in prison just for trying to provide the same relief to their loved ones. We can debate how strictly it should be regulated, from state-controlled stores to the current commercialized free-for-all, but there's absolutely no reason for cannabis to be illegal and criminalized.

One of my favorite uncles was an alcoholic. It stemmed from a catastrophic first marriage which involved him and his two young daughters being the recipient of nonstop, vitriolic abuse. My uncle was conflict avoidant, and the kids' mom was angry and troubled, with untreated bipolar disorder—a bad combination. She once took and threw every single piece of one of her daughter's clothing down the garbage shoot, where it emptied into an incinerator. This is not typical nurturing, maternal behavior.

As a child I remember visiting their home exactly once, even though they just lived right in New York, and we were in Boston. Their cramped, dingy apartment was in a building that was part of a large cluster of many identical towers, containing hundreds of equivalent apartments. It felt depressingly anonymous. We went for a walk, and my uncle shuffled next to us, chuckling at our suggestion that he quit smoking cigarettes. His attitude was, "Why would I do that? There's no other comfort or joy in my life." He looked haggard. I had no idea at the time that he was drinking himself to death with vodka.

My dad had studied and learned much about the benefits of cannabis over the preceding ten years. One indication that many people spoke of was as a "harm reduction" approach by substituting cannabis for more dangerous drugs, such as alcohol. My dad was always available to help anyone, anytime—you could call him in the middle of the night if you were upset and needed to talk. He discussed with his brother the possibility that, if he transitioned from vodka to weed, he might get off the alcohol and increase his ability to escape his miserable circumstances. My uncle was able to taper down on the alcohol and, as needed, use the cannabis as a substitute. Fairly quickly his drinking was no longer a significant factor in his life.

His circumstances steadily improved from that point on. His health stabilized, and he remained active and lucid until he died at the ripe old age of ninety. He ended up with a partner that he loved deeply and with whom he stayed for the final one-third century of his life. He was far more present and engaged with his family, and the extended family—we started seeing him again, and I just couldn't be more grateful to have had him, and his glorious, reborn sense of humor, back in our lives.

One of my most brilliant and successful relatives, a person that I've always been close to, suffers from lifelong ADHD. This didn't stop him from clawing his way through a PhD in mechanical engineering. He now studies and teaches artificial intelligence at a prestigious university. His ADHD partially manifests itself in a verbal delay, which makes it difficult for him to express his creative and complex thoughts with ease and fluidity. The large dose of Concerta that he has been put on by the psychiatrists makes him functional from a utilitarian "get your work done" perspective, but it doesn't alleviate the verbal delay or make him feel like himself.

With one modest puff of a sativa strain, his ADHD improves, and his verbal delay resolves for several hours. Immediately, he can express himself with a coherent articulateness and confidence that otherwise eludes him. In the teasing banter that my community is continuously participating in, the balance of power shifts, as he can verbally spar with the best of us. He describes it: "My brain gets unstuck and then it can function. I don't really get high." He can get his work done more easily, work that is far more complex than anything I do as a primary care doctor. He has said to me numerous times, "I wish I could use cannabis before work; I'd do better with [the] data and I'd be able to explain what I'm doing more clearly to my teammates."

One day I suspect that cannabinoids will much more openly be involved in many lines of work, especially tasks that involve the right hemisphere of our brains. This is especially true as we discover or develop more nonintoxicating medicinal cannabinoids.

The person in my family that was likely aided the most by cannabis, besides perhaps my brother Danny, was my dad. This is ironic and sort of poetic, given that my dad started out, in the late 1960s, intending to write a book about how irresponsibly destructive the use of cannabis was. He never could stop marveling at how off base he had been. What originally was intended as a heavy-hitting scientific call to alarm against cannabis transformed into an awareness that the legal consequences of prohibition were hurting people more than the (by no means entirely harmless) drug itself. Then he evolved a deep appreciation for how cannabis can help people flourish.

He didn't even try cannabis until the second half of his life. He never used it until well after he had completed his (first) book on the subject—*Marihuana Reconsidered*. As he aged, cannabis, along with a host of spectacular Boston-area doctors, helped him stay an inch or two ahead of the health conditions that were slowly closing in on him. He credited cannabis with facilitating enormous personal growth due to the insight and fellowship it provides. Cannabis helped him age and, ultimately, die with dignity and comfort. If you could ask him, from the ether (where it's been suggested that he's somewhere sharing a joint of the highly cognitive heirloom sativa strain named "Dr. Grinspoon" with his friend Carl Sagan), he would be the first to agree. I can just hear Carl's familiar resonant voice: "Look what you did, Lester. Legalization is spreading to billions and billions of people."

The fact that my dad lived until age ninety-two, in relatively good health, functional, able to walk slowly but independently (until close to the end), and able to intelligently and fluently (if forgetfully) converse until his final days, is a medical miracle. He had a Rasputin-like quality about him. Or maybe Houdini better describes it. To start, he had a rare bleeding disorder called Christmas disease, or hemophilia C, which tends to affect Ashkenazi Jews. It didn't come out until later in life, which is fortunate considering that one of his hobbies in his younger days was boxing, which he had the tall and lanky frame for. Boxing was how he kept the anti-Semites at bay when he was in the military—anti-Semitism was even more open back then. If they started taunting him, he'd challenge them to a boxing match, which they couldn't exactly decline. They soon learned not to taunt him.

It wasn't until he was in his middle age that he started having these spontaneous, dramatic, life-threatening bleeds due to his clotting system being compromised. Because of this bleeding disorder, he couldn't take anything except acetaminophen (Tylenol) for pain, which is much more effective at harming your liver than it is at treating serious pain. He hated opioids and avoided them like the plague—he had seen too many cases of addiction over his long and storied psychiatric career. On the road to ninety-two, there are inevitably surgeries, injuries, sprains, inflammations, fractures, arthritic joints, and many other assorted painful conditions. Whenever in discomfort, he would take a puff from his vaporizer, and the pain would lessen. He always felt comfortable doing this in public, as he believed in living his convictions. His attitude toward law enforcement, and the medical board, was along the lines of "make my day," especially as he got older. He was convinced that if he were ever arrested or disciplined, he would annihilate them in the court of public opinion. (He would have—it would have resulted in worse of a bloodbath than when he was boxing with the anti-Semites.) It's also difficult to picture the police arresting a ninety-year-old man for smoking a little bit of weed, in Massachusetts, in this day and age.

Cannabis was similarly helpful with one of his other main problems: sleeping. Insomnia runs deep throughout my family. As one ages, it becomes even more difficult to get a full night's restful sleep due to changes in our sleep cycle. He was a lifelong insomniac, and had tried a variety of sleeping pills, all of which have undesirable side effects, including memory loss, fatigue, grogginess, urinary retention, and dry mouth. Many of them can cause falls, which I was increasingly worried about as he aged and appeared progressively more rickety. With cannabis, he was able to lessen his use of many of these pills, the Ambiens and trazodones. He woke up feeling restful, not with a drug hangover.

When in his eighties, he developed metastatic prostate cancer and had to take androgen-blocking medications, the cannabis helped him get through the brutal hot flashes. He'd break out into drenching sweats in the middle of winter. Hot flashes are notoriously difficult to treat, but he said that one or two puffs from his trusty vaporizer broke the cycle.

As a wise psychiatrist once said to me, "aging isn't for sissies." My dad's experience with aging was significantly less painful and disruptive that it might have been because he had access to medical cannabis (which grateful legalization proponents sent him from around the world; I don't think he ever had to buy it). It was transformatively helpful to his experience. Seeing how profoundly it benefited my dad furthers my determination to see the day when everyone has access to the relief that cannabinoids provide in a safe, legal, and affordable manner.

My dad also attributed much of the personal growth that he enjoyed during the last half of his life to cannabis. By all accounts, he was an absolutely brilliant psychiatrist who took spectacular care of many patients, including some complex, high-profile patients who were specifically referred to him. He was a preternaturally good judge of character. Decades into retirement (from psychiatry—he probably *still* isn't retired from social justice activism, several years after his death), patients would still be sending him cards and gifts to express their gratitude. My mom continues to receive these tokens of appreciation.

Yet he always yearned to sand down the blunt edges that he had needed to climb from dirt-poor high school dropout, without two nickels to rub together, to graduating from Harvard Medical cum laude. He often said that he never "suffered fools gladly" and that he wished to evolve into someone who was more patient, tolerant, and diplomatic so that he could connect with all types of people better. About halfway through his lifespan, he discovered that cannabis was the key to his personal growth:

> I was 44 years old in 1972 when I experienced this first marijuana high. Because I have found it both so useful and benign I have used it ever since. . . . Only practiced cannabis users appreciate some of the other [beyond medical] ways in which it can be useful. It has been so useful to me that I cannot help but wonder how much difference it would have made had I begun to use it at a younger age. Because it has been so helpful in arriving at some important decisions and understandings, it is tempting to think that it might have helped me to avoid some "before cannabis era" bad decisions. In fact, now, when I have an important problem to solve or decision to make, I invariably avail myself of the opportunity to think about it both stoned and straight.[1]

Everyone who knew him marveled at how he personally transformed, far beyond "mellowing with age." He evolved from being the brutal taskmaster we grew up with—you have no idea—into an open, loving, and indulgent grandfather figure. He had always been generous, kind, and highly prosocial, but he used to also have a judgmental streak and, despite the poverty from which he came, a degree of academic snobbery. It was extraordinary how accepting he became of other people, as well as his own limitations, as his life progressed. Enlightened would be a good word for it. I am so glad that this patient, gentle, curious man is the grandfather that my kids got to know.

Along the way, I had so many cannabis-enhanced conversations with him about this process of aging and growth. I was fortunate enough to witness this growth in real time. He fully attributed these changes to the insight and gentle introspection, as well as to the person-to-person connections, that cannabis fosters. Even toward the very end, when his memory was failing, the cannabis brought him back out of the shadows of his pain and forgetfulness and enabled him to freely engage in open conversation, which he might not remember, but which he thoroughly enjoyed and freely contributed to. (People with dementia can be anxious, bitter, and confused; my dad was peaceful, accepting, and content—I truly believe the cannabis was partly responsible.)

As clinicians, in theory, we aren't encouraged to take care of family members under ordinary circumstances, as it might be difficult to be objective and to make tough decisions. This proscription was lifted in Massachusetts during the dark days of the COVID pandemic. This was a welcome change because it enabled me to provide care for many family members who were afraid to go to their doctor or to the hospital for fear of contracting the virus. As my father started heading toward the end of his life, in addition to being his health care proxy and primary medical decision maker, I took charge of the cannabinoid part of his care.

I'm only slightly exaggerating when I say that he was stitched together with cannabinoids during his last seven months. Less than a year before his death, in addition to his metastatic prostate cancer, he was suffering from inoperable colon cancer, which was causing daily rectal bleeding. His blood level was dropping and—with his bleeding disorder combined with the cancer—it looked like he wouldn't be with us for very much longer. From December to January, his blood level dropped more than ten points—a third of his blood. It seemed like it was a matter of days or weeks. It was time for a Hail Mary.

There are several cannabinoids that are extremely effective against colon cancer cells, as demonstrated in the lab and in some animal studies. They haven't been tried or rigorously studied in humans yet and aren't by any means considered mainstream practice. The following *has not been demonstrated to be effective in humans and it should not be tried in the place of chemotherapy*. In this circumstance, however, he was clearly dying, as was the case with my brother Danny so long ago, so what was there to lose?

With his consent—he would have jumped at the chance if he could still physically jump at that point, I bombarded his system with high doses of CBG (cannabigerol), CBN (cannabinol), and CBD, in addition to the THC he was freely using. Friends gave us samples for which I am profoundly grateful. The title of one 2014 paper describes that "colon carcinogenesis is inhabited by the TRPM8 antagonist cannabigerol, a *Cannabis*-derived non-psychotropic cannabinoid."[2] In another, CBG was reported to reduce cell proliferation in several cancer cell lines, including human breast, prostate, and colorectal carcinomas, as well as gastric adenocarcinomas.[3] There are a variety of studies showing this potential benefit, for CBG and many of the other "minor" cannabinoids, though not as a stand-alone or even, yet, as adjunct, disease-modifying treatment in humans (except possibly CBD in glioblastoma—see chapter 17). I figured, what is the counterargument? He loved taking cannabinoids, they are nontoxic (particularly if you are already dying), and they just might help. They also would help with other discomforts he had (CBD for anxiety and pain, CBG for anxiety and inflammation, CBN for inflammation and insomnia).

He dutifully continued to consume the THC part of the cocktail—we didn't have to twist his arm. I used to joke that I could navigate from across town directly to his apartment, in the senior living community, by smell, with my eyes closed. Or I could just drive toward the large mushroom cloud on the horizon—at times his apartment complex did somewhat resemble Bikini Atoll. (My mom hates these jokes . . . sorry, mom! She likes to pretend that my dad didn't hotbox the entire institution.) The only pragmatic difficulty was that he loved to have people to get high with. He usually wanted me to join him for companionship and conversation. When he offered, I often had to decline to consume because I usually had to drive home, not to mention finishing my work. I felt guilty about this, knowing he didn't have much time left.

Within a few days of starting this high-dose witches' brew of anti-inflammatory cannabinoids, his bleeding slowed to a trickle and then stopped. We rechecked his blood levels, four times, and throughout the next month, it remained rock stable—I never had it checked again. We were profoundly thankful for this, as we had run out of other options. He was too frail for any medical intervention. He lived another six months from the start of the high-dose cannabinoid therapy, in peace and comfort, at least a half year longer than we were expecting.

Could this have been coincidence? Of course. But the bleeding did stop shortly after I pushed the nuclear button on the high-dose cannabinoids, which have demonstrated anti-inflammatory and antitumor activity in colon cells, at least in the lab. This was the only intervention we made. So we'll never know. It does seem like an awfully big coincidence that he stopped bleeding within a few days of starting this regimen.

During the last few months of his life, the hospice team did a fantastic job of keeping him comfortable. They attentively ministered to each of his challenges and discomforts with well thought-out protocols. If he was too weak to get out of a chair, they even had a mechanical "person lifter" to hoist him out. It's amazing how much more patient centered and sophisticated hospice has become since I was in medical school.

My only complaint is that they kept wanting to load him up on morphine.

My dad typically wasn't in pain, especially with the cannabis and all the other cannabinoids, so I wasn't sure why he even needed such a strong painkiller. As it was, he was struggling to be awake and to communicate with us. The morphine just zonked him out—it made it seem as if he was already dead. There was nothing that my dad was experiencing that cannabis couldn't more comfortably treat. Aside from severe pain, the one advantage that morphine has is that it treats the "air hunger" when people have trouble breathing near the very end, such as if they are dying from a pulmonary issue. My dad was breathing fine, so I asked them to hold the morphine unless one of us specifically asked for it, or if he absolutely needed it.

The cannabis allowed him to continue to participate much more fully in life for the last few months, then weeks, then days. As far as I'm aware, he only received a handful of doses of morphine in total, due to the liberal use of cannabinoids.

His death can be a helpful blueprint for others who wish to leave this world with their faculties relatively intact, so that they can preserve the ability to connect with their loved ones as long as possible. It can usually be done without being opiated into oblivion, or at least with a lower dosage of opioids, as the cannabis and the opioids work well together. This is a gift to family members as well, who would rather interact with a slightly stoned loved one than an opiated lump.

All along, but particularly as he was nearing the end, he and I had involved conversations about the progress we've made toward legalization and the overarching role he played in all of it. It was clear, by the last few years of his life, that our society was coming to its senses about cannabis, and legalization was going to win the day. It gives me profound satisfaction that he got to witness, during his lifetime, the resounding success of at least one major component of his life's work. It is unfortunate that he couldn't stick around long enough to witness the similar thing happening with psychedelics, as he had urgently (and, back then, controversially) advocated for their study and usage in psychiatry as far back as 1979. The whole family shared his childlike excitement when cannabis finally became legal in Massachusetts. He even got to smoke the first joint that was legally sold in Massachusetts courtesy of family friend and veteran Stephen Mandile.

In many ways, this story comes around full circle, as my father passed away just as I was finishing up the proposal for this book. He read the proposal again and again and was tremendously excited about this project, though was regretful that he would not be around to celebrate its publication. The night before he passed, his entire family, including his grandchildren, celebrated his ninety-second birthday with a Zoom party, which was a wonderful way for him to say good-bye to all of us, even though we didn't know at that point that it was good-bye. As he often did, he spoke of how grateful he was for the life he lived, for his wonderful marriage of sixty-six years to my mother, for his children and his grandchildren, and for the opportunity to make a difference. His absolute favorite topic of conversation—even more than weed—had always been how lucky he was to have found my mom. During that night, he passed in complete comfort, with his wife of sixty-six years at his side. It was time to rejoin his son Danny, whom he had lost forty-seven years earlier. It was so odd for us to see this great man, so full of life, so much larger than life, lying there lifeless. He hadn't suffered (much) in the end.

My dad claimed, to his last breath, that cannabis strengthened and deepened his relationships with his family and his friends, helped ease the pains of aging, and helped prepare him, without fear, for what was coming. In his own words,

> In the meantime, Betsy and I are gradually being given the opportunity to explore another dimension of the ways in which cannabis can be valuable; we are discovering its usefulness in the task of achieving reconciliation with the aging process, including coming to terms with the inevitable physical and emotional aches, deficits and losses. Cannabis also enhances our appreciation of the time we have, now that we are both emeritus, to enjoy our children, grandchildren and friends, literature, music and travel, and our daily walks in the New England woods. Of still more importance, it helps us to realize the wisdom of Robert Browning's words, "Grow old along with me! The best is yet to be."[4]

Thank you, dad, on behalf of the millions who are no longer getting arrested or jailed, or penalized, or stigmatized, due to your life's work—and on behalf of the millions of others who now have access, worldwide, to cannabis as a vital medicine. Also, thank you for your brilliant, prescient contributions to psychiatry and to medicine, as well as to nuclear disarmament, drug policy, psychedelics, human rights, and to all of the other social issues that you cared so deeply about. Those profoundly inspiring conversations I eavesdropped on as a kid, fifty years ago in our living room, about the critical need for legalization, came true. You did it! You are proof that determined people can decide to change the world for the better, and with enough sustained effort, patience, collaboration, chutzpah, and creativity, the world can, in fact, be changed.

# NOTES

## Introduction

1. Kevin F. Boehnke et al., "Cannabis Use Preferences and Decision-Making among a Cross-Sectional Cohort of Medical Cannabis Patients with Chronic Pain," *Journal of Pain*, May 24, 2019.

## Chapter One

1. Jonathan P. Caulkins, "The Real Dangers of Marijuana," *National Affairs*, Winter 2016, https://www.nationalaffairs.com/publications/detail/the-real-dangers-of-marijuana.

2. Jon Weiner, "Art Linkletter and Richard Nixon: Alcohol vs. Pot," *The Nation*, May 27, 2010, https://www.thenation.com/article/archive/art-linkletter-and-richard-nixon-alcohol-vs-pot.

3. Jonathan P. Caulkins, *Marijuana Legalization: What Everyone Needs to Know* (New York: Oxford University Press, 2016).

## Chapter Two

1. William C. Woodward, MD (1937), https://medicalmarijuana.procon.org/historical-timeline/#1970-1989.

2. Christopher Ingraham, "A Maker of Deadly Painkillers Is Bankrolling the Opposition to Legal Marijuana in Arizona," *Washington Post*, September 9, 2016, https://www.washingtonpost.com/news/wonk/wp/2016/09/09/a-maker-of-deadly-painkillers-is-bankrolling-the-opposition-to-legal-marijuana-in-arizona.

3. "Insys Executives Used Rap Video to Push Sales of Potentially Lethal Opioid," CBS News, February 14, 2019, https://www.cbsnews.com/news/insys-executives-used-rap-video-to-push-sales-of-highly-addictive-opioid.

4. "Report: Aide Says Nixon's War on Drugs Targeted Blacks, Hippies," CNN Politics, March 23, 2016, https://www.cnn.com/2016/03/23/politics /john-ehrlichman-richard-nixon-drug-war-blacks-hippie/index.html.

5. Testimony of Robert L. DuPont, MD, to the House Committee on Government Reform, April 1, 2004, https://uk.sagepub.com/sites/default/files /upm-assets/116863_book_item_116863.pdf; https://www.ibhinc.org/medical -marijuana.

6. Jag Davies, "Marijuana Production Facility Hangs in Balance: DEA Administrative Law Judge Recommendation Expected . . . Any Day," *MAPS News*, Winter 2006–2007, https://maps.org/news-letters/v16n3-html/marijuana _production_facility.html.

7. Jessica Winter, "Weed Control Research on the Medicinal Benefits of Marijuana May Depend on Good Gardening—and Some Say Uncle Sam, the Country's Only Legal Grower of the Cannabis Plant, Isn't Much of a Green Thumb," *Boston Globe*, May 28, 2006, http://archive.boston.com/news/globe /ideas/articles/2006/05/28/weed_control.

8. Cathleen O'Grady, "Cannabis Research Database Shows How U.S. Funding Focuses on Harms of the Drug," *Science*, August 27, 2020, https://www .science.org/content/article/cannabis-research-database-shows-how-us-funding -focuses-harms-drug.

9. Robert Rizzuto, "DEA Rejects UMass Professor Lyle Craker's Bid to Grow Marijuana for Federally-Regulated Medical Research," MassLive, August 25, 2011, https://www.masslive.com/news/2011/08/dea_rejects_umass _amherst_prof.html.

10. "DEA Lawsuit Supporting Prof. Craker's Proposed UMass Amherst Marijuana Production Facility," MAPS, https://maps.org/research-archive/mmj /DEAlawsuit.html.

11. "Grinspoon, Reconsidered," *Harvard Crimson*, May 11, 2018, https:// www.thecrimson.com/article/2018/5/11/editorial-grinspoon-reconsidered.

## Chapter Three

1. "The LaGuardia Report—Sociological Study, Conclusions," Shaffer Library of Drug Policy, https://www.druglibrary.net/schaffer/Library/studies/lag /concl.htm.

2. "Marihuana: A Signal of Misunderstanding," Official Report of the National Commission on Marihuana and Drug Abuse, 1972, https://archive.org /details/marihuanasignalo0000unse.

3. "Historical Timeline: History of Marihuana as Medicine—2900 BC to Present," ProCon.org, May 12, 2022, https://medicalmarijuana.procon.org historical-timeline/#1970-1989.

4. Jordon McMahon, "Marijuana History and Legal Aspects in the United States," Murray State University, Spring 2017, https://digitalcommons.murray state.edu/cgi/viewcontent.cgi?article=1048&context=bis437.

5. "Grinspoon, Reconsidered," *Harvard Crimson*, May 11, 2018.

6. Jimmy Carter, "Drug Abuse Message to the Congress," August 2, 1977, https://www.presidency.ucsb.edu/documents/drug-abuse-message-the-congress.

7. Peter Bourne, interview, *Frontline*, n.d., https://www.pbs.org/wgbh /pages/frontline/shows/drugs/interviews/bourne.html.

8. "War on Drugs," *Britannica*, https://www.britannica.com/topic/war-on -drugs#ref1284289.

9. Kyle Swenson, "'We'll Never Be the Same': A Hydroponic Tomato Garden Led Police to Raid Kansas Family's Home," *Chicago Tribune*, July 29, 2017, https://www.chicagotribune.com/nation-world/ct-hydroponic-tomato-garden -police-raid-20170729-story.html.

10. Michael Isikoff, "Administrative Judge Urges Medicinal Use of Marijuana," *Washington Post*, September 7, 1988, https://www.washingtonpost.com /archive/politics/1988/09/07/administrative-judge-urges-medicinal-use-of-mari juana/e521d648-bfec-48a0-896b-6035722a8377.

11. Carey Goldberg, "Medical Marijuana Use Winning Backing," *New York Times*, October 30, 1996, https://www.nytimes.com/1996/10/30/us/medical -marijuana-use-winning-backing.html.

12. "Dr. Marcus Conant vs. John L Walters," *Drug Times*, December 17, 2020, https://www.drugtimes.org/medical-marijuana-laws/dr-marcus-conant-v -john-l-walters-no-0017222.html.

13. Ibid.

14. Kyle Jaeger, "Massachusetts Marijuana Tax Revenue Now Exceeds Alcohol by Millions," *Marijuana Moment*, January 24, 2022, https://www.mari juanamoment.net/massachusetts-marijuana-tax-revenue-now-exceeds-alcohol -by-millions.

15. Kyle Jaeger, "Seven in Ten Americans Back Marijuana Legalization, with Majorities Embracing Pro-Reform Politicians, Two New Studies Find," *Marijuana Moment*, April 25, 2022, https://www.marijuanamoment.net/seven -in-ten-americans-back-marijuana-legalization-with-majorities-embracing-pro -reform-politicians-two-new-polls-find.

## Chapter Four

1. "Dependence on Cannabis (Marijuana)," *Journal of the American Medical Association* 201, no. 6 (August 7, 1967): 368–71, https://jamanetwork.com/jour nals/jama/article-abstract/335058.

2. Kyle Jaeger, "American Medical Association Approves Marijuana Expungements Resolution and Addresses Over-Medicalization of Cannabis," *Marijuana Moment*, June 17, 2022, https://www.marijuanamoment.net/amer ican-medical-association-approves-marijuana-expungements-resolution-and -addresses-over-medicalization-of-cannabis.

3. Linda Girgis, "Is the AMA Really the Voice of Physicians in the US?," *Physicians Weekly*, June 9, 2015, https://www.physiciansweekly.com/is-the-ama -really-the-voice-of-physicians-in-the-us.

4. Dr. Lester Grinspoon, *Marihuana, the Forbidden Medicine* (New Haven, CT: Yale University Press, 1993).

5. Anastasia B. Evanoff et al., "Physicians-in-Training Are Not Prepared to Prescribe Medical Marijuana," *Drug and Alcohol Dependence* 180 (November 2017).

6. David B. Allen, MD, "Survey Shows Low Acceptance of the Science of the ECS (Endocannabinoid System) at American Medical Schools," *Outword Magazine*, n.d., http://www.outwordmagazine.com/inside-outword /glbt-news/1266-survey-shows-low-acceptance-of-the-science-of-the-ecs-endo cannabinoid-system.

7. Suhas Gondi and Andreas Mitchell, "Med Schools Need to Get with the Times on Medical Marijuana, Chronic Pain, and More," *STAT*, April 24, 2018, https://www.statnews.com/2018/04/24/medical-school-teaching-pain-medical -marijuana.

8. Evanoff et al., "Physicians-in-Training Are Not Prepared."

9. Lindsey Philpot et al., "A Survey of the Attitudes, Beliefs and Knowledge about Medical Cannabis among Primary Care Providers," BMC Family Practice, January 2019, https://www.researchgate.net/publication/330567640_A_survey _of_the_attitudes_beliefs_and_knowledge_about_medical_cannabis_among _primary_care_providers.

10. Jared M. Weisman, "A Systematic Review of Medical Students' and Professionals' Attitudes and Knowledge regarding Medical Cannabis," *Journal of Cannabis Research* 3 (October 12, 2021), https://www.ncbi.nlm.nih.gov/pmc/articles /PMC8507207.

11. Gillian L. Schauer et al., "Clinician Beliefs and Practices Related to Cannabis," *Cannabis and Cannabinoid Research*, April 26, 2021, https://www.lieber tpub.com/doi/10.1089/can.2020.0165.

12. Kenneth Finn, *Cannabis in Medicine: An Evidence-Based Approach* (Cham, Germany: Springer, 2020).

13. Wesley Boyd, "Using Marijuana Two Times a Month Cost This Doctor His License," *KevinMD*, March 23, 2018, https://www.kevinmd.com/2018/03/using-marijuana-2-times-month-cost-doctor-license.html.

14. Lester Grinspoon, *Marihuana Reconsidered* (Cambridge, MA: Harvard University Press, 1971).

15. Daily presidential briefing for President Richard Nixon, reproduced at the Richard Nixon Presidential Library and Museum, Yorba Linda, CA.

16. Grinspoon, *Marihuana, the Forbidden Medicine*.

## Chapter Five

1. Staci A. Gruber et al., "Splendor in the Grass? A Pilot Study Assessing the Impact of Medical Marijuana on Executive Function," *Frontiers in Pharmacology* 7 (2016), https://www.ncbi.nlm.nih.gov/pmc/articles/PMC5062916.

2. Peter Sterne, "Las Vegas Review-Journal Scales Back Marijuana Coverage," *Politico*, June 9, 2016, https://www.politico.com/media/story/2016/06/las-vegas-review-journal-scales-back-marijuana-coverage-004588.

3. IASP Presidential Task Force on Cannabis and Cannabinoid Analgesia, "International Association for the Study of Pain Presidential Task Force on Cannabis and Cannabinoid Analgesia Position Statement," *Journal of the International Association for the Study of Pain* 162 (July 2021), https://journals.lww.com/pain/Fulltext/2021/07001/International_Association_for_the_Study_of_Pain.1.aspx.

4. International Association for the Study of Pain, "IASP Position Statement on the Use of Cannabinoids to Treat Pain," March 18, 2021, https://www.iasp-pain.org/publications/iasp-news/iasp-position-statement-on-the-use-of-cannabinoids-to-treat-pain.

5. Kyle Jaeger, "Wells Fargo Analyst Says Marijuana Testing Mandate to Blame for Trucker Shortages and Rising Costs," *Marijuana Movement*, February 18, 2022, https://www.marijuanamoment.net/wells-fargo-analyst-says-federal-marijuana-testing-mandate-to-blame-for-trucker-shortages-and-rising-costs.

6. Christopher Moraff, "Jeff Sessions' Marijuana Adviser Wants Doctors to Drug Test Everyone," *Daily Beast*, January 3, 2018, https://www.thedailybeast.com/jeff-sessions-marijuana-adviser-wants-doctors-to-drug-test-everyone.

7. Moraff, "Jeff Sessions' Marijuana Adviser."

8. Teo Armus, "A Disabled Black Veteran Drove through Alabama with Medical Marijuana. Now He Faces Five Years in Prison," *Washington Post*,

July 14, 2020, https://www.washingtonpost.com/nation/2020/07/14/alabama
-veteran-marijuana-prison.

9. https://www.goodreads.com/quotes/21810-it-is-difficult-to-get-a-man
-to-understand-something.

10. Disclosure: I am an unpaid advisor to the Parabola Center.

11. https://www.parabolacenter.com.

12. Shaleen Title, "Big Tobacco Is Coming for Legal Marijuana," *Boston
Globe*, April 8, 2021.

## Chapter Six

1. ACLU, "Marijuana Arrests by the Numbers," n.d., https://www.aclu.org
/gallery/marijuana-arrests-numbers.

2. FBI, "Arrests Table: Drug Abuse Violations," 2019, https://ucr.fbi.gov
/crime-in-the-u.s/2019/crime-in-the-u.s.-2019/topic-pages/persons-arrested.

3. Dale W. Willits et al., "Racial Disparities in the Wake of Cannabis Legalization: Documenting Persistence and Change," *Race and Justice*, March 16,
2022, https://journals.sagepub.com/doi/abs/10.1177/21533687221087355.

4. Andrew Weil, MD, *The Natural Mind: An Investigation of Drugs and the
Higher Consciousness* (Boston: Houghton Mifflin, 1986).

5. Clayton Mosher and Scott Akins, *Drugs and Drug Policy: The Control of
Consciousness Alteration*, 2nd ed. (Los Angeles: SAGE, 2013).

6. Council on Mental Health and Committee on Alcoholism and Drug
Dependence, "Dependence on Cannabis (Marihuana)," *Journal of the American
Medical Association* 201, no. 6 (August 7, 1967), https://jamanetwork.com/jour
nals/jama/article-abstract/335058.

7. ACLU, "New ACLU Report: Despite Marijuana Legalization Black
People Still Almost Four Times More Likely to Get Arrested," April 20, 2020,
https://www.aclu.org/press-releases/new-aclu-report-despite-marijuana-lega
lization-black-people-still-almost-four-times.

8. "Life Sentence for Marijuana Possession Upheld in Mississippi," Equal
Justice Initiative, May 28, 2021, https://eji.org/news/life-sentence-for-mari
juana-possession-upheld-in-mississippi.

9. Ibid.

10. "Operation Green Merchant and H. W. Bush's War on Drugs," *High
Times*, February 2020.

11. Jesse Kornbluth, "Poisonous Fallout from the War on Marijuana," *New
York Times*, November 19, 1978, https://www.nytimes.com/1978/11/19/archives
/poisonous-fallout-from-the-war-on-marijuana-paraquat.html.

# Chapter Seven

1. "Cannabinopathic Medicine: Lester Grinspoon, M.D.'S New Coinage," Americans for Safe Access, March 14, 2013, https://www.safeaccessnow.or /cannabinopathic_medicine_lester_grinspoon_m_d_s_new_coinage.

2. Tom Frieden, "Evidence for Health Decision Making—Beyond Randomized, Controlled Trials," *New England Journal of Medicine* 377 (2017), https://www.nejm.org/doi/full/10.1056/NEJMra1614394.

3. Ibid.

4. Ibid.

5. Rishi Banerjee et al., "Real World Evidence in Medical Cannabis Research," *Therapeutic Innovation & Regulatory Science* 5, no. 6 (January 2022), https://pubmed.ncbi.nlm.nih.gov/34748204.

6. Ibid.

7. Ibid.

8. Ibid.

9. Personal communication with Dr. Mikael Sodergren.

10. Kevin Boehnke, "National Trends in Qualifying Conditions for Medical Cannabis," *Health Affairs* 38, no. 2 (2019), https://ajendomed.com/wp-content /uploads/2021/04/Qualifying-Conditions-for-Medical-Cannabis.pdf.

11. Hannah Balfour, "UK Regulator Publishes Guidance on Use of Real-World Data to Support Clinical Trials," *European Pharmaceutical Review*, December 17, 2021, https://www.europeanpharmaceuticalreview.com/news/166738/uk-regula tor-publishes-guidance-on-use-of-real-world-data-to-support-clinical-trials.

# Chapter Eight

1. Johànne Olivia Gronne Kuhl et al., "The Incidence of Schizophrenia and Schizophrenia-Spectrum Disorders in the Period 2000–2012. A Register-Based Study," *Schizophrenia Research* 176, nos. 2–3 (October 2016), https://www.science direct.com/science/article/abs/pii/S0920996416302900.

2. Michael Wainberg et al., "Cannabis, Schizophrenia Genetic Risk, and Psychotic Experiences: A Cross-Sectional Study of 109,308 Participants from the UK Biobank," *Translational Psychiatry* 11 (2021), https://www.nature.com /articles/s41398-021-01330-w.

3. Staci Gruber et al., "Prioritizing Mental Health in an Emerging Market: A Framework for Maintaining Public Health and Expanding Knowledge on Cannabis and Mental Health," Coalition for Cannabis Policy, Education, and Regulation, 2021, https://www.cpear.org/wp-content/uploads/2021/12 /CPEAR_Mental-Health_White-Paper_R5.pdf.

4. Marta Di Forti et al., "The Contribution of Cannabis Use to Variation in the Incidence of Psychotic Disorder across Europe (EU-GEI): A Multicenter Case-Control Study," *Lancet Psychiatry* 6, no. 5 (May 2019), https://pubmed.ncbi.nlm.nih.gov/30902669.

5. Christina Canon, "Psychosis, Addiction, Chronic Vomiting: As Weed Becomes More Potent, Teens Are Getting Sick," *New York Times*, June 23, 2022, https://www.nytimes.com/2022/06/23/well/mind/teens-thc-cannabis.html.

6. Di Forti et al., "The Contribution of Cannabis Use."

7. Ibid.

8. Iris E. Sommer et al., "High-Potency Cannabis and Incident Psychosis: Correcting the Causal Assumption," *Lancet Psychiatry* 6, no. 6 (June 2019), https://www.thelancet.com/journals/lanpsy/article/PIIS2215-0366(19)30130-0/fulltext.

9. Ibid.

10. Lester Black, "More and More Americans Are Smoking Pot. What Does That Mean for Their Health?," FiveThirtyEight, November 30, 2021, https://fivethirtyeight.com/features/more-and-more-americans-are-smoking-pot-what-does-that-mean-for-their-health.

11. Benjamin Murrie et al., "Transition of Substance-Induced, Brief, and Atypical Psychoses to Schizophrenia: A Systematic Review and Meta-analysis," *Schizophrenia Bulletin* 46, no. 3 (May 2020), https://academic.oup.com/schizophreniabulletin/article/46/3/505/5588638.

12. Kenneth S. Kendler et al., "Prediction of Onset of Substance-Induced Psychotic Disorder and Its Progression to Schizophrenia in a Swedish National Sample," *American Journal of Psychiatry* 176, no. 9 (September 2019), https://pubmed.ncbi.nlm.nih.gov/31055966.

13. Ibid.

14. Ibid.

15. R. A. Power et al., "Genetic Predisposition to Schizophrenia Associated with Increased Use of Cannabis," *Molecular Psychiatry* 19, no. 11 (November 2014), https://pubmed.ncbi.nlm.nih.gov/24957864.

16. Jonathan D. Schaefer et al., "Adolescent Cannabis Use and Adult Psychoticism: A Longitudinal Co-twin Control Analysis Using Data from Two Cohorts," *Journal of Abnormal Psychology* 130, no. 7 (October 2021), https://pubmed.ncbi.nlm.nih.gov/34553951.

17. L. Cinnamon Bidwell, "Association of Naturalistic Administration of Cannabis Flower and Concentrates with Intoxication and Impairment," *JAMA Psychiatry* 77, no. 8 (2020), https://jamanetwork.com/journals/jamapsychiatry/fullarticle/2767219.

## Chapter Nine

1. American Society of Addiction Medicine, "Public Policy Statement on Cannabis," October 2020, https://www.asam.org/advocacy/public-policy-stat ements/details/public-policy-statements/2020/10/10/cannabis.

2. German Lopez, "A Study Finding a Huge Increase in Alcoholism May Have Been Seriously Flawed," *Vox*, August 16, 2017, https://www.vox.com /science-and-health/2017/8/16/16150548/alcoholism-study.

3. American Psychiatric Association, *Diagnostic and Statistical Manual of Mental Disorders*, 5th ed. (Washington, DC: American Psychiatric Publishing, 2013).

4. Ibid.

5. Kyle Jaeger, "Top Federal Drug Official Says There's 'No Evidence' That Occasional Marijuana Use Is Harmful for Adults," *Marijuana Moment*, November 30, 2021, https://www.marijuanamoment.net/top-federal-drug-official-says -theres-no-evidence-that-occasional-marijuana-use-is-harmful-for-adults.

6. Maia Szalavitz, "Drug Dependence Is Not Addiction—and It Matters," *Annals of Medicine* 53, no. 1 (December 2021), https://pubmed.ncbi.nlm.nih .gov/34751058.

7. Anahad O'Connor, "Teenage Brains May Be Especially Vulnerable to Marijuana and Other Drugs," *New York Times*, June 1, 2021, https://www.ny times.com/2021/03/29/well/family/teenage-brain-marijuana.html.

8. Darshi Desai, "Increasing Trend of Cannabis Use Disorder among Young Patients Admitted Due to Myocardial Infarction," *Circulation* 144 (November 2021), https://www.ahajournals.org/doi/10.1161/circ.144.suppl_1.13627.

9. Ibid.

10. Megan Marples, "Young Adult Cannabis Consumers Nearly Twice as Likely to Suffer from a Heart Attack, Research Shows," CNN, September 8, 2021, https://www.cnn.com/2021/09/07/health/cannabis-heart-attack-young -adult-study-wellness.

11. Kelly Sagar et al., "Assessing Cannabis Use Disorder in Medical Cannabis Patients," *Cannabis* 4, no. 2 (2021), https://publications.sciences.ucf.edu/canna bis/index.php/Cannabis/article/view/91.

12. Ibid.

13. Ibid.

14. Ibid.

15. Deborah S. Hasin, "DSM-5 Criteria for Substance Use Disorders: Recommendations and Rationale," *American Journal of Psychiatry* 170, no. 8 (August 2013), https://www.ncbi.nlm.nih.gov/pmc/articles/PMC3767415.

16. Deborah S. Hasin et al., "Prevalence of Marijuana Use Disorders in the United States between 2001–2002 and 2012–2013," *JAMA Psychiatry* 72, no. 12 (December 2015), https://jamanetwork.com/journals/jamapsychiatry/full article/2464591.

17. Shaul Lev-Ran et al., "Gender Differences in Health-Related Quality of Life among Cannabis Users: Results from the National Epidemiologic Survey on Alcohol and Related Conditions," *Drug and Alcohol Dependence* 123, nos. 1–3 (June 2012), https://pubmed.ncbi.nlm.nih.gov/22143039.

18. Jodi M. Gilman et al., "Effect of Medical Marijuana Card Ownership on Pain, Insomnia, and Affective Disorder Symptoms in Adults: A Randomized Clinical Trial," *JAMA Network Open* 5, no. 3 (March 2022), https://pubmed .ncbi.nlm.nih.gov/35302633.

19. Janet E. Joy et al., *Marijuana and Medicine: Assessing the Science Base* (Washington, DC: National Academy Press).

20. Alan J. Budney et al., "An Update on Cannabis Use Disorder with Comment on the Impact of Policy Related to Therapeutic and Recreational Cannabis Use," *European Archives of Psychiatry and Clinical Neuroscience* 269, no. 1 (February 2019), https://pubmed.ncbi.nlm.nih.gov/30604051.

21. Ibid.

22. Christina A. Brezing, "The Current State of Pharmacological Treatments for Cannabis Use Disorder and Withdrawal," *Neuropsychoparmacology* 43, no. 1 (January 2018), https://pubmed.ncbi.nlm.nih.gov/28875989.

23. Daniel Finegold et al., "Probability and Correlates of Transition from Cannabis Use to DSM-5 Cannabis Use Disorder: Results from a Large-Scale Nationally Representative Study," *Drug and Alcohol Review* 39, no. 2 (February 2020), https://pubmed.ncbi.nlm.nih.gov/31916333.

24. Hasin et al., "Prevalence of Marijuana Use Disorders."

25. Sarah Wakeman, "Why Taking Drugs to Treat Addiction Doesn't Mean You're Still Addicted," *STAT*, May 18, 2017, https://www.statnews .com/2017/05/18/opioids-medication-assisted-therapy.

26. "ASAM Recommendations re: Cannabis," ASAM Board of Directors, October 10, 2020, https://nyscouncil.org/asam-recommendations-re-cannabis.

27. K. K. Aggarwal, "Previous Substance Use Disorder Is a Risk Factor for Future Development of Substance Use Disorder," MediNexus, October 12, 2018, https://www.emedinexus.com/post/7877.

28. Carlos Blanco et al., "Testing the Drug Substitution Switching-Addictions Hypothesis: A Prospective Study in a Nationally Representative Sample," *JAMA Psychiatry* 71, no. 11 (November 2014), https://pubmed.ncbi.nlm.nih.gov /25208305.

29. Mark A. Ware et al., "A Prospective Observational Study of Problematic Oral Cannabinoid Use," *Psychopharmacology* 235, no. 2 (December 2017), https://pubmed.ncbi.nlm.nih.gov/29250737.

30. Amna Zehra et al., "Cannabis Addiction and the Brain: A Review," *Journal of Neuroimmune Pharmacology* 13, no. 4 (2018), https://www.ncbi.nlm.nih.gov/pmc/articles/PMC6223748.

31. M. Price, "Marijuana Addiction a Growing Risk as Society Grows More Intolerant," *Monitor on Psychology* 42, no. 5 (May 2011), https://www.apa.org/monitor/2011/05/marijuana.

## Chapter Ten

1. Q. L. Brown et al., "Trends in Marijuana Use among Pregnant and Non-pregnant Reproductive-Aged Women, 2002–2014," *Journal of the American Medical Association* 317, no. 2 (2017), https://pubmed.ncbi.nlm.nih.gov/27992619.

2. Noah Daly, "Alabama Senate Committee Approves Bill to Force Women Who Want Medical Marijuana to Show Negative Pregnancy Tests," *Marijuana Moment*, March 31, 2022, https://www.marijuanamoment.net/alabama-senate-committee-approves-bill-to-force-women-who-want-medical-marijuana-to-show-negative-pregnancy-tests.

3. Melanie Dreher, "Nursing Is the Practice of Anthropology," *Beyond THC*, 2018, https://beyondthc.com/wp-content/uploads/2016/02/Dreher-Jamaica.pdf.

4. Ibid.

5. Daniel J. Corsi, "Association between Self-Reported Prenatal Cannabis Use and Maternal, Perinatal, and Neonatal Outcomes," *Journal of the American Medical Association* 322, no. 2 (June 2019), https://jamanetwork.com/journals/jama/fullarticle/2736583.

6. Ibid.

7. Ibid.

8. Michael Silverstein et al., "Cannabis Use in Pregnancy: A Tale of Two Concerns," *Journal of the American Medical Association* 322, no. 2 (June 2019), https://jamanetwork.com/journals/jama/article-abstract/2736581.

9. National Academies of Sciences, Engineering, and Medicine (NASEM), *The Health Effects of Cannabis and Cannabinoids: The Current State of Evidence and Recommendations for Research* (Washington, DC: National Academies Press, 2017), https://nap.nationalacademies.org/catalog/24625/the-health-effects-of-cannabis-and-cannabinoids-the-current-state.

10. Shayna N. Conner et al., "Maternal Marijuana Use and Adverse Neonatal Outcomes: A Systematic Review and Meta-analysis," *Obstetrics and Gynecology* 128, no. 4 (October 2016), https://pubmed.ncbi.nlm.nih.gov/27607879.

11. NASEM, *The Health Effects of Cannabis and Cannabinoids.*

12. Hanan El Marroun et al., "Preconception and Prenatal Cannabis Use and the Risk of Behavioural and Emotional Problems in the Offspring; a Multi-informant Prospective Longitudinal Study," *International Journal of Epidemiology* 48, no. 1 (February 2019), https://pubmed.ncbi.nlm.nih.gov/30239742.

13. Ibid.

14. Ibid.

15. Sarah E. Paul et al., "Associations between Prenatal Cannabis Exposure and Childhood Outcomes," *JAMA Psychiatry* 78, no. 1 (September 2020), https://pubmed.ncbi.nlm.nih.gov/32965490.

16. Alice Callahan, "To Justify Using Weed, Some Pregnant Women Cling to an Old and Dubious Study," *Scientific American*, September 2, 2019, https://www.scientificamerican.com/article/to-justify-using-weed-some-pregnant-women-cling-to-an-old-and-dubious-study.

17. Ciara A. Torres et al., "Totality of the Evidence Suggests Prenatal Cannabis Exposure Does Not Lead to Cognitive Impairments: A Systematic and Critical Review," *Frontiers in Psychology*, May 8, 2020, https://www.frontiersin.org/articles/10.3389/fpsyg.2020.00816/full.

18. Ibid.

19. Ibid.

20. Ibid.

21. Kathleen H. Chaput et al., "Commentary: Totality of the Evidence Suggests Prenatal Cannabis Exposure Does Not Lead to Cognitive Impairments: A Systematic and Critical Review," *Frontiers in Psychology*, August 21, 2020, https://www.frontiersin.org/articles/10.3389/fpsyg.2020.01891/full.

22. Ann Z. Bauer et al., "Paracetamol Use during Pregnancy: A Call for Precautionary Action," *Nature Reviews Endocrinology* 17, no. 12 (September 2021), https://pubmed.ncbi.nlm.nih.gov/34556849.

23. Daly, "Alabama Senate Committee Approves Bill."

24. Sheryl A. Ryan et al., "Marijuana Use during Pregnancy and Breastfeeding: Implications for Neonatal and Childhood Outcomes," *Pediatrics* 142, no. 3 (September 2018), https://pubmed.ncbi.nlm.nih.gov/30150209.

25. Ibid.

26. Katie Woodruff et al., "Pregnant People's Experiences Discussing Their Cannabis Use with Prenatal Care Providers in a State with Legalized Cannabis," *Drug and Alcohol Dependence* 227 (October 2021), https://www.sciencedirect.com/science/article/pii/S0376871621004932.

27. Ibid.

28. Cynthia L. Holland et al., "Obstetric Health Care Providers' Counseling Responses to Pregnant Patient Disclosures of Marijuana Use," *Obstetrics and Gynecology* 127, no. 4 (April 2016), https://www.ncbi.nlm.nih.gov/pmc/articles /PMC4805441.

## Chapter Eleven

1. Thomas D. Marcotte et al., "Driving Performance and Cannabis Users' Perception of Safety," *JAMA Psychiatry* 79, no. 3 (January 2022), https://jama network.com/journals/jamapsychiatry/fullarticle/2788264.

2. Tim J. Gelmi et al., "Impact of Smoking Cannabidiol (CBD)-Rich Marijuana on Driving Ability," *Forensic Sciences Research* 6, no. 3 (May 2021), https:// www.tandfonline.com/doi/full/10.1080/20961790.2021.1946924.

3. Ole Rogeberg et al., "The Effects of Cannabis Intoxication on Motor Vehicle Collision Revisited and Revised," *Addiction* 111, no. 8 (2016), https:// pubmed.ncbi.nlm.nih.gov/26878835.

4. Jean-Louis Martin et al., "Cannabis, Alcohol and Fatal Road Accidents," *PLOS One* 12, no. 11 (2017), https://www.ncbi.nlm.nih.gov/pmc/articles /PMC5678710.

5. Danielle McCartney et al., "Determining the Magnitude and Duration of Active $\Delta^9$-Tetrahydrocannabinol ($\Delta^9$-THC)-Induced Driving and Cognitive Impairment: A Systematic and Meta-analytic Review," *Neuroscience Biobehavioral Reviews* 126 (July 2021), https://pubmed.ncbi.nlm.nih.gov/33497784.

6. Michael A. White et al., "The Risk of Being Culpable for or Involved in a Road Crash after Using Cannabis: A Systematic Review and Meta-analyses," *Drug Science, Policy and Law*, December 2021, https://journals.sagepub.com/doi /full/10.1177/20503245211055381.

7. Mark Asbridge et al., "Acute Cannabis Consumption and Motor Vehicle Collision Risk: Systematic Review of Observational Studies and Meta-analysis," *BMJ Clinical Research*, February 2012, https://www.bmj.com/content/344/bmj .e536.

8. Ibid.

9. J. H. Lacey et al., "Drug and Alcohol Crash Risk: A Case-Control Study," National Highway Traffic Safety Administration, 2016, https://www.nhtsa.gov /document/drug-and-alcohol-crash-risk-case-control-study.

10. Russell C. Callaghan et al., "Canada's Cannabis Legalization and Drivers' Traffic-Injury Presentations to Emergency Departments in Ontario and Alberta,

2015–2019," *Drug and Alcohol Dependence* 228 (November 2021), https://www
.sciencedirect.com/science/article/abs/pii/S0376871621005032.

11. Daniel Perkins et al., "Medicinal Cannabis and Driving: The Intersection of Health and Road Safety Policy," *International Journal of Drug Policy* 97 (November 2021), https://www.sciencedirect.com/science/article/pii/S09553 95921002127.

12. Ibid.

13. Ibid.

14. Cameron Ellis, "Medical Cannabis and Automobile Accidents: Evidence from Auto Insurance," *Health Economics*, June 12, 2022, https://onlinelibrary .wiley.com/doi/10.1002/hec.4553.

15. Thomas R. Arkell et al., "The Failings of *Per Se* Limits to Detect Cannabis-Induced Driving Impairment: Results from a Simulated Driving Study," *Traffic Injury Prevention* 22, no. 2 (February 2021), https://pubmed.ncbi.nlm .nih.gov/33544004.

16. Jodi M. Gilman et al., "Identification of Δ9-Tetrahydrocannabinol (THC) Impairment Using Functional Brain Imaging," *Neuropsychopharmacology* 47 (January 2022), https://www.nature.com/articles/s41386-021-01259-0.

17. Ibid.

## Chapter Twelve

1. Josiane Bourque et al., "Cannabis and Cognitive Functioning: From Acute to Residual Effects, from Randomized Controlled Trials to Prospective Designs," *Frontiers in Psychiatry*, June 10, 2021, https://www.frontiersin.org /articles/10.3389/fpsyt.2021.596601/full.

2. National Academies of Sciences, Engineering, and Medicine, *The Health Effects of Cannabis and Cannabinoids: The Current State of Evidence and Recommendations for Research* (Washington, DC: National Academies Press, 2017), https://nap.nationalacademies.org/catalog/24625/the-health-effects-of-canna bis-and-cannabinoids-the-current-state.

3. Helen Shen, "Cannabis and the Adolescent Brain," *Proceedings of the National Academy of Sciences* 117, no. 1 (January 7, 2020), https://www.pnas.org/doi /10.1073/pnas.1920325116.

4. Laura Dellazizzo et al., "Residual Neurocognitive Effects of Cannabis Use in Adolescents and Adults: A Systematic Meta-review of Meta-analyses," *Addiction* 117, no. 1 (July 2022), https://pubmed.ncbi.nlm.nih.gov/35048456.

5. Ibid.

6. Ibid.

7. Bourque et al., "Cannabis and Cognitive Functioning."

8. Ibid.

9. J. Cobb Scott et al., "Cannabis Use in Youth Is Associated with Limited Alterations in Brain Structure," *Neuropsychopharmacology* 44, no. 8 (July 2019), https://pubmed.ncbi.nlm.nih.gov/30780151.

10. Ibid.

11. Carl L. Hart, "Exaggerating Harmful Drug Effects on the Brain Is Killing Black People," *Neuron* 107, no. 2 (July 2020), https://www.cell.com/neuron/pdf /S0896-6273(20)30473-6.pdf.

12. Carl Hart, *Drug Use for Grown-Ups* (New York: Penguin, 2021).

13. Hart, "Exaggerating Harmful Drug Effects."

14. L. Koenders et al., "Longitudinal Study of Hippocampal Volumes in Heavy Cannabis Users," *Journal of Psychopharmacology* 31, no. 8 (August 2017), https://pubmed.ncbi.nlm.nih.gov/28741422.

15. Barbara J. Weiland et al., "Daily Marijuana Use Is Not Associated with Brain Morphometric Measures in Adolescents or Adults," *Journal of Neuroscience* 35, no. 4 (January 2015), https://www.ncbi.nlm.nih.gov/pmc/articles /PMC4308597.

16. Ibid.

17. Ibid.

18. Ibid.

19. Rachel E. Thayer et al., "Preliminary Results from a Pilot Study Examining Brain Structure in Older Adult Cannabis Users and Nonusers," *Psychiatry Research, Neuroimaging* 285 (March 2019), https://pubmed.ncbi.nlm.nih.gov/30785022.

20. Staci A. Gruber et al., "The Grass Might Be Greener: Medical Marijuana Patients Exhibit Altered Brain Activity and Improved Executive Function after 3 Months of Treatment," *Frontiers of Pharmacology* 8 (January 2018), https:// pubmed.ncbi.nlm.nih.gov/29387010.

21. Ibid.

22. Kelly A. Sagar et al., "An Observational, Longitudinal Study of Cognition in Medical Cannabis Patients over the Course of 12 Months of Treatment: Preliminary Results," *Journal of the International Neuropsychological Society* 27, no. 6 (July 2021), https://pubmed.ncbi.nlm.nih.gov/34261553.

## Chapter Thirteen

1. Helen Shen, "Cannabis and the Adolescent Brain," *Proceedings of the National Academy of Sciences* 117, no. 1 (January 2020), https://www.pnas.org /doi/10.1073/pnas.1920325116.

2. National Academies of Sciences, Engineering, and Medicine, *The Health Effects of Cannabis and Cannabinoids: The Current State of Evidence and Recommendations for Research* (Washington, DC: National Academies Press, 2017), https://nap.nationalacademies.org/catalog/24625/the-health-effects-of-cannabis-and-cannabinoids-the-current-state.

3. Lena Kristin Wendel, "Residual Effects of Cannabis-Use on Neuropsychological Functioning," *Cognitive Development* 59 (July–September 2021), https://doi.org/10.1016/j.cogdev.2021.101072.

4. Ibid.

5. Ibid.

6. J. Cobb Scott, "Association of Cannabis with Cognitive Functioning in Adolescents and Young Adults: A Systematic Review and Meta-analysis," *JAMA Psychiatry* 75, no. 6 (June 2018), https://pubmed.ncbi.nlm.nih.gov/29710074.

7. Randi Melissa Schuster et al., "One Month of Cannabis Abstinence in Adolescents and Young Adults Is Associated with Improved Memory," *Journal of Clinical Psychiatry* 79, no. 6 (October 2018), https://www.ncbi.nlm.nih.gov/pmc/articles/PMC6587572.

8. Ibid.

9. Shen, "Cannabis and the Adolescent Brain."

10. Ashley A. Knapp et al., "Psychometric Assessment of the Marijuana Adolescent Problem Inventory," *Addictive Behaviors* 79 (April 2018), https://www.sciencedirect.com/science/article/abs/pii/S0306460317304665.

11. Madeline H. Meier et al., "Persistent Cannabis Users Show Neuropsychological Decline from Childhood to Midlife," *Proceedings of the National Academy of Sciences* 109, no. 40 (July 2012), https://www.pnas.org/doi/10.1073/pnas.1206820109.

12. Ibid.

13. Ole Rogeberg, "Correlations between Cannabis Use and IQ Change in the Dunedin Cohort Are Consistent with Confounding from Socioeconomic Status," *Proceedings of the National Academy of Sciences* 110, no. 11 (March 2013), https://pubmed.ncbi.nlm.nih.gov/23319626.

14. Madeline H. Meier et al., "Associations between Adolescent Cannabis Use and Neuropsychological Decline: A Longitudinal Co-twin Control Study," *Addiction* 113, no. 2 (February 2018), https://pubmed.ncbi.nlm.nih.gov/28734078.

15. Amna Zehra et al., "Cannabis Addiction and the Brain: A Review," *Journal of Neuroimmune Pharmacology* 13, no. 4 (March 2018), https://www.ncbi.nlm.nih.gov/pmc/articles/PMC6223748.

16. Ibid.

17. C. Mokrysz et al., "Are IQ and Educational Outcomes in Teenagers Related to Their Cannabis Use? A Prospective Cohort Study," *Journal of Psy-*

*chopharmacology* 30, no. 2 (February 2016), https://www.ncbi.nlm.nih.gov/pmc /articles/PMC4724860.

18. Jonathan D. Schaefer et al., "Associations between Adolescent Cannabis Use and Young-Adult Functioning in Three Longitudinal Twin Studies," *Proceedings of the National Academy of Sciences* 118, no. 14 (April 2021), https:// pubmed.ncbi.nlm.nih.gov/33782115.

19. Madeline H. Meier, "Cannabis Use and Psychosocial Functioning: Evidence from Prospective Longitudinal Studies," *Current Opinion Psychology* 38 (April 2021), https://pubmed.ncbi.nlm.nih.gov/32736227.

20. Carl Hart, *Drug Use for Grown-Ups* (New York: Penguin, 2021).

21. Madeline Meier, "Long-Term Cannabis Use and Cognitive Reserves and Hippocampal Volumes in Midlife," *American Journal of Psychiatry* 179, no. 5 (March 8, 2022), https://ajp.psychiatryonline.org/doi/full/10.1176/appi .ajp.2021.21060664.

22. Ryan Grim, "A White House Drug Deal Gone Bad," *Slate*, September 7, 2006, https://slate.com/technology/2006/09/a-white-house-drug-deal-gone -bad.html.

23. Ibid.

## Chapter Fourteen

1. Kevin F. Boehnke et al., "Qualifying Conditions of Medical Cannabis License Holders in the United States," *Health Affairs* 38, no. 2 (February 2019), https://www.healthaffairs.org/doi/full/10.1377/hlthaff.2018.05266.

2. S. C. Smith, "Clinical Endocannabinoid Deficiency (CECD) Revisited: Can This Concept Explain the Therapeutic Benefits of Cannabis in Migraine, Fibromyalgia, Irritable Bowel Syndrome and Treatment-Resistant Conditions?," *Neuroendocrinology Letters* 35, no. 3 (January 1, 2014), https://europepmc.org /article/med/24977967.

## Chapter Fifteen

1. Amanda Reiman et al., "Cannabis as a Substitute for Opioid-Based Pain Medication: Patient Self-Report," *Cannabis and Cannabinoid Research* 2, no. 1 (June 2017), https://www.ncbi.nlm.nih.gov/pmc/articles/PMC5569620.

2. Kevin F. Boehnke et al., "Pills to Pot: Observational Analyses of Cannabis Substitution among Medical Cannabis Users with Chronic Pain," *Journal of Pain* 20, no. 7 (July 2019), https://pubmed.ncbi.nlm.nih.gov/30690169.

3. Ziva D. Cooper et al., "Impact of Co-administration of Oxycodone and Smoked Cannabis on Analgesia and Abuse Liability," *Neuropsychopharmacology*

43, no. 10 (September 2018), https://www.ncbi.nlm.nih.gov/pmc/articles /PMC6098090.

4. Suzanne Nielsen et al., "Opioid-Sparing Effect of Cannabinoids: A Systematic Review and Meta-Analysis," *Neuropsychopharmacology* 42, no. 9 (August 2017), https://pubmed.ncbi.nlm.nih.gov/28327548.

5. Caroline A. MacCallum et al., "Practical Strategies Using Medical Cannabis to Reduce Harms Associated with Long Term Opioid Use in Chronic Pain," *Frontiers of Pharmacology* 12 (April 2021), https://www.frontiersin.org /articles/10.3389/fphar.2021.633168/full.

6. Ed Mahon, "Turned Away," *Spotlight PA*, June 28, 2021, https://www .spotlightpa.org/news/2021/06/pa-medical-marijuana-insurance-drug-treat ment-confusion.

7. Stephanie Lake and Michelle St. Pierre, "The Relationship between Cannabis Use and Patient Outcomes in Medication-Based Treatment of Opioid Use Disorder: A Systematic Review," *Clinical Psychology Review* 82 (December 2020), https://pubmed.ncbi.nlm.nih.gov/33130527.

8. Stephanie Lake et al., "Frequency of Cannabis and Illicit Opioid Use among People Who Use Drugs and Report Chronic Pain: A Longitudinal Analysis," *PLOS Medicine*, November 2019, https://journals.plos.org/plosmedicine /article?id=10.1371/journal.pmed.1002967.

9. "Patients and Caregivers," PA.gov, https://www.health.pa.gov/topics/pro grams/Medical%20Marijuana/Pages/Patients.aspx.

10. Chelsea Shover, "Association of State Policies Allowing Medical Cannabis for Opioid Use Disorder with Dispensary Marketing for This Indication," *JAMA Network Open* 3, no. 7 (July 1, 2020), https://pubmed.ncbi.nlm.nih .gov/32662844.

## Chapter Sixteen

1. Jodi M. Gilman, "Effect of Medical Marijuana Card Ownership on Pain, Insomnia, and Affective Disorder Symptoms in Adults: A Randomized Clinical Trial," *JAMA Network Open* 5, no. 3 (March 2022), https://pubmed.ncbi.nlm .nih.gov/35302633.

2. Jennifer H. Walsh et al., "Treating Insomnia Symptoms with Medicinal Cannabis: A Randomized, Crossover Trial of the Efficacy of a Cannabinoid Medicine Compared with Placebo," *Sleep* 44, no. 11 (November 2021), https:// www.ncbi.nlm.nih.gov/pmc/articles/PMC8598183.

3. National Academies of Sciences, Engineering, and Medicine, *The Health Effects of Cannabis and Cannabinoids: The Current State of Evidence and Recom-*

*mendations for Research* (Washington, DC: National Academies Press, 2017), https://nap.nationalacademies.org/catalog/24625/the-health-effects-of-canna bis-and-cannabinoids-the-current-state.

4. Marcus Bachhuber et al., "Use of Cannabis to Relieve Pain and Promote Sleep by Customers at an Adult Use Dispensary," *Journal of Psychoactive Drugs* 51, no. 5 (November–December 2019), https://www.ncbi.nlm.nih.gov/pmc /articles/PMC6823130.

5. Jacob M. Vigil et al., "Effectiveness of Raw, Natural Medical Cannabis Flower for Treating Insomnia under Naturalistic Conditions," *Medicines* 5, no. 3 (July 2018), https://pubmed.ncbi.nlm.nih.gov/29997343.

6. Sharon R Sznitman et al., "Medical Cannabis and Insomnia in Older Adults with Chronic Pain: A Cross-Sectional Study," *BMJ Support Palliative Care* 10, no. 4 (December 2020), https://pubmed.ncbi.nlm.nih.gov/31959585.

7. Rita Kukafka, "The Use of Cannabinoids for Insomnia in Daily Life: Naturalistic Study," *Journal of Medical Internet Research* 23, no. 10 (October 2021), https://www.ncbi.nlm.nih.gov/pmc/articles/PMC8581757.

8. Carl Sagan in Lester Grinspoon's *Marihuana Reconsidered* (Cambridge, MA: Harvard University Press, 1971).

9. Thomas Megelin and Imad Ghorayeb, "Cannabis for Restless Legs Syndrome: A Report of Six Patients," *Sleep Medicine* 36 (August 2017), https:// pubmed.ncbi.nlm.nih.gov/28655453.

10. Imad Ghorayeb, "More Evidence of Cannabis Efficacy in Restless Legs Syndrome," *Sleep and Breathing* 24, no. 1 (March 2020), https://pubmed.ncbi .nlm.nih.gov/31820197.

11. Jaime M. Monti et al., "Clinical Management of Sleep and Sleep Disorders with Cannabis and Cannabinoids: Implications to Practicing Psychiatrists," *Clinical Neuropharmacology* 45, no. 2 (March–April 2022), https://pubmed.ncbi .nlm.nih.gov/35221321.

## Chapter Seventeen

1. Ilana M. Braun et al., "Medical Oncologists' Beliefs, Practices, and Knowledge Regarding Marijuana Used Therapeutically: A Nationally Representative Survey Study," *Journal of Clinical Oncology* 36, no. 19 (July 2018), https://pubmed .ncbi.nlm.nih.gov/29746226.

2. Timothy S. Sannes et al., "United States Oncologists' Clinical Preferences Regarding Modes of Medicinal Cannabis Use," *Cancer Communications* 41, no. 6 (June 2021), https://www.ncbi.nlm.nih.gov/pmc/articles/PMC8211351.

3. Ran Abuhasira et al., "Epidemiological Characteristics, Safety and Efficacy of Medical Cannabis in the Elderly," *European Journal of Internal Medicine* 49 (March 2018), https://pubmed.ncbi.nlm.nih.gov/29398248.

4. Lihi Bar-Lev Schleider et al., "Prospective Analysis of Safety and Efficacy of Medical Cannabis in Large Unselected Population of Patients with Cancer," *European Journal of Internal Medicine* 49 (March 2018), https://pubmed.ncbi.nlm.nih.gov/29482741.

5. Ibid.

6. Ibid.

7. Craig Marine, "The Good Doctor: He's Been in on the AIDS Battle since the Beginning, but It's the Feds Donald Abrams Fights When It Comes to Scoring Marijuana," *SFGate*, August 12, 2001, https://www.sfgate.com/health/article/THE-GOOD-DOCTOR-He-s-been-in-on-the-AIDS-battle-2891131.php.

8. Donald Abrams, "Short Term Effects of Cannabinoids in HIV Infection," *MAPS Medical Marijuana*, 2000, https://maps.org/research-archive/mmj/mjabrams.html.

9. Marine, "The Good Doctor."

10. Jenny G. Turcott et al., "The Effect of Nabilone on Appetite, Nutritional Status, and Quality of Life in Lung Cancer Patients: A Randomized, Double-Blind Clinical Trial," *Support Care Cancer* 26, no. 9 (September 2018), https://pubmed.ncbi.nlm.nih.gov/29550881.

11. Gil Bar-Sela et al., "The Effects of Dosage-Controlled Cannabis Capsules on Cancer-Related Cachexia and Anorexia Syndrome in Advanced Cancer Patients: Pilot Study," *Integrative Cancer Therapies* 18 (January–December 2019), https://pubmed.ncbi.nlm.nih.gov/31595793.

12. Tarek Taha et al., "Cannabis Impacts Tumor Response Rate to Nivolumab in Patients with Advanced Malignancies," *Oncologist* 24, no. 4 (April 2019), https://pubmed.ncbi.nlm.nih.gov/30670598.

13. Gil Bar-Sela et al., "Cannabis Consumption Used by Cancer Patients during Immunotherapy Correlates with Poor Clinical Outcome," *Cancers* 12, no. 9 (August 2018), https://pubmed.ncbi.nlm.nih.gov/32872248.

14. National Academies of Sciences, Engineering, and Medicine, *The Health Effects of Cannabis and Cannabinoids: The Current State of Evidence and Recommendations for Research* (Washington, DC: National Academies Press, 2017), https://nap.nationalacademies.org/catalog/24625/the-health-effects-of-cannabis-and-cannabinoids-the-current-state.

15. Sean D. McAllister et al., "Cannabinoid Cancer Biology and Prevention," *Journal of the National Cancer Institute Monographs*, November 2021, https://pubmed.ncbi.nlm.nih.gov/34850900.

16. Ibid.

17. Chris Twelves et al., "A Phase 1b Randomised, Placebo-Controlled Trial of Nabiximols Cannabinoid Oromucosal Spray with Temozolomide in Patients with Recurrent Glioblastoma," *British Journal of Cancer* 124 (February 2021), https://www.nature.com/articles/s41416-021-01259-3.

18. Thomas M. Clark, "Scoping Review and Meta-Analysis Suggests that *Cannabis* Use May Reduce Cancer Rick in the United States," *Cannabis Cannabinoid Research* 6, no. 5 (October 2021), https://pubmed.ncbi.nlm.nih.gov/33998861.

## Chapter Eighteen

1. Jill Simonian, "A Critical Narrative Review of Medical Cannabis in Pediatrics beyond Epilepsy, Part 1: Background," *Pediatric Medicine* 3 (August 2020), https://pm.amegroups.com/article/view/5632/html#B52.

2. American Academy of Child and Adolescent Psychiatry, "Use of Medical Marijuana in Children and Adolescents with Autism Spectrum Disorder for Core Autism Symptoms or Co-Occurring Emotional or Behavioral Problems," May 2019, https://www.aacap.org/aacap/Policy_Statements/2019/Use_of_Medical_Marijuana_in_Children_and_Adolescents_with_Autism_Spectrum_Disorder_for_Core_Autism_S.aspx.

3. Don Wei et al., "Endocannabinoid Signaling Mediates Oxytocin-Driven Social Reward," *Proceedings of the National Academy of Sciences* 112, no. 45 (2015), https://pubmed.ncbi.nlm.nih.gov/26504214.

4. Debra S. Karhson et al., "Plasma Anandamide Concentrations Are Lower in Children with Autism Spectrum Disorder," *National Library of Medicine* (2018), https://pubmed.ncbi.nlm.nih.gov/29564080/#:~:text=In%20keeping%20with%20this%20notion,concentrations%20in%20children%20with%20ASD.

5. Adi Aran et al., "Lower Circulating Endocannabinoid Levels in Children with Autism Spectrum Disorder," *Molecular Autism* 10 (January 2019), https://pubmed.ncbi.nlm.nih.gov/30728928.

6. Joshua J. Green and Eric Hollander, "Autism and Oxytocin: New Developments in Translational Approaches to Therapeutics," *Neurotherapeutics* 7, no. 3 (July 2010), https://pubmed.ncbi.nlm.nih.gov/20643377.

7. Estacio Amaro da Silva Junior et al., "Evaluation of the Efficacy and Safety of Cannabidiol-Rich Cannabis Extract in Children with Autism Spectrum Disorder: Randomized, Double-Blind and Controlled Placebo Clinical Trial," *Trends in Psychiatry and Psychotherapy* 44 (May 2022), https://pubmed.ncbi.nlm.nih.gov/35617670.

8. Serap Bilge and Baris Ekici, "CBD-Enriched Cannabis for Autism Spectrum Disorder: An Experience of a Single Center in Turkey and Reviews of the Literature," *Journal of Cannabis Research* 3, no. 1 (December 2021), https://pubmed.ncbi.nlm.nih.gov/34911567.

9. Ibid.

10. Paulo Fleury-Teixeira et al., "Effects of CBD-Enriched Cannabis Sativa Extract on Autism Spectrum Disorder Symptoms: An Observational Study of 18 Participants Undergoing Compassionate Use," *Frontiers of Neurology* 10 (October 2019), https://pubmed.ncbi.nlm.nih.gov/31736860.

11. Ibid.

12. Ibid.

13. Lihi Bar-Lev Schleider et al., "Real Life Experience of Medical Cannabis Treatment in Autism: Analysis of Safety and Efficacy," *Nature*, January 2019, https://www.nature.com/articles/s41598-018-37570-y.

14. Adi Aran et al., "Brief Report: Cannabidiol-Rich Cannabis in Children with Autism Spectrum Disorder and Severe Behavioral Problems: A Retrospective Feasibility Study," *Journal of Autism and Developmental Disorders* 49, no. 3 (March 2019), https://pubmed.ncbi.nlm.nih.gov/30382443.

15. Mojdeh Mostafavi and John Gaitanis, "Autism Spectrum Disorder and Medical Cannabis: Review and Clinical Experience," *Seminars in Pediatric Neurology* 35 (October 2020), https://pubmed.ncbi.nlm.nih.gov/32892960.

16. Dana Barchel et al., "Oral Cannabidiol Use in Children with Autism Spectrum Disorder to Treat Related Symptoms and Co-morbidities," *Frontiers of Pharmacology* 9 (January 2019), https://pubmed.ncbi.nlm.nih.gov/30687090.

17. V. Nezgovorova, "Potential of Cannabinoids as Treatments for Autism Spectrum Disorders," *Journal of Psychiatric Research* 137 (May 2021), https://www.sciencedirect.com/science/article/abs/pii/S0022395621001266.

## Chapter Nineteen

1. Gabriella Gobbi et al., "Association of Cannabis Use in Adolescence and Risk of Depression, Anxiety, and Suicidality in Young Adulthood: A Systematic Review and Meta-analysis," *JAMA Psychiatry* 76, no. 4 (2019), https://jamanetwork.com/journals/jamapsychiatry/fullarticle/2723657.

2. Ibid.

3. Ibid.

4. Kevin P. Hill et al., "Risks and Benefits of Cannabis and Cannabinoids in Psychiatry," *American Journal of Psychiatry* 179, no. 2 (December 2021), https://pubmed.ncbi.nlm.nih.gov/34875873.

5. Board of Trustees of the American Psychiatric Association, "Position Statement in Opposition to Cannabis as Medicine," American Psychiatric Association, July 2019, https://www.psychiatry.org/File%20Library/About-APA/Organization-Documents-Policies/Policies/Position-Cannabis-as-Medicine.pdf.

6. Hill et al., "Risks and Benefits."

7. Ibid.

8. Ibid.

9. Lester Grinspoon, "The Use of Cannabis as a Mood Stabilizer in Bipolar Disorder: Anecdotal Evidence and the Need for Clinical Research," *Journal of Psychoactive Drugs* 30, no. 2 (September 6, 2011), https://www.tandfonline.com/doi/abs/10.1080/02791072.1998.10399687.

10. Hill et al., "Risks and Benefits."

11. https://www.lexico.com/en/definition/sophistry.

12. Nahid M. Abed Faghri et al., "Understanding the Expanding Role of Primary Care Physicians (PCPs) to Primary Psychiatric Care Physicians (PPCPs): Enhancing the Assessment and Treatment of Psychiatric Conditions," *Mental Health Family Medicine* 7, no. 1 (March 2010), https://www.ncbi.nlm.nih.gov/pmc/articles/PMC2925161.

13. Staci Gruber et al., "Prioritizing Mental Health in an Emerging Market: A Framework for Maintaining Public Health and Expanding Knowledge on Cannabis and Mental Health," Coalition for Cannabis Policy, Education, and Regulation, 2021, https://www.cpear.org/wp-content/uploads/2021/12/CPEAR_Mental-Health_White-Paper_R5.pdf.

14. Ibid.

15. Carrie Cuttler et al., "A Naturalistic Examination of the Perceived Effects of Cannabis on Negative Affect," *Journal of Affective Disorders* 235 (August 2018), https://pubmed.ncbi.nlm.nih.gov/29656267.

16. Ibid.

17. Board of Trustees of the APA, "Position Statement."

18. C. Hindocha et al., "The Effectiveness of Cannabinoids in the Treatment of Posttraumatic Stress Disorder (PTSD): A Systematic Review," *Journal of Dual Diagnosis* 16, no. 1 (January–March 2020), https://pubmed.ncbi.nlm.nih.gov/31479625.

19. Marcel O. Bonn-Miller et al., "Using Cannabis to Help You Sleep: Heightened Frequency of Medical Cannabis Use among Those with PTSD," *Drug and Alcohol Dependence* 136 (March 2014), https://pubmed.ncbi.nlm.nih.gov/24412475.

20. Colin Cameron et al., "Use of a Synthetic Cannabinoid in a Correctional Population for Posttraumatic Stress Disorder–Related Insomnia and Nightmares, Chronic Pain, Harm Reduction, and Other Indications," *Journal of Clinical*

*Psychopharmacology* 34, no. 5 (October 2014), https://pubmed.ncbi.nlm.nih .gov/24987795.

21. George A. Fraser, "The Use of a Synthetic Cannabinoid in the Management of Treatment-Resistant Nightmares in Posttraumatic Stress Disorder (PTSD)," *CNS Neuroscience & Therapeutics* 15, no. 1 (Winter 2009), https:// pubmed.ncbi.nlm.nih.gov/19228182.

22. Yasir Rehman et al., "Cannabis in the Management of PTSD: A Systematic Review," *AIMS Neuroscience* 8, no. 3 (May 2021), https://pubmed.ncbi.nlm .nih.gov/34183989.

23. Ibid.

24. National Academies of Sciences, Engineering, and Medicine, *The Health Effects of Cannabis and Cannabinoids: The Current State of Evidence and Recommendations for Research* (Washington, DC: National Academies Press, 2017), https://nap.nationalacademies.org/catalog/24625/the-health-effects-of-canna bis-and-cannabinoids-the-current-state.

25. Ibid.

26. Mallory Je Loflin et al., "Cannabinoids as Therapeutic for PTSD," *Current Opinion in Psychology* 14 (April 2017), https://pubmed.ncbi.nlm.nih .gov/28813324.

27. Samuel T. Wilkinson et al., "Marijuana Use Is Associated with Worse Outcomes in Symptom Severity and Violent Behavior in Patients with Posttraumatic Stress Disorder," *Journal of Clinical Psychiatry* (September 2015), https:// www.ncbi.nlm.nih.gov/pmc/articles/PMC6258013.

28. Ibid.

29. Ibid.

30. Emily M. LaFrance et al., "Short and Long-Term Effects of Cannabis on Symptoms of Post-Traumatic Stress Disorder," *Journal of Affective Disorders* 274 (September 2020), https://pubmed.ncbi.nlm.nih.gov/32469819.

31. Stephanie Lake et al., "Does Cannabis Use Modify the Effect of Posttraumatic Stress Disorder on Severe Depression and Suicidal Ideation? Evidence from a Population-Based Cross-Sectional Study of Canadians," *Journal of Psychopharmacology* 34, no. 2 (February 2020), https://pubmed.ncbi.nlm.nih .gov/31684805.

32. Marcel O. Bonn-Miller et al., "The Long-Term, Prospective, Therapeutic Impact of Cannabis on Post-Traumatic Stress Disorder," *Cannabis Cannabinoid Research* 7, no. 2 (April 2022), https://pubmed.ncbi.nlm.nih.gov/33998874.

33. Hill et al., "Risks and Benefits."

34. Bonn-Miller et al., "The Long-Term, Prospective, Therapeutic Impact."

35. Holly Mansell et al., "Cannabis for the Treatment of Attention Deficit Hyperactivity Disorder: A Report of 3 Cases," *Medical Cannabis Cannabinoids* 5, no. 1 (January 2022), https://pubmed.ncbi.nlm.nih.gov/35224434.

36. Eva Maria Milz et al., "Successful Authorised Therapy of Treatment Resistant Adult ADHD with Cannabis: Experience from a Medical Practice with 30 Patients," *International Cannabinoid in Medicine & Research Conference*, September 2015, https://www.researchgate.net/publication/331629710_Suc cessful_authorised_therapy_of_treatment_resistant_adult_ADHD_with_Can nabis_experience_from_a_medical_practice_with_30_patients.

37. Mallory Loflin, "Subtypes of Attention Deficit-Hyperactivity Disorder and Cannabis Use," *Substance Use & Misuse* 49, no. 4 (2014), https://pubmed .ncbi.nlm.nih.gov/24093525.

38. Jeffrey Y. Hergenrather et al., "Cannabinoid and Terpenoid Doses Are Associated with Adult ADHD Status of Medical Cannabis Patients," *Rambam Maimonides Medical Journal* 11, no. 1 (January 2020), https://pubmed.ncbi.nlm.nih .gov/32017685.

39. Leanne Tamm et al., "Impact of ADHD and Cannabis Use on Executive Functioning in Young Adults," *Drug and Alcohol Dependence* 133, no. 2 (December 2013), https://pubmed.ncbi.nlm.nih.gov/23992650.

40. Ruth E. Cooper et al., "Cannabinoids in Attention-Deficit/Hyperactivity Disorder: A Randomised-Controlled Trial," *European Neuropsychopharmacology* 27, no. 8 (May 2017), https://pubmed.ncbi.nlm.nih.gov/28576350.

41. Amanda Stueber and Carrie Cuttler, "Self-Reported Effects of Cannabis on ADHD Symptoms, ADHD Medication Side Effects, and ADHD-Related Executive Dysfunction," *Journal of Attention Disorders* 26, no. 6 (April 2022), https://pubmed.ncbi.nlm.nih.gov/34632827.

42. Gruber et al., "Prioritizing Mental Health."

## Chapter Twenty

1. Anees Bahji et al., "Cannabinoids in the Management of Behavioral, Psychological, and Motor Symptoms of Neurocognitive Disorders: A Mixed Studies Systematic Review," *Journal of Cannabis Research* 4, no. 1 (March 2022), https:// pubmed.ncbi.nlm.nih.gov/35287749.

2. Emilio Perucca, "Critical Aspects Affecting Cannabidiol Oral Bioavailability and Metabolic Elimination, and Related Clinical Implications," *CNS Drugs* 34 (June 5, 2020), https://link.springer.com/article/10.1007/s40263-020-00741-5.

3. Lucile Rapin et al., "Cannabidiol Use and Effectiveness: Real-World Evidence from a Canadian Medical Cannabis Clinic," *Journal of Cannabis Research* 3,

no. 1 (June 2021), https://jcannabisresearch.biomedcentral.com/articles/10.1186/s42238-021-00078-w.

4. Shankar Tumati et al., "Medical Cannabis Use among Older Adults in Canada: Self-Reported Data on Types and Amount Used, and Perceived Effects," *Drugs and Aging* 39, no. 2 (February 2022), https://pubmed.ncbi.nlm.nih.gov/34940961.

5. Mateus M. Bergamaschi et al., "Cannabidiol Reduces the Anxiety Induced by Simulated Public Speaking in Treatment-Naïve Social Phobia Patients," *Neuropsychopharmacology* 36, no. 6 (May 2011), https://pubmed.ncbi.nlm.nih.gov/21307846.

6. Nobuo Masataka, "Anxiolytic Effects of Repeated Cannabidiol Treatment in Teenagers with Social Anxiety Disorders," *Frontiers in Psychology*, November 8, 2019, https://www.frontiersin.org/articles/10.3389/fpsyg.2019.02466/full.

7. Graham Gulbransen et al., "Cannabidiol Prescription in Clinical Practice: An Audit on the First 400 Patients in New Zealand," *BJGP Open* 4, no. 1 (May 2020), https://pubmed.ncbi.nlm.nih.gov/32019776.

8. M. J. De Vita et al., "The Effects of Cannabidiol and Analgesic Expectancies on Experimental Pain Reactivity in Healthy Adults: A Balanced Placebo Design Trial," *Experimental and Clinical Psychopharmacology*, April 22, 2021, https://pubmed.ncbi.nlm.nih.gov/34251840.

9. Scott Shannon et al., "Cannabidiol in Anxiety and Sleep: A Large Case Series," *Permanente Journal* 23 (2019), https://www.ncbi.nlm.nih.gov/pmc/articles/PMC6326553.

10. Yasmin L. Hurd et al., "Cannabidiol for the Reduction of Cue-Induced Craving and Anxiety in Drug-Abstinent Individuals with Heroin Use Disorder: A Double-Blind Randomized Placebo-Controlled Trial," *American Journal of Psychiatry* 176, no. 11 (May 2019), https://ajp.psychiatryonline.org/doi/10.1176/appi.ajp.2019.18101191.

11. Ibid.

12. Christopher Kudrich et al., "Adjunctive Management of Opioid Withdrawal with the Nonopioid Medication Cannabidiol," *Cannabis Cannabinoid Research*, October 22, 2021, https://pubmed.ncbi.nlm.nih.gov/34678050.

13. Chandni Hindocha et al., "Cannabidiol Reverses Attentional Bias to Cigarette Cues in a Human Experimental Model of Tobacco Withdrawal," *Addiction* 113, no. 9 (May 2018), https://pubmed.ncbi.nlm.nih.gov/29714034.

14. Celia J. A. Morgan et al., "Cannabidiol Reduces Cigarette Consumption in Tobacco Smokers: Preliminary Findings," *Addictive Behaviors* 38, no. 9 (September 2013), https://pubmed.ncbi.nlm.nih.gov/23685330.

15. Tom P. Freeman et al., "Cannabidiol for the Treatment of Cannabis Use Disorder: Phase IIa Double-Blind Placebo-Controlled Randomised Adap-

tive Bayesian Dose-Finding Trial," *Lancet Psychiatry* 7, no. 10 (October 2020), https://www.ncbi.nlm.nih.gov/pmc/articles/PMC7116091.

16. Celia J. A. Morgan et al., "Impact of Cannabidiol on the Acute Memory and Psychotomimetic Effects of Smoked Cannabis: Naturalistic Study," *British Journal of Psychiatry* 197, no. 4 (January 2018), https://www.cambridge.org/core journals/the-british-journal-of-psychiatry/article/impact-of-cannabidiol-on-the -acute-memory-and-psychotomimetic-effects-of-smoked-cannabis-naturalistic -study/54EB46D7698008BA4A9E5A27A57AA281.

17. Laurel P. Gibson et al., "Effects of Cannabidiol in Cannabis Flower: Implications for Harm Reduction," *Addiction Biology* 27, no. 1 (January 2022), https://pubmed.ncbi.nlm.nih.gov/34467598.

18. Alberto Sainz-Cort et al., "Opposite Roles for Cannabidiol and δ-9-Tetrahydrocannabinol in Psychotomimetic Effects of Cannabis Extracts: A Naturalistic Controlled Study," *Journal of Clinical Psychopharmacology* 41, no. 5 (September–October 2021), https://pubmed.ncbi.nlm.nih.gov/34412109.

19. Elizabeth Robinson et al., "Knowledge, Attitudes, and Perceptions of Cannabinoids in the Dermatology Community," *Journal of Drugs in Dermatology* 17, no. 12 (December 2018), https://pubmed.ncbi.nlm.nih.gov/30586258.

## Chapter Twenty-One

1. Kyle Jaeger, "Top Federal Drug Official Says There's 'No Evidence' That Occasional Marijuana Use Is Harmful for Adults," *Marijuana Moment*, November 30, 2021, https://www.marijuanamoment.net/top-federal-drug-official-says -theres-no-evidence-that-occasional-marijuana-use-is-harmful-for-adults.

2. Cathleen O'Grady, "Cannabis Research Data Reveals a Focus on Harms of the Drug," *Science* 369, no. 6508 (September 2020), https://www.science.org /doi/10.1126/science.369.6508.1155.

3. Pauline Anderson, "Most Addiction Specialists Support Legalized Therapeutic Psychedelics," *Medscape*, December 16, 2021, https://www.medscape .com/viewarticle/964987.

4. "From the Desk of Rick Doblin, Ph.D.," *MAPS Bulletin* 31, no. 3 (2021), https://maps.org/news/bulletin/from-the-desk-of-rick-doblin-ph-d-3.

5. Kevin Boehnke, "Medical Cannabis Use Is Associated with Decreased Opiate Medication Use in a Retrospective Cross-Sectional Survey of Patients with Chronic Pain," *Journal of Pain* 17, no. 6 (March 19, 2016), https://pubmed.ncbi .nlm.nih.gov/27001005.

6. Marcus Bachhuber et al., "Use of Cannabis to Relieve Pain and Promote Sleep by Customers at an Adult Use Dispensary," *Journal of Psychoactive Drugs*

51, no. 5 (November–December 2019), https://www.ncbi.nlm.nih.gov/pmc/articles/PMC6823130.

7. Charles T. Tart, "Marijuana Intoxication: Common Experiences," *Nature* 226 (1970), https://www.nature.com/articles/226701a0.

8. Ibid.

9. Lester Grinspoon, *Marihuana Reconsidered* (Cambridge, MA: Harvard University Press, 1977).

10. Ibid.

11. Ibid.

12. Ibid.

13. Carl Sagan, *Dragons of Eden: Speculations on the Evolution of Human Intelligence* (New York: Random House, 1977).

## Chapter Twenty-Two

1. Ilana M. Braun et al., "Cancer Patients' Experiences with Medicinal Cannabis-Related Care," *Cancer* 127, no. 1 (January 2020), https://pubmed.ncbi.nlm.nih.gov/32986266.

2. Ashley Bradford, "Medical Marijuana Laws Reduce Prescription Medication Use in Medicare Part D," *Health Affairs* 35, no. 7 (July 2016), https://www.healthaffairs.org/doi/10.1377/hlthaff.2015.1661.

3. Jonathan P. Caulkins, "The Real Dangers of Marijuana," *National Affairs*, Winter 2016, https://www.nationalaffairs.com/publications/detail/the-real-dangers-of-marijuana.

4. Ibid.

5. Naomi Martin, "Marijuana in Mass. Should Come with Warnings about Psychosis, Group Says," *Boston Globe*, June 5, 2019, https://www.bostonglobe.com/metro/2019/06/05/marijuana-mass-should-come-with-warnings-about-psychosis-group-says/LlJrfKslcpIQgcXMO5JPAO/story.html.

6. Jonathan P. Caulkins, "The Real Dangers of Marijuana," *National Affairs*, Winter 2016, https://www.nationalaffairs.com/publications/detail/the-real-dangers-of-marijuana.

## Afterword

1. Lester S. Grinspoon, "A Cannabis Odyssey," *Harvard Crimson*, September 15, 2003, https://www.thecrimson.com/article/2003/9/15/a-cannabis-odyssey-my-improbable-cannabis.

2.  Francesca Borrelli et al., "Colon Carcinogenesis Is Inhibited by the TRPM8 Antagonist Cannabigerol, a *Cannabis*-Derived Non-psychotropic Cannabinoid," *Carcinogenesis* 35, no. 12 (December 2014), https://academic.oup.com/carcin/article/35/12/2787/335166.

3.  Alessia Ligresti et al., "Antitumor Activity of Plant Cannabinoids with Emphasis on the Effect of Cannabidiol on Human Breast Carcinoma," *Journal of Pharmacology and Experimental Therapeutics* 318, no. 3 (September 2006), https://pubmed.ncbi.nlm.nih.gov/16728591.

4.  Lester Grinspoon, "A Cannabis Odyssey: To Smoke or Not to Smoke, by Lester Grinspoon," entry posted to Dr. Grinspoon's marijuana-uses.com website on Monday, April 20, 2009, https://www.northernstandard.com/a-cannabis-odyssey-to-smoke-or-not-to-smoke-by-lester-grinspoon.

# ACKNOWLEDGMENTS

I would like to acknowledge, and thank, the following people for their love, support, and assistance. First—my immediate family: my amazing, now-adult children, Zach, Emma, and Jacob, and my brilliant wife, Lizzi, who is always there for me, and also my brothers, Josh and David, and my kind, patient, and quietly brilliant mom, Betsy, who is truly the bedrock of all of our accomplishments, particularly my dad's.

I'd like to thank my spectacular agent Linda Konner, who believed in this project from the start, and my fabulously talented editor Jake Bonar, as well as the rest of the generous, helpful, and competent staff at Prometheus.

I'd like to acknowledge the following people who helped me with this project, in no particular order:

Allen St. Pierre whose generosity in answering all of my questions and whose knowledge of the legalization movement (which he has been integral to) is unparalleled. Dick Evans and Keith Stroup who shared their vast knowledge of, and experiences with, the War on Cannabis with me. Andy Weil—thanks for the thoughtful foreword and for your great work in this field, along with Ethan Nadelmann and Rick Doblin, who tirelessly worked with my dad, at different points in the last half century, to make this all happen. Staci Gruber, for your brilliance, friendship and inspiration, and feedback, and to all of Staci's spectacular associates such as Kelly Sagar, who was incredibly generous in answering all of my questions. To my colleagues at Doctors for Cannabis Regulation who read chapters and provided invaluable feedback, particularly David Nathan, Bryon Adinoff, Godfrey Pearlson, and especially Genester Wilson-King, who also gave such an eloquent talk at the recent University of

ACKNOWLEDGMENTS

Massachusetts conference in honor of my dad. To David Fink who helped me with epidemiology. To Mikael Sodergren for insightful comments on real-world evidence. To Shaleen Title—a profoundly inspiring warrior for social justice—for her comments and support. To Dan Adams for all of the great background material he dug up about my dad and Nixon, and for all of his fantastic reporting. To Jake Bakalar, my dad's close friend and coauthor, over decades, who read my entire manuscript and provided much-needed critical commentary. To Donald Abrams for comments and inspiration. To Steve DeAngelo for his historical perspective on the War on Cannabis. To Kenneth Finn for collegially discussing areas where we can all (hopefully) find common ground—I know that somewhere you have an inner flower child. To my writing group partners Ron Elliott and Fred Dalzell, and, especially, to my oldest friend, Dr. Andrew Budson, a brilliant memory specialist whom I've been bouncing these ideas off of, in one way or another, for about forty years and who has always been incredibly patient and generous with comments. To my good friend Tom Leckrone, for his support and tremendous insight into these issues. I would also like to acknowledge Stephen Mandile, Marion McNabb, Nancy Ferrari, Benji Grinspoon, Audrey "Snodgrass" Grinspoon, Dr. Anthony Portnoy, Lucas Perrier, Carl Sagan, Dr. Mark Eisenberg, and, finally, my coach, Barrett McBride, for keeping me sane and on task.

There are far too many other people in the cannabis, addiction, harm reduction, and medical communities who have helped me, through discussions, correspondence, and working together on these issues, to thank individually.

Most of all, I'd like to thank and acknowledge my late father, the original Dr. G., who got this all started and kept it going—against the odds—and who patiently mentored me on cannabis medicine and policy, with love and an unfailing belief in me, over my entire life.

# INDEX

INDEX

referenda, 73–75
regulation: and ASD use, 271; of
   CBD, 303; and pregnancy use,
   158; recommendations for, 343–45;
   of strains, need for, 228–29; and
   teen use, 219–20
rehab industry, 19; and drug testing,
   69; views of, 72, 144–45
Reiman, Amanda, 238–39
REM sleep, 254
reparations, 86, 345, 356–57
reporting requirements, changing, on
   cannabis use during pregnancy,
   159, 173
research. *See* scientific research
respiratory center, 232–33
restless legs syndrome (RLS), 248,
   254–55
retrograde transmission, 234
revenge sleep procrastination, 251–52
Rice, Andrew, 67
Rick Simpson Oil (RSO), 268
rimonabant, 232
Ritalin, 270
Russell, Allen, 82
Russo, Ethan, 234

safe banking bills, 345–46
safety, recommendations for, 118–19,
   356
Sagan, Carl, 4–5, 48, 61, 63, 252,
   331–33, 337–38
Sagar, Kelly, 288
SAMHSA. *See* Substance Abuse
   and Mental Health Services
   Administration
Sativex, 230, 300, 304, 310. *See also*
   nabiximols
Schedule I, 31, 37–38, 97–98, 303
schizophrenia, 102–5

scientific research: on addiction,
   121–23; on ADHD, 299–300; on
   autism effects, 269, 273–77; on
   cancer symptom relief, 257–58;
   on cancer treatment, 266–68; on
   cannabis-related care, 346–47; on
   CBD, 305; on cognitive effects,
   185–200, 211–15; and confusion,
   65–66; currency of, issues with,
   212–13; on driving while stoned,
   175–81; on endocanabinoid
   system, 226–27; Grinspoon
   (Lester) and, 61–62; issues in, 53,
   92, 141, 186–87, 283; LaGuardia
   Committee, 28–29; misdiagnosis
   of CUD and, 135–36; negative
   pressure on, 18–26, 105, 161,
   194, 262–63, 323–24; on opioid
   withdrawal and cannabis, 243; on
   pregnancy effects, 159–70; progress
   in, 48–53, 151–52; on psychosis,
   103, 105–13; recommendations for,
   67, 344, 351–53; on recreational
   use, 328–30; Sagan on, 48; on
   sleep effects, 249–51; standards
   for evidence and, 89–101; on teen
   use, 203–8; on veterans and PTSD,
   292–96
screen time, and insomnia, 249
self-medication: and psychosis, 106;
   teens and, 219; veterans and, 294
Seroquel, 253
serotonin receptors, 304
set and setting, 234, 290, 328–29,
   336
sexual experiences, 61, 216, 329, 332,
   335, 338
Shafer, Raymond, 29
Shafer Commission, 29–30
Sinclair, Upton, 71–72

422

# AUTHOR'S NOTE

This book, and the contents herein, are not intended to in any way constitute medical advice or to serve as a substitute for, or adjunct to, medical or professional advice given by one's own providers or otherwise. For any and all medical issues, or other issues, including lifestyle and health issues, the reader is instructed to consult his or her own personal physician and to not take anything in this book as intended to be specific medical advice that pertains to his or her specific circumstances or conditions, which only they and their personal physicians are aware of. While this book may mention the use of cannabis, CBD, or other cannabinoids in the context of hypothetically treating specific medical conditions or with regard to popular recreational uses, this is not to be construed as specific advice for any particular patient or person or any inducement to try or use cannabinoids. Anyone interested in treatment with cannabinoids or the use of cannabinoids for any reason, recreational or otherwise, must work with his or her own caregivers and personal support network independent of anything they read in this text. The state of cannabinoid medicine and science is evolving rapidly, and while the author has made good faith efforts to ensure that the information discussed in this book was accurate at the time of its publication, he cannot represent and warrant to its accuracy in perpetuity.